HEALTH COMMUNICATION

HEALTH COMMUNICATION
A Handbook for Health Professionals

PETER GUY NORTHOUSE, Ph.D.
Department of Communication Arts and Sciences
Western Michigan University

LAUREL LINDHOUT NORTHOUSE, R.N., M.S.N.
Ph.D. Candidate, Clinical Nursing Research
University of Michigan

PRENTICE-HALL, INC., *Englewood Cliffs, New Jersey 07632*

Library of Congress Cataloging in Publication Data

Northouse, Peter G.
　　Health communication.

　　Includes bibliographies and index.
　　1. Communication in medicine—Handbooks, manuals,
etc.　2. Allied health personnel and patient—Handbooks,
manuals, etc.　3. Interpersonal communication—Handbooks,
manuals, etc.　4. Nonverbal communication (Psychology)—
Handbooks, manuals, etc.　I. Northouse, Laurel L.
II. Title.　[DNLM: 1. Communication—handbooks.
2. Delivery of Health Care—handbooks.　3. Professional-
Patient Relations—handbooks.　W 39 N876h]
R118.N67　1985　　　610'.141　　　84-17859
ISBN　0-13-384835-3 (pbk.)

Editoral/production supervision:
　Zita de Schauensee
Cover design: Wanda Lubelska Design
Manufacturing buyer: John Hall

Printed in the United States of America

10　9　8　7　6　5　4　3　2　1

ISBN　0-13-384835-3　01

Prentice-Hall International, Inc., *London*
Prentice-Hall of Australia Pty. Limited, *Sydney*
Editora Prentice-Hall do Brasil, Ltda., *Rio de Janeiro*
Prentice-Hall Canada Inc., *Toronto*
Prentice-Hall of India Private Limited, *New Delhi*
Prentice-Hall of Japan, Inc., *Tokyo*
Prentice-Hall of Southeast Asia Pte. Ltd., *Singapore*
Whitehall Books Limited, *Wellington, New Zealand*

TO SCOTT AND OUR FAMILIES

Contents

Preface

Health Communication has been written for people interested in understanding and improving the communication between health professionals and between health professionals and clients. The book recognizes that the increasingly complex and multifaceted nature of health care delivery will require professionals to have a broader understanding of communication. It also recognizes that the changing nature of relationships among professionals and clients will necessitate more effective interpersonal communication in health care settings.

Health Communication includes several unique features. First, selected concepts and theories of human communication are directly applied to communication problems and situations in health care settings. Second, pertinent research that helps to explain human interaction in health care is incorporated throughout the text. Third, the book approaches health communication primarily from a descriptive, rather than a prescriptive, orientation that recognizes the ability of the reader to take the information provided and use it in her or his own practice. Fourth, special emphasis is given to communication issues unique to professional-professional, professional-client, professional-family, and client-family member relationships (Chapter 3). Finally, the book synthesizes one author's orientation to the communication field and the other author's orientation to the field of nursing.

In the first chapter an overview of various models of communication highlights the transactional, multidimensional aspects of human communication. Chapter 2 describes five selected communication variables and discusses how the appliction of these variables can enhance communication in health care settings. Each variable is considered from the client's and the professional's perspective. Chapter 3 describes the major types of relationships in health care settings and identifies problems that can block effective communication in these relationships. Chapter 4 highlights the importance of nonverbal communication in effective health communication. In addition, this chapter dispels several common myths about nonverbal communication and explains specific dimensions of the nonverbal process.

The last four chapters focus more directly on specific kinds of communication activities in which health professionals engage. Chapter 5 describes the communication dimensions of interviews in health care relationships. The preparation, initiation, exploration, and termination phases of an interview are discussed, and techniques that can be used by professionals to make health care interviews more effective are suggested. Chapter 6 describes the properties of small groups and discusses practical ways to make communication in small groups more effective. Chapter 7 addresses communication that occurs in health care organizations and describes different ways of viewing leader-follower interactions in health care settings. The last chapter focuses on human conflict, including some sources of interpersonal conflict and ways of dealing with it.

Health Communication is written primarily for nurses and other health professionals such as administrators, health educators, physicians, chaplains, social workers, dietitians, and occupational and physical therapists. The book is intended for college-level courses in nursing, health care administration, health psychology, public health, social work, communication, and other health-related areas. This book would also be useful as a text in continuing education, in-service training, and other health education programs.

ACKNOWLEDGMENTS

We are indebted to many individuals who played an important role in the development of this book. We would like to thank Robert Weisman, field representative for Prentice-Hall, for his kind assistance at the beginning of this project and throughout its development. David Gordon, Nursing and Allied Health Editor, deserves special recognition for his valuable guidance and direction during the many phases of the publication process. We would also like to acknowledge the competent editorial assistance of Joan

Kmenta and the excellent production contributions of Zita de Schauensee A special thanks goes to Terry Hammink for his substantive feedback on each chapter of the book in its formative stages.

For comprehensive reviews of the text, we would like to thank Marcia Andersen, Wayne State University; Paul Arntson, Northwestern University; Beverly Henry, University of Florida; Shirley P. Hoeman, Kessler Institute for Rehabilitation; Imogene M. King, University of South Florida; Teddy Langford, Texas Technical University. These reviewers offered us salient critiques and suggestions that helped to focus our thinking and improved the overall quality of the text.

For their encouragement and interest in this project we would also like to thank our colleages at the University of Michigan and Western Michigan University. We are grateful to Cinda Swinsick for her efficient typing, Judy Copeman for her thoroughness in word processing, and Rene Rossman for her conscientious efforts in preparing the index. Finally, we express our deepest appreciation to our families who have stood by us, allowed us time to work, and gave us full support during the long process of manuscript preparation.

Peter Guy Northouse
Laurel Lindhout Northouse

Kalamazoo, Michigan

1

An Introduction
to Health Communication

*One necessary condition for human communication is an
interdependent relationship between the source and the
receiver. Each affects the other.*   —Berlo, 1960

This is a book about communication between people in health care organizations. It is an attempt to answer such questions as, How can better communication be created in health care settings? Is it possible to eliminate the problems that lead to communication breakdowns? What changes are needed to make interpersonal communication more effective in professional-client and professional-professional relationships? To address these questions and the issues related to them, we will present selected concepts and theories of human communication and apply them to the communication that occurs in health care settings.

To begin, it is important to have a common understanding of what is meant by the word *communication*. Communication is a complex and multifaceted process. Although the word *communication* is often used in a general way to describe a variety of events, it is actually a term that refers to an identifiable process that has specific characteristics. Explaining the process of communication and how communication functions among individuals in health care organizations is the focus of this book.

In this chapter, we define different kinds of communication and then describe basic assumptions about human communication. In addition, we present several models that have been developed to explain communication and health-related processes. These models provide the background for the developmental model of health communication that appears in the final section of this chapter.

DEFINITIONS OF COMMUNICATION

In some ways, the word *communication* is similar to universal words such as *freedom, love,* or *democracy*. Although each of us intuitively knows what he or she means by such words, they can have different meanings for different people. Because communication has multiple meanings, it is important to identify a specific meaning and also to distinguish between different kinds of communication. Proceeding from general to specific, we now turn to definitions of communication, human communication, and health communication.

Communication

Since the late 1940s many definitions have been used by researchers in their attempts to capture the precise meaning of the phenomenon called communication. Researchers have defined communication from their own individual perspectives, often emphasizing aspects of the communication process that are most related to their own scientific interests. Nevertheless, the following examples show that there are features common to all the various definitions of communication.

An inclusive yet straightforward definition of communication is provided by linguist George A. Miller (1951): "Communication means that information is passed from one place to another" (p. 6). This definition stresses the idea that something (information) is being transferred from one point to another point. It includes what happens when one person talks to another on the telephone; it includes what happens between the input and output of a complicated computer program; and it includes what happens when news is transferred from one country to another via satellite.

A second definition of communication is supplied by Clevenger (1959): "Communication is a term used to refer to any dynamic, information-sharing process" (p. 5). This definition includes the "transfer of information" notion found in Miller's definition, but it also emphasizes the idea that communication is a process that involves sharing. Sharing implies that a common set of meanings exists between a source and a receiver. In the health care setting, an example of the source and the receiver sharing meanings is illustrated by the ongoing exchange of information between a social worker and a nurse who collaborate to work out rehabilitation plans that will promote the quality of life of a patient with a spinal cord

Injury. In such a case, it is crucial that the meaning of the concept *quality of life* is shared among the social worker, the nurse, and the patient if the communication process is to be successful. These individuals need to articulate and share their viewpoints in an effort to agree on treatment plans designed to promote the patient's quality of life.

A third approach to defining communication is taken by Cherry (1966), who defines it as "a sharing of elements of behavior, or modes of life, by the existence of a set of rules" (p. 6). This definition includes the idea of transferring information, as the Miller and Clevenger definitions did, but Cherry also stresses the notion that a common set of rules is needed for communication. In our interactions, the rules can be explicit or implicit; and they can vary from being broad-based rules, such as the professional language we use to describe certain characteristics or events (e.g., decubitus ulcer, schizophrenia), or narrower rules, such as the idiosyncratic customs that govern our personal relationships (e.g., nicknames used for close co-workers, or unique nonverbal gestures).

Taken together, these definitions provide a representative picture of the approach researchers have taken toward defining the nature of communication. Keeping these definitions in mind, we will be using the following definition of communication in this text: *Communication is the process of sharing information through a set of common rules.* This definition incorporates the major elements of previous definitions, including transfer of information, shared meaning, and rules. In later chapters we will discuss how various factors influence the communication process as we define it here. For example, situational pressures can interfere with the transfer of information; differences between the client's perspective and the professional's perspective can get in the way of shared meanings; and certain inappropriate responses can change the rules of the communication process.

Human Communication

Human communication is a special case, or subset, of communication (see Fig. 1.1). As Dance (1967) has pointed out, "although all human communication is communication, not all communication is human communication" (p. 289). Human communication refers to the interactions *between people*. Human communication differs from some forms of communication (e.g., animal communication) because it involves the use of symbols and language. Cronkhite (1976) suggests that "human communication has occurred when a human being responds to a symbol" (p. 20). The ability to use symbols or other representational language is unique to the communication behavior of human beings. Brown and Keller (1979) also emphasize use of symbols in defining human communication. Their definition is as follows:

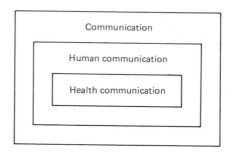

FIGURE 1.1   Relationship between three kinds of communication.

Communication [is] symbolic interaction. By interaction we mean what happens when one person says something and the other responds to it. . . . we have to have at least *one response to one initiation* before we can say we have established a connection, a hook-up, a relatedness—a tie of communication (p. 4).

These definitions suggest that human communication has to do with how individuals interact with each other through the use of symbolic behavior—through language. The process is transactional and affective in nature (Burgoon & Ruffner, 1978): In other words, it is ongoing, not static, and it involves human feelings and attitudes as well as information.

Before proceeding to define health communication, we would like to identify several contexts (situations) in which human communication typically occurs (see Fig. 1.2). These categories are presented to give you a frame of reference for the areas into which human communication is usually subdivided. You will see in Figure 1.2 that categories are based on the number of persons usually present in a given situation. The categories can be thought of as a sequence, beginning with communication contexts that have the fewest individuals (e.g., intrapersonal or interpersonal communication) and moving through contexts that include many individuals, with mass communication contexts at the other extreme. The nature of each context influences the human communication process. Although we will address issues related to all the contexts represented in Figure 1.2, our discussions will be focused more on the interpersonal, small group, and organizational contexts of communication.

Health Communication

Health Communication is narrower in scope than human communication (see Fig. 1.1). Health communication is a subset of human communication that is concerned with how individuals in a society seek to maintain health and deal with health-related issues. In health communication the fo-

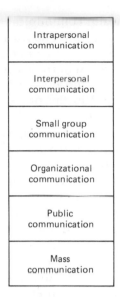

FIGURE 1.2 Basic human communication contexts. (Adapted from M. Ruffner and M. Burgoon, *Interpersonal Communication*. New York: Holt, Rinehart & Winston, 1981, p. 2.)

cus is on specific health-related transactions and factors that influence these transactions (Pettegrew, 1982). Transactions that occur between health professionals and between professionals and clients are of particular interest in health communication. Transactions can be verbal or nonverbal, oral or written, personal or impersonal, and issue oriented or relationship oriented, to name a few of their characteristics. In general, health communication is concerned with the application of communication concepts and theories to transactions that occur among individuals on health-related issues.

Health communication occurs in many of the human communication contexts discussed in the previous section. At the level of mass communication, health communication refers to areas such as national and world health programs, health promotion, and public health planning. In the area of public communication, health communication refers to presentations, speeches, and public addresses made by individuals on health-related topics. In organizational contexts, health communication may be involved with areas such as hospital administration, staff relations, and organizational communication climates. Within small group contexts, health communication refers to areas such as treatment planning meetings, staff reports, and health team interactions. Health communication in interpersonal contexts includes those variables in the human communication process that directly affect professional-professional and professional-client interaction. Finally, health communication in the intrapersonal context would refer to our inner thoughts, beliefs, and feelings, and our "self-talk" about health issues that influence our health-directed behaviors. It is apparent that communication in these contexts has a common health-related focus; however, the specific aims of the communication as well as the number of people involved in the process may vary considerably.

As Friedman and DiMatteo (1979) point out, research on interpersonal relations in health care settings is still in its infancy. The discipline of health communication is also a new area of study that parallels several other newer fields of study including health psychology, medical sociology, biomedical communication, behavioral medicine, behavioral health, and medical communications. These newer fields are building on the groundwork laid by professional disciplines such as nursing, social work, psychology, sociology, medicine, and public health. Health communication can be viewed as overlapping these other fields, while the focus is more specifically on *communication issues* in health care settings. Information and knowledge generated in health communication research contribute to the development of theory in these other fields, and research findings emerging from these fields contribute to the development of theory in health communication. In this sense, health communication is truly interdisciplinary in nature.

Although the term *health communication* is more specific than *communication* and *human communication,* it still encompasses a large body of information. In this book we will not be able to address ourselves to all the aspects of health communication nor to all the contexts in which it occurs. However, we will be able to discuss in depth some selected concepts and theories of human communication that play an essential role in health communication. Our underlying aim is to encourage communication that is sensitive to clients' and professionals' needs. We believe that effective health communication can facilitate the client's ability to cope, and enhance the professional's efforts to provide quality care.

BASIC ASSUMPTIONS ABOUT HUMAN COMMUNICATION

In studying how people communicate with each other, researchers have found that human communication has several identifiable properties (Berlo, 1960; Watzlawick, Beavin & Jackson, 1967). In constructing models and theories of human communication, these properties represent the fundamental assumptions or axioms upon which subsequent theories are built. As you read about these basic assumptions, think of how they apply to your own experiences in communicating with others. Are these assumptions valid for you? Do they make sense from your view of how human communication functions?

Human Communication Is a Process

To many persons, the word *communication* triggers an image of an individual talking to someone else on the telephone. This image of one person sending a message along a channel to another person is based on a linear approach to communication, which might be compared to a "hypodermic needle" model of human communication (Burgoon, Heston, & McCroskey, 1974). In this approach, person A instills his or her message into person B. Communication occurs in one direction, with one person directly influencing a second person through the use of specific messages. This approach is too restrictive because human communication is more than a one-way or linear event.

In fact, human communication is an ongoing, continuous, dynamic, and ever-changing process. "It does not have *a* beginning, *an* end, *a* fixed sequence of events. It is not static, at rest. It is moving" (Berlo, 1960, p. 24). This implies that communication between person A and person B should be viewed as a "continuous interaction of an extremely large number of variables" (Miller, 1972, p. 35), all of which continually change during a communication event. Stated another way, communication as a process means that when person A communicates with person B, the physical, emotional, and social states of A and B may change during their communication; these changes in turn induce further changes in their interaction.

The assumption that human communication is a process is important because it forces us to recognize the complexity of human communication and the many interrelationships that it involves. In health care, the process assumption of communication directs our attention to professional-professional and professional-client communication as ongoing dynamic processes rather than one-way, fixed sequences of events. The process assumption directs us not only to look at factors that affect the client but also to analyze factors that affect the nurse, social worker, or physical therapist, and to examine how the ongoing interchange between all of these people will vary depending on the nature of the situation. Of course it is important to analyze the impact of a single message created by one person and sent to another. However, analysis of communication as a process is even more important, because it provides us with a richer understanding of how messages interact with and are mediated by many other variables involved in the human communication process.

Human Communication Is Transactional

A second assumption about human communication, which is an extension of the first assumption, is that human communication is transactional. When we say human communication is transactional, we mean that both individuals in an interaction affect and are affected by each other (Wilmot, 1979). Transactional communication implies that the communication between two individuals is interactional and involves reciprocal influence (Mortensen, 1972). Each individual is both a source and a receiver at the same time. As person A constructs a message for person B, A is receiving cues from B that influence how A formulates the message. A transactional approach forces us to look at the simultaneous interplay between the sender and the receiver of a message.

If we accept a transactional perspective, we shift our focus away from an analysis of the ways in which one person affects another; instead we focus on the relationships between individuals that are developed and maintained through their mutual influence on one another. When we talked about the process assumption, we said that communication is not a one-way event. It is also an interaction. To study communication as a transactional process involves emphasizing the communication behavior of individuals *in relationships*. The transactional viewpoint focuses on the combined properties of the participants in an interaction, not on their individual characteristics (Millar & Rogers, 1976, p. 90). When describing human communication from a transactional perspective, it is important that we think of individuals together in a relationship rather than separately (Wilmot, 1979, p. 12).

To illustrate this point, consider what occurs in a health care situation when a health professional is having a conversation with a client. Each individual perceives the other in the context of what occurs in the interaction. If the nurse, for example, chooses to be dominant with a client, it may be because the nurse desires to be dominant, or it may be because the nurse picks up cues from the client that seem to indicate the client would prefer to be submissive. In other words, the nature of the interaction could be influenced by the desires of the nurse or client, by their perceptions of the other person's desires, or by both of these factors working together simultaneously.

We are saying that in relationships communication outcomes are mutually determined. Human communication in relationships is a *two-person process*. Health professionals do not make clients submissive and they do not make themselves dominant. Clients and health professionals engage in human interaction, and by doing so they establish how they are related and how they want to communicate.

Human Communication Is Multidimensional

A third assumption is that human communication is multidimensional. When human communication takes place, it occurs on two levels. One level can be characterized as the *content dimension* and the other as the *relationship dimension* (Watzlawick, Beavin, & Jackson, 1967, p. 54). In human communication, these two dimensions are inextricably bound together. The content dimension of communication refers to the words, language, and information in a message; the relationship dimension refers to the aspect of a message that defines how participants in an interaction are connected to each other.

To illustrate the two dimensions, consider the following hypothetical statement made by a nurse to a patient: "Please take this medication." The content dimension of this message refers to taking medication. The relationship dimension of this message refers to how the nurse and the patient are affiliated—to the nurse's authority in relation to the patient, the nurse's attitude toward the patient, the patient's attitude toward the nurse, and their feelings about one another. It is the relationship dimension that implicitly suggests how the content dimension should be interpreted, since the content alone can be interpreted in many ways. The exact meaning of the message emerges for the nurse and patient as a result of their interaction. If a caring relationship exists between the nurse and the patient, then the content ("please take this medication") will probably be interpreted by the patient as a helpful suggestion from a nurse who is concerned about the patient's well-being. However, if the relationship between the nurse and the patient is distant or strained, the patient may interpret the content of the message as a rigid directive, delivered by a nurse who enjoys giving orders. These two interpretations illustrate how the meanings of messages are not in words alone but in individuals' interpretations of the messages in light of their relationships.

The content and relationship dimensions of messages are illustrated further in the following example of professional-professional communication. A physician says to a nurse, "Why didn't Mr. Jones get the sleeping pill I prescribed last night?" The content dimension of the physician's question could be interpreted in different ways depending on the nature of the nurse-physician relationship. If the physician and nurse have an effective, collegial relationship, the nurse could interpret the content of the question as a request for factual information about the patient. If, however, a competitive relationship marked by repeated power struggles exists between the physician and the nurse, then the content of the same question could be interpreted by the nurse as an attempt by the physician to challenge the nurse's judgment or as an attempt to exert control over the nurse. Although the content dimension of a message is often easier to identify than the relationship dimension, it is often the relationship dimension that is critical to the ultimate interpretation of the message.

Wilmot (1979) has proposed several postulates about the content and relationship dimensions of messages which are illustrated in Table 1.1. The postulates emphasize that both the content and relationship dimensions influence the development of meaning in human interaction.

Watzlawick, Beavin, and Jackson (1967) argue that in healthy relationships, the relationship dimension of communication recedes into the background and the content dimension of messages becomes more impor-

TABLE 1.1   Content and Relationship Postulates

Human communication has both a content and a relationship dimension. These dimensions are interconnected. Meaning in interaction depends on the interplay between the content and relationship dimensions of communication.

POSTULATES

1. Every content statement has relational meaning.
2. Each participant in the dyad (relationship) translates the relational messages in a unique way.
3. Successful dyads (relationships) negotiate and work through their different relational translations of content statements and actions.
4. We develop rituals as ways to assure ourselves that the relational translations are similar.
5. A relationship develops explicitly on the content level, and simultaneously builds implicitly on the relational level.
6. Content competence is not equal to relational competence.
7. Every relational definition has content implications.
8. Relationships cannot be constructed or maintained only by relational talk.

Adapted from William W. Wilmot, *Dyadic Communication*, Second Edition, © 1979, Addison Wesley Pub. Co. Inc., Reading, Mass. Page 98, postulates 1–8. Reprinted with permission.

tant to the participants. In troubled relationships the opposite occurs: There is a continuous struggle on the relationship dimension, while the content dimension recedes into the background (p. 52).

Think for a moment about some of the relationships you have established with others. In healthy relationships, the conversations flow smoothly and there is little discussion or struggle about how participants are related. In these relationships we focus more on *what* is being said—we may ask for details or describe at length events that have happened to us. We spend little time discussing who is right or who is wrong. The opposite occurs in troubled relationships in which things are not going well. In these relationships we spend a lot of energy on relationship talk—on trying to figure out such things as who is in control in the relationship, who is dominant, or who is going to be the submissive participant. Our conversations do not flow smoothly and we feel conflicted about how we see our relationship. In these relationships we may mistakenly think that we differ with another person on content issues, when the conflict may really arise from subtle problems in the relationship that are influencing and hindering the interaction. Given the choice, most of us prefer to have our interpersonal communication free of the conflict caused by relationship struggles.

For many reasons, which we will discuss in more detail in Chapter 3, health professionals do not spend much time developing relationships with clients and with other health professionals. Yet it is important that health professionals recognize that the relationships they develop with clients and with other health professionals significantly influence the effectiveness of their interpersonal communication. The *meaning* in health transactions emerges from the interplay between the content and relationship dimensions of messages. Developing relationships is important because it influences how content will be interpreted. Given the multidimensional assumption of human communication, effective communication is more likely to be achieved when health professionals are equally attentive to both the content and the relationship dimensions of messages.

SELECTED MODELS OF COMMUNICATION

Researchers have constructed many models in attempts to reduce the complexity of the human communication process. These models, which are primarily word-picture diagrams, try to impose some pattern on a process that is intricate and complex. The value of these models is that they help us to more easily understand the underlying structure of the communication process. By highlighting certain aspects of the communication process, models show how these aspects are interconnected with one another. In essence, models help us to understand abstract events by representing these events in ways that have structure and clarity.

Building models to represent complex theories has certain limitations. Models are never perfect. Because of their very nature, models cannot include *all* the elements of the process they are supposed to represent. Selecting certain attributes to be a part of a model unavoidably results in excluding other attributes. In addition, because models are attempts to represent complex events in a simplified way, there is a tendency for models to oversimplify the process or the event being described. This limitation of oversimplification is inherent in building models that represent theories of human behavior.

Recognizing the advantages and the limitations of models, we have chosen to present and discuss four models that represent the complexity of human communication in ways that illuminate and clarify the process without oversimplifying it. The four are (1) the Shannon-Weaver model, (2) the SMCR model, (3) the speech communication model, and (4) the Leary model. These models encompass the major thoughts, concepts, and theories set forth by communication researchers to explain how the communication process operates.

Shannon-Weaver Model

One of the first models of communication, and in many ways one of the most influential, was a linear model developed by Shannon and Weaver in 1949. In the Shannon-Weaver model (see Fig. 1.3), communication is represented as a system in which a *source* selects information that is formu-

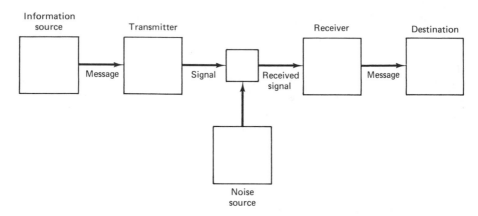

FIGURE 1.3 Shannon-Weaver communication model. (Reprinted from C. E. Shannon and W. Weaver, *The Mathematical Theory of Communication*. Copyright 1949 by The University of Illinois Press. Champaign, Ill.: University of Illinois Press, p. 98.)

lated (encoded) into a message. This message is then *transmitted* by a signal through a *channel* to a *receiver*. The receiver interprets (decodes) the message and sends it to some *destination*. A unique feature in this model is the concept of *noise*. Noise refers to those factors that influence or disturb messages while they are being transferred along the channel from the source to the destination. For Shannon and Weaver, who were interested in telecommunications, noise referred to static, which creates errors between the input and output of the message in the system. In a human communication model, noise could refer to any disturbance, such as audible sound, perceptual distortions, or psychological misinterpretations, that changes the meaning of a message as it is sent from one person to another.

One strength of this early model is the uniform manner in which it attempts to describe the pathway of a communication message from source to receiver. A limitation of this model, however, is that it does not show the transactional relationship between the source and the receiver. Because the model is linear, it implies that communication is a one-way event. As later communication theorists have noted, and as we discussed earlier in this chapter, communication in human relationships is an interactional process. Another feature omitted from the Shannon-Weaver model, but which is present in subsequent communication models, is the principle of feedback—a link from the receiver back to the source that acts to regulate and monitor the flow of information within the system. The use of the Shannon-Weaver model in health care settings would only show us the communication pathway from a nurse to a patient, or from a physician to a nurse. The interaction component or feedback between the two people would be missing.

SMCR Model

In his book *The Process of Communication* (1960), Berlo presented what is now a classic model of communication—one that emphasizes, as the title of the book suggests, that communication is a process. Berlo's model is called the SMCR model, standing for the first letter in the words *source*, *message*, *channel*, and *receiver* (see Fig. 1.4). Berlo views these four components as being intertwined.

The SMCR model represents a communication process that occurs as a *source* formulates messages based on his or her communication skills, attitudes, knowledge, and sociocultural system. These *messages*, which have unique elements, structure, content, treatment, and codes, are transmitted along *channels*, which can include seeing, hearing, touching, smelling, and tasting. A *receiver* interprets messages based on her or his own communication skills, attitudes, knowledge, and sociocultural system.

The strength of this model is the manner in which it represents the complexity of communication and treats communication as a process rather than a static event. The model is limited by omitting the feedback component of communication, and by not vividly illustrating the process function. If this model is applied to health care settings, it would enable us to see the many factors that influence a client's communication, such as his or her attitudes and sociocultural background. However, the ways in which a health professional's feedback to a client's message affects subsequent communication would not be indicated in this model. Similarly, this model helps explain how experience and education affect professional-professional communication (e.g., the communication between a *new* baccalaureate nurse and an *experienced* practical nurse) but is less helpful in highlighting how feedback influences ongoing professional-professional dialogue.

Source	Message	Channel	Receiver
Communication skills	Elements	Seeing	Communication skills
Attitudes	Structure	Hearing	Attitudes
Knowledge	Content	Touching	Knowledge
Social system	Treatment	Smelling	Social system
Culture	Code	Tasting	Culture

FIGURE 1.4 SMCR model. (Adapted from David K. Berlo, *The Process of Communication: An Introduction to Theory and Practice*, p. 72. Copyright © 1960 by Holt, Rinehart and Winston, Inc. Reprinted by permission of Holt, Rinehart and Winston, CBS College Publishing.)

Speech Communication Model

Miller (1972) developed a model to represent speech communication (see Fig. 1.5) that illustrates the feedback feature of communication not represented in the SMCR model. In Figure 1.5, speech communication is represented by three factors: the speaker, the receiver, and feedback. The speaker *encodes* (formulates) messages based on his or her *attitudes*; the messages are *decoded* (translated) by a receiver on the basis of her or his *attitudes*. Then the receiver gives either *positive* or *negative feedback* to the speaker, who then is able to modify subsequent messages.

We have included this model of the speech communication process because it represents, in an uncomplicated fashion, the central factors in human communication. However, this model may be almost too simple to capture the complexity of the entire communication process. For example, this model's simplicity may not allow us to fully understand communication in health care settings, where such factors as the context or the setting may significantly influence the process of communication. On the other hand, unlike the SMCR model, this model makes it easier to understand the important transactional and feedback components that exist between client and professional in the communication process.

Leary Model

The reflexive model of human interaction developed by Leary is quite different from the previous models we have discussed. Leary's model, which first appeared in the mid-1950s, has received considerable attention in recent years. It is truly a transactional and multidimensional model, stressing relationships and the interactional aspects of interpersonal communication. It states, in effect, that human communication is a two-person process in which both individuals influence and are influenced by each other.

Leary developed this model as a result of his experiences as a therapist with patients in psychotherapy. He observed that his own behavior was different in his sessions with different patients—that is, he found that patients influenced the way he behaved toward them. Leary concluded that individuals actually train others to respond to them in particular ways—

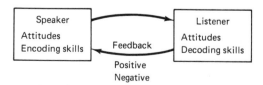

FIGURE 1.5 A simple model of the speech communication process. (Reprinted from G. R. Miller, *An Introduction to Speech Communication* (2nd ed.). Indianapolis: The Bobbs-Merrill Co., Inc., 1972, p. 58.)

ways that are pleasing for the individual's own preferred interpersonal behavior. For example, if we like to be submissive, we condition others to behave in dominant ways toward us; conversely, if we like to be dominant, we condition others to behave submissively.

Leary's model is designed to classify certain aspects of interpersonal behavior used in interpersonal communication. Figure 1.6 gives a simplified version of the Leary model. (See Leary's article "The Theory and Measurement Methodology of Interpersonal Communication" [1955] for an extended description of the theory.)

From the perspective of the Leary model, every communication message can be viewed as occurring along two dimensions: dominance-submission and hate-love. Both of these dimensions occur on the relationship level of interaction. When we interact with someone else, each of our messages has a dominant-submissive quality and a hate-love quality. Responses that others make to our messages are based on how they perceive and interpret these dimensions in our messages.

Two rules govern how these dimensions function in human interaction. *Rule 1*: Dominant or submissive communicative behavior usually stimulates the *opposite* behavior in others. Stated in another way, acting autocratically (dominantly) usually stimulates others to act submissively, and acting powerlessly usually stimulates others to act dominantly. *Rule 2*: Hateful or loving behavior usually stimulates the *same* behavior from others. This means that being kind usually encourages kindness from others, while being hostile usually stimulates aggressiveness from others. Leary states that these rules operate reflexively—our responses toward each other are involuntary and immediate in interpersonal situations. Our own

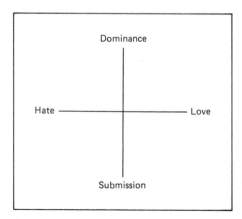

FIGURE 1.6   Leary's reflexive model. (Based on T. Leary, "The Theory and Measurement Methodology of Interpersonal Communication." *Psychiatry,* 1955, *18,* 152. Copyright © 1955 by the William Alanson White Psychiatric Foundation, Inc.)

communication behaviors automatically stimulate dominant or submissive and love or hate reactions in others.

The Leary model can be directly applied to communication in health care settings. As we will discuss in Chapter 3, patients in acute care settings often assume or are placed in the submissive role, while health professionals often assume a dominant role. The strength of the Leary model is the transactional way in which he describes these power and affiliation issues in human interactions. If we are really going to understand our communication with others, we need to look at the qualities that both persons bring to the interaction. Two weaknesses of the Leary model, as described here, are that it does not portray the ongoing, fluid process of human communication; and it omits other important variables that arise from the environment.

SELECTED HEALTH-RELATED MODELS

To this point we have been primarily concerned with models of human communication. However, we believe that it is important to look specifically at the health-related fields and see how these fields have portrayed communication in their models. Obviously, the focus of these models will not be solely on the common elements of communication, but on the broader goal of maximizing health outcomes. For this reason, we need to examine both communication models *and* health-related or clinically based models in order to develop a model for health communication.

As we discussed in the previous section, diagrams or word-pictures to explain human behavior are never perfect or fully complete. Nevertheless, for our discussion we have selected three widely accepted models developed by researchers to explain human behavior as it pertains to health and illness. The three are (1) the therapeutic model, (2) the health belief model, and (3) the King interaction model. There are many other health-related models that could have been selected. These three models were chosen because each provides a very different focus or emphasis in health care and each has a direct relationship to human communication.

Therapeutic Model

The therapeutic model emphasizes the important role *relationships* play in assisting clients and patients to adjust to their circumstances and to move in the direction of health and away from illness. Communication that is therapeutic is not significantly different from ordinary human exchanges (Ruesch, 1961, p. 31). Effective human communication is by its nature therapeutic. When used by health professionals, *therapeutic communication* can be defined as a skill that helps people to "overcome temporary stress, to get along with other people, to adjust to the unalterable, and to overcome psychological blocks which stand in the way of self-realization" (Ruesch, 1961, p. 7). Although therapeutic communication appears to be a term that describes communication in traditional psychotherapeutic settings, it also describes communication between health professionals and clients in other health care contexts.

Although many models have been developed to describe the various kinds of psychotherapeutic theories, not all of these therapeutic models are pertinent to health-related interaction. One model that *is* pertinent and has proved useful in explaining the interactions that occur in health care settings is the Rogerian model. Carl Rogers (1951) believes that if a therapist communicates honest, caring understanding to the client, it will help the client adjust in a healthy way to his or her circumstances. This Rogerian model is labelled *client-centered* because the focus of the interaction is on the client. In this model, the helper is encouraged to communicate with empathy, positive regard, and congruence. These three behaviors, together, comprise the necessary conditions to help the client successfully. We have depicted these components in Figure 1.7.

For Rogers, *empathy* is the process of communicating to clients the feeling of being understood; it is standing in the shoes of the client (see Chapter 2 in this book). *Positive regard* is the process of communicating support to the client in a caring and nonjudgmental way. It is communication that is genuine, unthreatening, and unconditional. Communicating *congruence* involves the honest expression of the helper's own thoughts and feelings. Congruence requires that the helping professional will respond honestly to the client and attempt to be real in his or her relationship with the client.

The therapeutic model illustrated in the Rogerian client-centered approach is extremely valuable in identifying some of the necessary conditions for productive interactions. However, its main emphasis is on the relationship between two people, so the influences of the setting and the

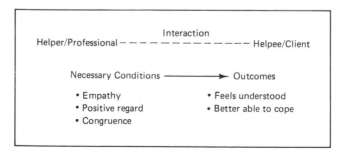

FIGURE 1.7 A therapeutic model. (Adapted from C. Rogers *Client-Centered Therapy*. Boston: Houghton Mifflin Company, 1951.)

situation on the professional-client interaction are noticeably absent from this model. The Rogerians, however, would probably remind us that even the best settings for interactions will not be as important as an honest *interpersonal transaction* between the professional and client.

In health care settings, the therapeutic model can be directly applied to professional-client communication. The Rogerian model describes how health professionals should communicate if they choose to be client-centered. According to the Rogerian model, when health professionals communicate empathy, positive regard, and congruence, clients are better able to confront and cope with their illnesses.

Health Belief Model

The health belief model, formulated by Rosenstock and his colleagues (1966, 1974), is broader, more complex, and has a very different focus from the therapeutic model. The frequent use of this model in health care settings and its heavy emphasis on the client's perceptions are two reasons that it is being examined for its potential contributions to a developmental model of health communication. This model was designed to explain the nature of individuals' preventive health actions. Since the model appeared in the late 1950s, it has been the focus of a great deal of research; it has come to be recognized as one of the most influential social-psychological theories formulated to explain how healthy individuals seek to avoid illness (Cockerham, 1978; Becker, 1979).

As Figure 1.8 illustrates, the health belief model consists of three major elements: (1) an individual's perception of susceptibility to and severity of the disease, (2) an individual's perception of the benefits and barriers to taking a preventive health action to prevent disease, and (3) the cues available to an individual that would stimulate him or her to engage in preventive health activity (Becker & Maiman, 1975). At the top of the diagram a fourth element of the model appears containing demographic and social-psychological variables. These variables, called modifying factors, indirectly influence individuals' perceptions and beliefs, but they are not viewed as causal predictors of health behavior (Becker & Maiman, 1975). In essence, the health belief model is designed to predict the likelihood of individual health behavior as a function of perceived threat and perceived benefit (Stone, 1979, p. 73).

Although many aspects of the health belief model involve communication, two aspects are distinctively communication centered. First, the Cues to Action element of the model includes mass media campaigns, advice from others, newspaper articles, and similar message-related variables, all of which are types of communication. Communication is essential if individuals are to receive cues that have potential for motivating them to take health action. For example, newspaper articles on the importance of fas-

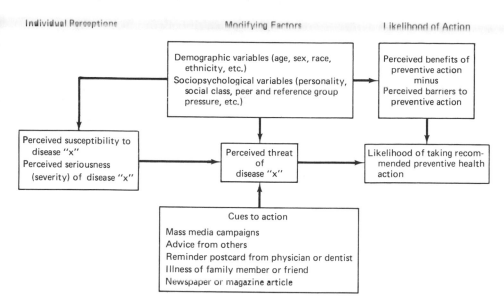

FIGURE 1.8 The health belief model as predictor of preventive health behavior. (Reprinted from M. H. Becker and L. A. Maiman "Sociobehavioral Determinants of Compliance with Health and Medical Care Recommendations." *Medical Care*, 1975, *13* (1), 12.)

tening seat-belts may persuade people to buckle-up while driving their cars. In the same way, messages on the radio about cancer and cigarette smoking may influence persons to quit smoking. A second element of the model that is particularly relevant to health communication pertains to Modifying Factors, which include social-psychological variables. Many of these variables are important elements in the communication process. Becker and Maiman (1975) refer to a series of studies showing that compliance behavior in patients is associated with the communication in health professional-client relationships. Patients' failure to comply has been found to be related to communication patterns in which the health professional is described as formal, rejecting, or controlling; the professional strongly disagrees with the patient; the professional interviews the patient at length without allowing for feedback, or engages in nonreciprocal interaction; and the health care worker fails to make clear the purpose of treatment. Clearly, communication has an impact on the health behavior of clients.

The health belief model has certain merits and also certain limitations. On the positive side, the model illustrates the importance of broader modes of communication, such as the impact of mass media, on health behavior. The health belief model also focuses on the perceptions and beliefs of clients that can be altered to enhance certain health behaviors (Becker, 1979). This model is instructive because it helps to predict and explain why clients seek health services and why their health behavior may or may not

be compliant. On the negative side, the health belief model has been criticized for placing too much emphasis on abstract, conceptual beliefs (Safer
et al., 1979). Another problem, identified by Stone (1979), is that not all the
research results have supported the predictions of the health belief model.
Individuals do not always follow up on health recommendations that have
alerted them to a potential health threat. Overall, this model highlights the
clients' perceptions of preventive health care measures rather than the
transactional nature of the client-professional interaction in promoting
health care.

King Interaction Model

King's work (1971, 1981) on the development of a conceptual framework for nursing provides the basis for a third health-related model, which
can be described as an interaction model. King's model places strong emphasis on the communication process between nurses and clients and,
therefore, was selected as an important model for understanding health
communication. King uses a systems perspective to describe how health
professionals (nurses) assist clients to maintain health. She provides a conceptual framework that discusses the interrelationships among personal,
interpersonal, and social systems. Although King describes the nature of
each of these three systems, she gives particular emphasis to interpersonal
systems in health care.

The paradigm King employs to discuss the role of interpersonal systems in health care is represented in Figure 1.9. King (1971) describes the
nature of this model as follows:

> In the interactive process, as nurse and patient assess goals to be
> achieved, and mutually define health goals, a transaction occurs. This
> mutual agreement has an effect on the actions and judgment of the
> nurse and patient and influences each one's perception. A series of
> these kinds of acts takes place as the nurse and patient interact in a
> nursing situation (p. 92).

The King model illustrates vividly the process and transactional assumptions of human communication that we discussed earlier in this chapter. In addition, the interaction model incorporates the feedback concept.
Essentially the model suggests that in nurse-patient interactions both the
nurse and the patient simultaneously make *judgments* about their circumstances and about each other, based on their *perceptions* of the situation.
Judgments, in turn, lead to verbal or nonverbal *actions* that stimulate *reactions* in the nurse and the patient. At this point new perceptions are established and the process repeats itself. *Interaction* is the dynamic process that
includes the reciprocal interplay between the nurse's and the client's perceptions, judgments, and actions. *Transactions* are the result of the recipro-

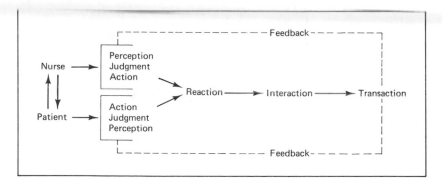

FIGURE 1.9   An interaction model. An approach to the nurse-client communication process. (Reprinted from I. M. King, *Toward a Theory of Nursing: General Concepts of Human Behavior*, p. 92. Copyright © 1971 by John Wiley & Sons, Inc.)

cal relationships established by nurses and clients as they participate together in determining mutual health-related goals.

King's model has many assets as a model for explaining communication between a health professional and client. It represents the nurse-patient interaction process in a manner similar to the models formulated by the communication theorists. This model encompasses the important dimensions of relationship, process, and transaction that have been identified as crucial elements in the communication process. The feedback loop in the model also indicates the importance of shared meaning between the nurse and client. Although King does not show in this diagram how interpersonal relations are affected by situational factors, nor how interpersonal relations are related to the patient's health behavior, she does explain these issues in *A Theory For Nursing* (1981).

A DEVELOPMENTAL MODEL OF HEALTH COMMUNICATION

The communication and health-related models we have described in the previous sections provide the foundation for constructing a model of health communication. To describe the health communication process, we present a developmental model in Figure 1.10 that illustrates health communication as we presently conceptualize it. We have labeled this model *developmental* because we see the field of health communication as unfolding in its initial stages of development. As we pointed out earlier, health communication is a relatively young discipline. Because it is a newer area of study, we believe our model is only a first step toward the construction of a refined model of health communication.

Health communication refers specifically to transactions between par-

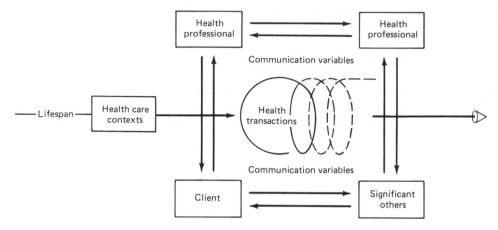

FIGURE 1.10   Health communication model.

ticipants in health care about health-related issues. Our primary focus is on the health communication that occurs within various kinds of relationships in health care settings. In contrast to previously described models, this model of health communication takes a broader systems view of communication, and it emphasizes the way in which a series of factors can impact on the interactions in health care settings. The health communication model (HCM) in Figure 1.10 illustrates the three major factors of the health communication process: participants, transactions, and contexts. Included within each major factor are several subelements that describe the composition of each factor more fully.

Participants

Health professionals, clients, and significant others are the primary participants in health communication. When an individual is engaged in health communication he or she is participating from the perspective of one of these three roles.

The category of health professionals includes a wide range of individuals—nurses, health administrators, social workers, physicians, health educators, occupational and physical therapists, pharmacists, chaplains, public health personnel, health psychologists, technicians, and other specialists. Many individuals performing a variety of functions participate in health communication as health professionals.

We use the term *health professional* to identify any individual who has the education, training, and experience to provide health services to others. Each health professional brings to health care settings unique characteristics, beliefs, values, and perceptions that will affect how he or she interacts with clients and with members of the health care team. For example, beliefs about what motivates clients to adhere to treatment regimens or opinions about how much choice clients should have in health care decisions are factors that will influence health professionals' interactions with others. Similarly the age, sociocultural background, and past experiences of the health professional will affect the way in which he or she responds to clients and co-workers. Although these issues will be addressed in more detail in Chapters 3 and 4, the health communication model presented here encompasses not only the role of the health professional, but also the beliefs and values that are unique to that person and that influence the person's interactions with others.

Clients are individuals toward whom health services are directed. In acute care settings the client is usually, but not always, referred to as the *patient*. In other health care settings, the individuals who are receiving services are simply referred to as *clients*. In the HCM, the term *client* is used to designate the individuals who are the focus of the health care services that are being provided. At one time or another, all of us have participated as clients in health communication, whether as a patient in a hospital or as an individual attending a clinic or agency.

For our purposes, the term *client* in the health communication model will also encompass the specific characteristics, values, and beliefs that these individuals bring to the health care setting. Just as the personal characteristics of health professionals influence *their* interactions, the unique characteristics of clients influence the interactions clients have with others. For example, as the health belief model pointed out, the perceptions of the client can affect whether or not these persons even seek out the help of health care professionals. Similarly, whether a client has values oriented more toward quality of life or toward quantity of life will also influence his or her choices and interactions with others. These are only a few of the numerous intrapersonal factors that can affect clients in the health communication model.

The social network of the client includes a third set of individuals who are participants in health communication. Clients' significant others have been found to be most essential in supporting clients as they seek to maintain health. These social networks include family members (spouses, sisters, brothers, and other relatives), roommates, friends, co-workers, and other individuals connected in a significant way to the person utilizing health services. In short, clients' social networks are composed of all those individuals who are significant others in a client's life, but who are not health professionals.

Too often in the past health professionals have overlooked the important role played by family members and other significant individuals in enhancing the health of the ill person. We have included the client's significant others in our model of health communication because we believe that these persons are frequent and essential participants in the health communication process.

Transactions

Transactions are a second major element in the health communication model. *Transactions* refer to the health-related interactions that occur between participants in the health communication process. Transactions are represented in the model in four kinds of relationships: professional-professional, professional-client, client-significant other, and professional-significant other. Health communication is concerned with the health transactions that occur in these relationships.

The model also indicates that these interpersonal relationships can influence other types of relationships in the health care setting. For example, how health professionals communicate with each other can affect how health professionals and clients interact. Similarly, how a client reacts with members of his or her social network can influence later interaction between the client and health professionals.

Health transactions involve any interaction between individuals about health-related information. This includes seemingly unimportant relationship-building communication on topics such as the weather, sports, and so on, to more important communication on topics such as diagnoses, treatment plans, or prescribed health behavior changes. All human communication in health care settings is not health communication. But if human communication in some way influences individuals in maintaining health, it is related to health communication.

In the HCM, health transactions include both verbal and nonverbal communication behavior. Both types of communication are equally important, and health transactions are most effective when verbal and nonverbal aspects of messages are compatible with each other. In Chapter 4 we will discuss the unique role that nonverbal communication plays in health care transactions.

Health transactions also include both the content and relationship dimensions of messages. Health transactions deal with health-related content—how a client seeks to attain and maintain health over a lifespan. The relationship dimension of health transactions is established within the various relationships represented by the model and influences how the content of the messages should be interpreted.

In the center of the health communication model, health transactions are represented by a circle from which an unending spiral emerges. This illustrates the ongoing, transactional nature of health communication. Health communication is not a static event but an interactive process that occurs at various points in time during the course of a person's life. It includes continual feedback, which allows participants to adjust and readjust their communication. Health transactions are constantly moving forward *and* turning back to make changes and alterations in the message.

At the top and bottom of the HCM, there are many communication variables that influence the participants and their messages. In Chapter 2, we will discuss selected communication variables that have a significant impact on health communication.

Contexts

A third major element of the health communication process is health care *contexts*—the settings in which health communication takes place and the systemic properties of these settings. Health care contexts actually have a great influence on the communication among health professionals, clients, family members, and others involved in the process.

At one level, health care contexts refer to health care settings, such as hospitals, nursing homes, and outpatient clinics. Health communication may be affected by the specific setting in which it occurs, such as a hospice, a hospital room, a physician's office, a clinic, or a waiting room, to name a few possibilities. For example, an intensive care unit, with its accelerated pace and lack of privacy, will affect patterns of communication in a different way from an ambulatory care unit where private office space is available and the pace may be less hectic. Each particular health care setting affects the dynamics of health transactions that take place within it.

At another level, health care contexts can refer to the number of participants within a particular health care setting. Health communication may take place in a one-to-one situation, in triads, in small groups, and among larger collections of individuals. The number of persons present within a given context also influences interactions in the context.

Together, the components of our health communication model include participants, transactions, and contexts; they provide a systems perspective on communication in health care. In the HCM, we have attempted to integrate elements of human communication from the communication models and place them within the goals of care proposed by the health-related models. It is our belief that as the complexity of health care continues to increase, health communication can be better understood from this broader systems perspective. This is not to negate the importance of messages, channels, or characteristics of the source and receiver of the message, but rather to propose that these factors be studied while keeping in mind the many contextual factors and relationships that affect the health transaction.

SUMMARY

For purposes of our discussion, communication is the process of sharing information according to a common set of rules. When information is shared between individuals using a common system of symbols and language, the process is called human communication. Health communication refers to health-related transactions between individuals who are attempting to maintain health and avoid illness.

There are three basic assumptions that can be made concerning human communication. First, human communication is a process, which means it is ongoing, dynamic, and ever changing. Second, human communication is transactional, which means each participant in an interaction is simultaneously affected by each other participant. Third, human communication is multidimensional, which means it has both a content and relationship dimension. Both dimensions (content and relationship) are inextricably bound together in human interaction.

Selected models of communication provide ways of illustrating different aspects of the process. Shannon and Weaver's model depicts communication as a one-way, linear event. Berlo's SMCR model indicates elements that affect the source, message, channel, and receiver in the communication process. Miller's speech communication model emphasizes the important role of feedback in human communication. Leary's reflexive model illustrates how dominance-submission and hate-love are central in each human communication interaction.

Although they are widely different in form and structure, the selected health-related models we presented are useful in describing issues of communication as they pertain to health. Rogers's therapeutic model sets forth ways of communicating that are effective for health professionals who choose to be client-centered. A paradigm that is useful in explaining why individuals do or do not engage in certain health-related behaviors is found in Rosenstock's health belief model. King's interaction model designates what occurs in nurse-patient interactions and emphasizes the transactional and feedback features of health professional–client communication.

Together, the selected communication and health-related models provide the basis for a developmental health communication model (HCM). The HCM has three major elements: participants, health transactions, and contexts. Considered together, these elements illustrate that health communication is a transactional multidimensional process by which individuals (both health professionals and clients) interact with each other on health-related issues in a mutual effort to maintain the client's health.

REFERENCES

Becker, M. H. Psychosocial aspects of health-related behavior. In H. E. Freeman, S. Levine, & L. G. Reeder (Eds.), *Handbook of medical sociology* (3rd ed.), Englewood Cliffs, N.J.: Prentice-Hall, Inc., 1979.

Becker, M. H., & Maiman, L. A. Sociobehavioral determinants of compliance with health and medical care recommendations. *Medical Care,* 1975, *13*(1), 10–24.

Berlo, D. K. *The process of communication.* New York: Holt, Rinehart & Winston, 1960.

Brown, C. T., & Keller, P. W. *Monologue to dialogue: An exploration of interpersonal communication* (2nd ed.), Englewood Cliffs, N.J.: Prentice-Hall, Inc., 1979.

Burgoon, M., Heston, J. K., & McCroskey, J. *Small group communication: A functional approach.* New York: Holt, Rinehart & Winston, Inc., 1974.

Burgoon, M., & Ruffner, M. *Human communication.* New York: Holt, Rinehart & Winston, 1978.

Cherry, C. *On human communication.* Cambridge, Mass.: M.I.T. Press, 1966.

Clevenger, T. What is communication? *Journal of Communication,* 1959, *9,* 2–10.

Cockerham, W. C. *Medical sociology.* Englewood Cliffs, N.J.: Prentice-Hall, Inc., 1978.

Cronkhite, G. *Communication and awareness.* Menlo Park, Calif.: Cummings Publishing Company, 1976.

Dance, F. E. X. Toward a theory of human communication. In F. E. X. Dance (Ed.), *Human communication theory: Original essays.* New York: Holt, Rinehart & Winston, Inc., 1967, 288–309.

Friedman, H. S., & DiMatteo, M. R. Health care as an interpersonal process. *Journal of Social Issues,* 1979, *35*(1), 1–11.

King, I. M. *Toward a theory for nursing: General concepts of human behavior.* New York: John Wiley & Sons, Inc., 1971.

King, I. M. *A theory for nursing: Systems, concepts, process.* New York: John Wiley & Sons, Inc., 1981.

Leary, T. The theory and measurement methodology of interpersonal communication. *Psychiatry,* 1955, *18,* 147–161.

Millar, F. E., & Rogers, L. E. A relational approach to interpersonal communication. In G. R. Miller (Ed.), *Explorations in interpersonal communications.* Beverly Hills, Calif.: Sage Publications, 1976, 87–103.

Miller, G. A. *Language and communication.* New York: McGraw-Hill Book Company, 1951.

Miller, G. R. *An introduction to speech communication* (2nd ed.). New York: The Bobbs-Merrill Co., Inc., 1972.

Mortensen, C. D. *Communication: The study of human interaction.* New York: McGraw-Hill Book Company, 1972.

Pettegrew, L. S. Some boundaries and assumptions in health communication. In L. S. Pettegrew, P. Arntson, D. Bush, and K. Zoppi (Eds.), *Explorations in provider and patient interaction.* Louisville, Ky.: Humana Inc., 1982.

Rogers, C. R. *Client-centered therapy.* Boston: Houghton Mifflin Company, 1951.

Rosenstock, I. M. Why people use health services. *Milbank Memorial Fund Quarterly,* 1966, *44*(3), 94–124.

Rosenstock, I. M. Historical origins of the Health Belief Model. *Health Education Monographs,* 1974, *2*(4), 354–386.

Ruesch, J. *Therapeutic communication.* New York: W. W. Norton & Co., 1961.

Ruffner, M., & Burgoon, M. *Interpersonal communication.* New York: Holt, Rinehart & Winston, 1981.

Safer, M. A., Tharps, Q. J., Jackson, T. C., and Leventhal, H. Determinants of three stages of delay in seeking care at a medical clinic. *Medical Care,* 1979, *17*(1), 11–29.

Shannon, C. E., & Weaver, W. *The mathematical theory of communication.* Champaign: University of Illinois Press, 1949.

Stone, G. C. Psychology and the health system. In G. C. Stone, F. Cohen, N. E. Adler, and Associates (Eds.). *Health psychology—A handbook: theories, applications, and challenges of a psychological approach to the health care system.* San Francisco: Jossey-Bass, Inc., Publishers, 1979.

Watzlawick, P., Beavin, J., & Jackson, D. D. *Pragmatics of human communication.* New York: W. W. Norton & Co., Inc., 1967.

Wilmot, W. W. *Dyadic communication: A transactional perspective* (2nd ed.). Reading, Mass.: Addison-Wesley Publishing Co., Inc., 1979.

2 Communication Variables in Health Care

*There are certain communicative aspects in all social
situations, and these bear most directly on the interaction
of the respective parties.*   —Mortensen, 1972

The communication process includes numerous variables, each of them
important to an understanding of the overall process of communication.
As illustrated in the health communication model discussed in Chapter 1,
these variables affect the health transactions that occur in various health
care relationships. Because it is not possible to discuss all of the variables,
we have chosen to consider five which we think are *central* to effective
health communication. We are aware that we have selected only a few out
of many possible variables, and that our readers might have chosen different variables. However, the variables we discuss can be studied in light of
communication research and can be directly applied to health care settings.

We have chosen to examine the following variables: (1) empathy, (2)
control, (3) trust, (4) self-disclosure, and (5) confirmation. In our discussion, we will describe each variable, present a conceptual framework for
it, and then apply the variable to health care settings. In keeping with our
belief that communication is a transactional process, based on the thoughts
and feelings that both individuals bring to the interaction, the application
section will consider each variable from the client's and the health professional's perspective.

EMPATHY

Of all the variables used to explain health communication, empathy is regarded as one of the most essential and at the same time one of the most complex variables operating in the communication process (Forsyth, 1980; Gagan, 1983; Kalisch, 1973; LaMonica, 1981). Empathy is believed to affect communication outcomes in all types of relationships—from our everyday social relationships to intense therapeutic encounters. It is well established that empathy plays an important role in effective, interpersonal communication (Cronkhite, 1976; Miller & Steinberg, 1975; Rogers, 1975). Without empathy, the communication between people lacks the essential quality of understanding.

The term *empathy* is credited to Theodor Lipps (1909), who defined *Einfuhlung* as the process of "feeling into." However, much of the recent interest in empathy is a result of Carl Rogers' pioneering work (1951, 1959) on client-centered therapy. In his description of empathy, Rogers defines empathy as a process that involves

> entering the private perceptual world of the other and becoming thoroughly at home in it. It involves being sensitive, moment to moment, to the changing felt meanings which flow in this other person, to the fear or rage or tenderness or confusion or whatever, that he is experiencing. It means temporarily living in his life, moving about in it delicately without making judgments, sensing meanings of which he is scarcely aware, but not trying to uncover feelings of which the person is totally unaware, since this would be too threatening. It includes communicating your sensings of his world as you look with fresh and unfrightened eyes at elements of which the individual is fearful. It means frequently checking with him as to the accuracy of your sensings, and being guided by the responses you receive. . . .
>
> To be with another in this way means that for the time being you lay aside the views and values you hold for yourself in order to enter another's world without prejudice. . . . (Rogers, 1975, p. 4)

This extensive definition indicates the complexity of the empathic process.

Other researchers have defined empathy in ways that differ from Rogers; some of the definitions focus on empathy as emotional sensitivity, accuracy of understanding, intuition, or a personality trait, to name a few. Although different definitions emphasize different aspects of the empathic process, all of the definitions include the element of *understanding*. Some representative definitions are as follows:

> (Empathy is) intellectualistic endeavor to understand by mimicry and inference those activities not immediately intelligible. (Freud, 1948, p. 66)

(Empathy is the) imaginative transporting of oneself into the thinking, feeling and acting of another and so structuring the world as he does. (Dymond, 1950, p. 343)

(Empathy is) the ability to perceive accurately the feelings of another person and to communicate this understanding to him. (Kalisch, 1971, p. 714)

(Empathy is) a vicarious emotional response to the perceived emotional experiences of others. (Mehrabian & Epstein, 1972, p. 525)

(Empathy is) the degree to which the therapist is successful in communicating his awareness and understanding of the client's feelings in language that is attuned to that client. (Lambert, DeJulio, & Stein, 1978, p. 468)

From these definitions, we see that the phenomenon of empathy may involve different processes whereby an individual comes to understand the thoughts and feelings of another individual. Empathy is *not* sympathy. These two words are frequently used interchangeably although their meanings are very different. Sympathy is the concern, sorrow, or pity shown by an individual for another individual. It is the expression of one's *own* feelings about another person's predicament. Empathy is an attempt to feel *with* another person, to understand the other's feelings from the *other's* point of view. Empathy is the sharing of another's feelings and not the expression of one's own feelings. In empathy the focus is on the client with the problem, whereas with sympathy the focus shifts away from the client to the listener. In short, empathy is observing the world from another person's point of view.

Conceptual Frameworks of Empathy

To further understand empathy, we need to examine how researchers and theoreticians have studied this important but elusive concept. What are the major components of empathy and can we explain its effects? There are primarily four basic ways of approaching and explaining empathy: (1) a Rogerian framework, (2) an interpersonal perception framework, (3) a personality framework, and (4) a perceived empathy framework. In fact, most research on empathy has been conducted from the Rogerian conceptual framework.

Rogers contends that empathy is one of the core conditions of successful psychotherapy (1957) and one of the major elements in establishing a helping relationship (1958, 1961). For Rogers, empathy involves cognitive, affective, and communication components. The *cognitive* perceptual process involves observing a client's behavior and processing the obtained information. The *affective* process involves being sensitive to a client's feelings.

The *communication* component, which has been of special interest to researchers and clinicians in the helping professions, focuses on the language and responses of the therapist. By focusing on the communication dimension of empathy, researchers have been able to design specific strategies and techniques to assist professionals in developing and enhancing their empathic skill (Carkhuff, 1969; Gazda, et al., 1973; Hammond, Hepworth, & Smith, 1977). Many of the common therapeutic techniques (reflection, restatement, and paraphrasing) are actually communication skills.

A second way of looking at empathy, although more limited in scope than the Rogerian approach, is the conceptual framework called the interpersonal perception perspective. In this approach, empathy is thought of as a *perceptual process* that occurs *in* an individual as she or he attempts to understand (perceive) the beliefs, attitudes, and values of another (Dymond, 1948; Gage & Cronbach, 1955; Hobart & Fahlberg, 1965; Northouse, 1979). From this orientation, empathy is seen as a general ability that all people have in varying degrees (Cline & Richards, 1960; Dance & Larson, 1972). A strength of this approach is its emphasis on measuring how accurately one person's perceptions of another person's attitudes match that other person's *actual* attitudes. On the other hand, one limitation of this approach is its narrower view of empathy—that it is only a perceptual process—which omits the important communicative dimension found in the Rogerian approach.

A third perspective is provided by the personality theorists, who view empathy as one personality trait among many other traits, such as dogmatism, introversion-extroversion, or dominance-submission. Like other individual personality traits, empathy may be exhibited by different persons in varying degrees. In this view, an empathic person is one who displays a relatively high degree of understanding of another person. Personality theorists do not concern themselves with the aspects of communication skill or accuracy of perception, both of which are important in the other two conceptual frameworks for viewing empathy.

A fourth approach to empathy focuses on the client's point of view (Barrett-Lennard, 1981; Laing, Phillipson, & Lee, 1966). *Perceived empathy* is one individual's belief or feeling that another individual perceives his or her perspective accurately. In many ways, perceived empathy is one of the major goals in the helping process. Stated in another way, our primary purpose in responding to others is to help them, by communicating to them that we understand some of the dimensions of the world as they see it. Perceived empathy occurs entirely within the *receiver*, making this approach different from the first three we discussed.

By looking at these different conceptual frameworks, the reader can see that empathy is not a simple *unitary* variable but a *complex* variable. Empathy may occur within the source, within the receiver, and in transmitted messages between the source and the receiver (Northouse, 1981). For example, the therapist (source) makes an empathic statement that is sent (message-channel) to the patient (receiver). These four frameworks focus on different aspects of the communication process. The personality viewpoint examines the empathic traits of the *source*; the Rogerian approach focuses on the empathic *message* or content component; the interpersonal perception framework for empathy focuses on the accuracy of the source's perceptions related to the receiver's thoughts and feelings (channel). Perceived empathy focuses only on the *receiver* and the receiver's feelings of being understood. These conceptual frameworks are classified under the traditional communication categories—source, message-channel, and receiver—in Figure 2.1.

Empathy is indeed complex and may occur at several points within the communication process. Because of this, many qualities—observational skill, communication skill, perceptual skill, emotional sensitivity, and caring, to mention just a few—are needed by those who are asked to exhibit empathy.

Applications of Empathy in Health Care

Given the complexity of the empathic process, how can theoretical information about empathy best be applied in health care settings? We believe that it is important to address empathy both from the client's perspective and from the professional's perspective. The common premise to both perspectives is that understanding is achieved through empathy. In fact, it is an essential factor in effective interpersonal communication. For clients, empathy is important because illness is confusing and frightening, and being understood helps clients cope with these emotions. For professionals, empathy is essential because it helps professionals to understand clients

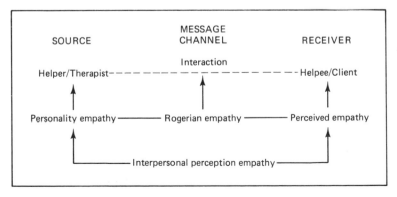

FIGURE 2.1 Classification of kinds of empathy within the framework of traditional communication categories.

and their problems, as well as to understand other professionals and themselves.

Empathy: The client's perspective

Clients in health care settings have many needs that range from physiological to psychosocial. One of their strongest psychosocial needs is the need to be understood. Yet the impersonal nature of health care organizations makes this need the hardest to fulfill. Many things (e.g., availability of time, advanced technology, staff shortages, demands for efficiency, etc.) may hinder and prevent health professionals from attending fully to clients. Nonetheless, clients' negative reactions to the strange and highly technological health care system are reduced significantly when health professionals are sensitive to clients' points of view. Expressing empathy helps clients satisfy their need for understanding.

Researchers have established that showing empathy produces positive therapeutic outcomes for clients (Bergin & Strupp, 1972; Traux & Mitchell, 1971). First, showing empathy reduces clients' feelings of alienation (Rogers, 1975) and of being "all alone" with their predicament. When clients feel understood, they feel connected to others and a part of life. Empathy breaks down the sense of being an isolated island that people with illness often experience, and it also provides clients with a sense of confirmation. When health professionals empathize with clients, clients feel understood; they know that they exist and that their point of view has value (Kalisch, 1973).

At times, however, health professionals may become too caught up in their own feelings and expectations and fail to see the values and expectations of the client. The following example illustrates this problem.

John is a 25-year-old man, who was hospitalized for numerous diagnostic tests to rule out the possibility of Hodgkin's disease. John and his new wife of two months anxiously awaited the results of a biopsy of a neck node. They expressed much relief and hope when the pathology report returned and showed that the results were negative.

The thoracic surgeon who did the biopsy, however, was convinced that John's symptomology was still characteristic of Hodgkin's disease and suggested that another biopsy from a different location be done. When the pathology report from this second biopsy was completed, the surgeon accompanied by two residents and a nurse rushed into John's room and loudly announced, with a wide smile on his face, "I found the specific cell that confirms my diagnosis. I was right—it is Hodgkin's disease." Possibly noting the look on John's face, the physician said, "You should be glad it's Hodgkin's disease; it could have been a lot worse! You've got a good ten years ahead of you." John and his wife thanked the physician for being so thorough and persistent that an accurate diagnosis could be made.

However, moments after the health team left the room, John and his wife burst into tears. Later, when he recalled the incident, John said, "I was mystified by the situation. I felt such shock, fear, horror—yet it seemed inappropriate to have these feelings—it would have spoiled the surgeon's celebration of having found what he was searching for. Thank God that the nurse in the background had tears in her eyes, although she never said anything. It was the only thing that let me know that my inner feelings weren't crazy."

This surgeon became preoccupied with the diagnostic process and failed to be sensitive to the meaning of the diagnosis to the patient and his family. In this case, the surgeon was oblivious to the patient's anxiety and fear about the results of the pathology report on the second biopsy. On the other hand, the nurse in the example was sensitive to the patient's feelings, and she did communicate her understanding of the patient's feelings by her actions. As the patient said, it was the empathic response of the nurse that validated his own emotions.

In addition, empathy helps clients feel that others care about them, which leads to greater self-acceptance (Rogers, 1975). Empathy enhances clients' feelings of being understood and facilitates their adjustment to very stressful situations. Being understood in a nonjudgmental way assists clients in feeling positive about their own value and worth. Finally, empathy promotes the feelings of control within clients. If professionals have listened to them without making judgments, clients gain a sense of control by expressing their own thoughts without opposition or evaluation. They become less dependent on others and feel more in charge of the way they want to respond to life events (Kalisch, 1973).

Empathy: The professional's perspective

Empathy also has an impact on health professionals, who, like clients, have a need to be understood. Health professionals desire understanding not because they are confronting an illness but rather because they desire to be more effective helpers to clients and also to have better interpersonal relationships with co-workers. Empathy, then, enables health professionals to improve the accuracy of their communication with clients and to reduce communication problems with other health professionals.

When a professional is able to empathize with another, he or she adopts a new frame of reference for the other. This new frame of reference in turn increases the probability that the professional will be able to interpret the other person's communication more accurately because the professional has been sensitized to the uniqueness and nuances of the other's point of view. Empathy assists professionals to see the problems of clients and other professionals more clearly.

In addition, empathy helps professionals to build effective

interpersonal relationships with each other—an almost universally desired goal. Many examples can be cited to illustrate how professionals have a need for empathic communication. In hospitals, pharmacists wish nurses understood the pressures pharmacists face when asked to fill a certain prescription immediately when at the same time they must fill thousands of daily hospital prescriptions. Nurses wish patients and families understood why it takes time to respond to call lights when there are staff shortages. Nurses wish physicians would acknowledge the nurses' unique areas of expertise. Physicians wish nurses understood the responsibility they feel for patient care. Staff in radiology departments would like personnel on the floors to understand the importance of preparing patients properly for complex X-ray procedures. In nursing homes, administrators wish families understood staffing difficulties and why there are sometimes delays in having patients ready for visitation hours. Staff members wish administrators would understand their desire for fair scheduling. Public health nurses would like clients to understand the importance of programs to prevent communicable diseases.

These examples illustrate only a few of the many situations in which health professionals desire understanding. In each situation, the wish being expressed by the professionals is for others to accurately perceive them and what they are doing in the health care setting. Health professionals are justified in wanting to be fully understood by other health professionals, because the misunderstandings between professionals often lead to communication breakdowns, interpersonal conflict, personal stress, and, in the end, to ineffective patient care.

Health professionals at all levels within the health care system need to share in the responsibility for giving empathic understanding to others. Several techniques can be employed in showing empathy. The techniques themselves will not automatically result in empathic communication, but they will assist professionals in improving their empathic skills. Empathic behavior is complex, but it can be learned. In Chapter 5, we will present specific communication approaches that can increase your ability to empathize with clients and others.

CONTROL

The second major communication variable is control—a subtle but powerful factor in health communication. Control is an integral part of every communication event and an intrinsic component of human interaction. Whenever an individual is influenced by or influences another person or event, aspects of control are present. Previous work on control in health care has analyzed control primarily from the perspective of the individual. Does the client have a sense of control over life events? Does he or she desire more control in health matters? How can clients' health-related behaviors be controlled? In this section we will take a new approach to looking at control: We will consider not only the individual perspective, which we have called *personal control,* but also the interpersonal or transactional perspective, which we have called *relational control.* This approach will allow us to discuss more fully the issues involving control in health care.

Personal control is the perception people have that they can influence the way in which circumstances affect their lives. Personal control, in effect, increases people's feelings of potency about their actions and minimizes their feelings of powerlessness. It is important for people to see their environments as controllable and predictable (Wortman, 1976). Control does *not* need to be exercised, or even be real, to have an effect on the individual; it only needs to be *perceived* (Thompson, 1981). Although both clients and professionals express a need for personal control, most of the research on personal control has been done from the perspective of the client.

Relational control refers to the perception individuals have about how they are connected to others, and it includes the degree to which they feel able to influence the nature and development of relationships. This type of control resides within interpersonal relationships, rather than as a characteristic of individuals. Through communication, individuals in professional-professional and professional-client relationships establish who is in control, that is, who is most able to influence the relationship in a given situation. If individuals within a relationship share similar definitions of relational control, more effective interpersonal communication will result (Morton, Alexander, & Altman, 1976).

Conceptual Frameworks of Control

Personal control

Researchers have identified many aspects of control including perceived control, actual control, reactance, power, and learned helplessness, to name a few (Chanowitz & Langer, 1980). Two fields of research are particularly useful to us in our discussion of personal control.

First, Thompson (1981) has devised a typology of control that categorizes personal control into four separate areas: (1) *behavioral control,* (2) *cognitive control,* (3) *informational control,* and (4) *retrospective control. Behavioral control* is the belief that one can utilize one's own behavior to alter the probability, intensity, or duration of a threatening event. An example of behavioral control might be an orthopedic patient who is experiencing pain in one position, who shifts his or her body weight into a new position, and thereby relieves the pain. *Cognitive control* is the belief that one can develop mental strategies that will influence the circumstances that affect one's life. Cognitive control could be demonstrated by a patient who is anxious about an upcoming procedure but can practice distraction (such as thinking about a pleasant event) to reduce some of the anxiety. *Informational control* is the belief that an individual can acquire knowledge about external events that affect that person's situation. Teaching preoperative patients about forthcoming procedures and sensations would be one means of assisting them to increase their informational control. *Retrospective control* is the belief that a person can accept responsibility for events in the past, thus mastering the situation after it has happened. Accident victims who have a need to understand what caused their accident and to determine if it could have been prevented may be exercising retrospective control. Many researchers believe that the way individuals exhibit these different types of control is related to the way they handle life stress and illness (Seligman, 1975; Thompson, 1981; Wortman & Brehm, 1975).

Second, personal control has been studied from the *locus of control* perspective. Research on locus of control originated with Rotter (1954) and social learning theory. According to this theory, individuals develop certain expectations about the influences or impact of their own behaviors through a learning process. For individuals who believe that their own behavior determines what happens to them, the locus of control is said to be *internal*. For individuals who believe that outside forces or factors primarily determine what occurs in their lives, the locus of control is called *external*. For example, the person who believes that engaging in exercise routines and diet alterations will limit the occurrence of heart problems is operating from an internal control perspective. Conversely, the person who assumes that heart problems are due to heredity and nothing can be done to prevent them is operating from an external perspective. Locus of control, then, is a personality variable that discriminates between internally oriented and externally oriented individuals.

Locus of control in general has been measured by Rotter's Internal-External (I-E) scale (1966). More specifically, the locus of control of an individual's health beliefs has been measured by the Health Locus of Control (HLC) scale (Wallston, et al. 1976) and by a more current refined version of this scale, the Multidimensional Health Locus of Control (MHLC) scale (Wallston, Wallston, & DeVellis, 1978). The items on the MHLC instrument directly assess individuals' beliefs about whether responsibility for health-related matters lies within themselves, with others, or in external events.

Research on locus of control has been of interest to health professionals because it is believed that locus of control may contribute to an understanding of individuals' health-related behavior. For example, control has been studied as a factor related to the following behaviors: learning health information, influencing health care professionals' decisions, receiving feedback, seeking help from experts, complying with others' wishes, and responding to threats (Arakelian, 1980). However, research on locus of control has its limitations (Lewis, 1982a; Lowery, 1981). First, internal-external locus of control is regarded as a personality variable, and it is therefore questionable whether or not individuals can learn to change their locus of control even if they would benefit from doing so. Second, there is a tendency for researchers to imply that it is good to be "internal" and bad to be "external" (Rotter, 1975). Yet there *may* be situations in which it is not always healthy to maintain a high internal perspective (Lowery, 1981) or in which it may be realistic to relinquish some personal control in health matters (Lewis, 1982b). For example, to assume that a client could have prevented certain progressive diseases or natural disasters could be unrealistic and could generate a great deal of guilt or self-blame in the client. Wortman and Brehm (1975) have suggested that overemphasizing a person's sense of control in these types of situations may be maladaptive, and they recommend that an accurate assessment of a person's potential for control in a specific situation is more useful for individuals. A final criticism of locus of control, or the personal control perspective, is that measures of locus of control have not been reliable predictors of health-related behaviors (Lewis, 1982a; Lowery, 1981). That is, these measures have not added to our understanding of clients' health behavior.

Relational control

Relational control differs from personal control in that it focuses on relationship or interpersonal characteristics, whereas personal control focuses on characteristics of individuals. Relational control is regarded as a transactional process—an interaction that occurs between individuals in a relationship—and is thus part of the relationship dimension of messages (Bateson, 1958; Haley, 1963; Jackson, 1959; Watzlawick, Beavin, & Jackson, 1967).

As we discussed in Chapter 1, every message has two dimensions: a content dimension and a relationship dimension, inextricably bound together. In interpersonal communication, participants determine where they stand with each other on the *relationship* dimension through the sharing of information on the *content* dimension. For example, when individuals talk about seemingly unimportant matters such as school, weather, sports, or general news, they are in essence finding out how they feel about their relationship. The point is that individuals decide how they are related to each other and decide who is in control in a relationship through interaction. Healthy relationships are based on a mutual agreement, either spoken or unspoken, regarding the issues of control between the participants (Morton, Alexander, & Altman, 1976). Good relationships are free of constant conflict regarding who is dominant or who is in charge in the relationship.

The kinds of relationships that individuals establish through relational control can be complementary, symmetrical, or parallel (see Fig. 2.2).

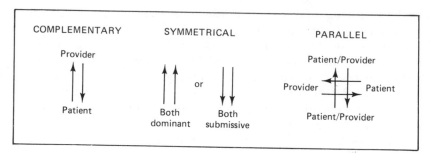

FIGURE 2.2   Kinds of relationships established through relational control.

In *complementary relationships,* the control is unequally distributed (Millar & Rogers, 1976; Watzlawick, Beavin, & Jackson, 1967, p. 68): One person is dominant and the other is submissive. In the classic medical model, health providers are typically the individuals with the control and patients are encouraged to be submissive and without control (Krantz & Schulz, 1980). In other health care models, clients are taking more responsibility for health-related decisions; it is no longer the norm for the provider to be in the dominant position in complementary provider-client relationships.

In *symmetrical relationships* control is shared equally by participants, and the differences between individuals are minimized (Watzlawick, Beavin, & Jackson, 1967, p. 69). Symmetrical relationships are sometimes characterized by competition for control or submission (Parks, 1977; Rogers & Farace, 1975). It is not always clearly established who is in control in symmetrical relationships; the relationship may constantly be redefined (Wilmot, 1979). In health care settings, professional-professional relationships are frequently symmetrical. However, because professionals want to be perceived as competent and they desire to have their opinions accepted by others, competition for control may develop as professionals interact with each other in a symmetrical relationship.

A third kind of relationship is a *parallel relationship* in which control is transferred back and forth between participants. This kind of relationship may shift between being complementary and being symmetrical. Parallel relationships result in communication patterns that are more flexible and less likely to result in dysfunctional interaction (Wilmot, 1979). Health professionals who take turns at holding and giving control, depending on the situation, rather than competing for control would be an example of a parallel relationship.

Applications of Control in Health Care

Issues involving personal and relational control constantly confront both the client and the professional in health care settings. Control is important to clients primarily because they are experiencing the loss of it. For professionals, control is important because it is through the negotiation of control that they are able to effectively work with clients and with other health professionals. In the previous section we discussed personal and relational control. Now we would like to answer the obvious next question: How can health professionals utilize these concepts regarding control to improve their communication with clients and other professionals?

Control: The client's perspective

Loss of personal control is a major obstacle that confronts every client, whether the individual has a serious illness, such as cancer or kidney disease, or a less serious ailment. As Cantor (1978) points out

> Most of us need to experience some sense of control over our destinies. We need to feel that what we do and say will have substantial effect on the events of our lives. We need to make sense of ourselves and our surroundings (p. 10).

But illness makes clients confront the reality that they do not always have mastery of their destinies. Illness induces uncertainty into the lives of clients—and with uncertainty comes the loss of control, which in turn leads to feelings of fright, anger, helplessness, and incompetence. Losing control takes from clients a primary means of ascribing meaning to their lives. Unless individuals feel potent, and able to influence events in their lives, they will feel victimized by outside forces, see life as senseless, and view their own lives as insignificant (Cantor, 1978, p. 11).

Although clients may experience loss of control in many health care settings, it is even more pronounced in a hospital setting. S. E. Taylor (1979) has suggested that "the hospital is one of the few places where an individual forfeits control over virtually every task he or she customarily performs" (p. 157). In her research on hospital patient behavior, Taylor found that loss of control results in depersonalization in patients and that patients typically respond to depersonalization by acting helpless (a "good patient" role) or by acting angry (a "bad patient" role). In addition, Taylor reports that hospital patients may react to the loss of control through heightened sensitivity to their physiological response to illness or by seeking information from numerous people in an indiscriminate manner.

As health professionals, it is important that we be sensitive to the effect that loss of control has on clients in health care settings. To help clients cope with this, health professionals need to address not only the causes for feelings of loss of control but also ways to restore clients' sense of control. An essential element in the treatment process is assessing whether clients are more internally or externally oriented in their preferences for control (Shillinger, 1983). For example, a nurse could ask a patient if he or she normally likes to "take charge" of events (internally oriented) or if he or she prefers to take a "wait and see" attitude and generally lets events run their own course (externally oriented). In addition, assessment is needed of the patient's environment, the patient's illness, and other factors that may affect the amount of control that is realistically available to the patient. Giving patients free control in areas they can manage alone and a participant role with a health professional in areas they cannot manage alone would be the outcome of this assessment process.

By utilizing behavioral, cognitive, informational, and retrospective dimensions of personal control, professionals may encourage clients to become more involved in their own care, and to learn new behaviors or skills that will enable them to be less dependent on health professionals. Other clients may gain a sense of cognitive control by learning to control their attitudes to their circumstances, although they may not be able to control specific health outcomes. Providing clients with information about treatments and procedures will help them to experience some sense of predictability (McIntosh, 1974). Finally, being with clients and encouraging them to express their thoughts and feelings as they struggle with the meaning of illness in their lives may enable them to gain a degree of retrospective control.

The fundamental advantage of giving patients a chance to exercise legitimate control is that it allows patients to feel more independent, to feel less helpless, and thereby to feel more worthwhile. Secondly, patient participation appears to improve the physical and psychological adjustments of patients (Egbert et al., 1964; Schulman, 1979). There is some evidence to suggest that when patients are given control over aspects of care that they can manage, "symptom incidence and complaints are reduced, morale is higher, there is a reduced need for medication, and patients often leave the hospital sooner" (S. E. Taylor, 1979, p. 180). Finally, it can be argued that there may be a decrease in malpractice litigation and a decrease in health care costs when patients are encouraged to be active participants in their care (Blum, 1960; Vaccarino, 1977).

Control: The professional's perspective

The issues of control that professionals confront are different from those confronting clients. For professionals, *loss* of control is not as crucial a problem as finding effective ways to *share* control with other professionals and clients. Thus relational control becomes the predominant issue for health professionals.

Learning to share control in professional-professional relationships is not an easy process. Over the years health care organizations have functioned with hierarchical lines of authority clearly established. Sharing control was not common. It was usually clear who had control, how much control they had, as well as who did not have control. More recently, this has changed, and health care professionals now confront the issue of how to share control. Many factors (patient rights, changing roles of health professionals, self-help groups, holistic orientations) have put pressure on the authoritarian structures of health care systems to become more democratic and allow greater participation. Not only has this resulted in a breakdown of traditional roles, but it also has created an increased need for negotiations and communication to clarify issues of control in relationships.

Agreement regarding who is in control is the key to effective professional-professional and professional-client relationships, and arriving at this agreement takes place through interaction. Sometimes the content of interaction may be an important issue, such as the need for a CAT scan, or it can be a less important issue, such as parking problems. Whatever the issue, in interactions with each other, professionals have a need to feel that their ideas and opinions are of value and that they are competent. Through sharing information, professionals are able to define where they stand with each other. If they can do this in mutually acceptable ways, more productive interpersonal communication is likely to result.

The difficulties that health professionals experience in learning to share control are compounded by the nature of the environment in which they are required to practice. Much of what occurs in health settings has a life and death dimension. Health professionals who function under these critical conditions "believe they require total control in order that the environment in which they attempt to save lives be maximally efficient and predictable" (Friedman & DiMatteo, 1979, p. 8). Yet health professionals also practice in organizations in which professionals must depend on one another if they are to function with the most effectiveness. It seems then that the task for health professionals is to learn how to share control, because through *sharing* control interdependence can be achieved without any individuals *losing* control.

How control is shared depends on the nature of the relationships, that is, whether they are complementary, symmetrical, or parallel. In the following example, examine the responses to determine what the nature of the relationships may be.

> PHYSICIAN TO NURSE: I want the most recent lab reports on Mr. Johnson. Could you find them for me?
> NURSE TO PHYSICIAN:
> RESPONSE A: No, I'm doing meds. You'll have to find them yourself.
> RESPONSE B: Yes, I'll look them up for you right now.
> RESPONSE C: No . . . But perhaps you could find them over there (*nods head*) on the latest printout from the lab.

Obviously there are numerous responses that could be made to the physician's request in this example. We have chosen these three hypothetical responses to illustrate how the control dimensions of a message are negotiated depending on the nature of the relationship. Response A represents a straightforward rejection of the physician's assertion of control. Although the physician would like to be in control in this situation, the nurse exerts his or her own control. This characterizes a symmetrical relationship. This symmetrical relationship (in which both people seek dominance) can lead to interpersonal conflict, however, as they compete for control. In response B, on the other hand, the nurse accepts the physician's request for control. The nurse is this case essentially accepts the physician's definition of the relationship, which places the physician in the dominant controlling position and the nurse in the submissive controlled position. This represents the complementary relationship. Who has control in this case is clearly established and also agreed upon mutually. Although this response may preserve harmony in their relationship, it can also negate the importance of the nurse role or place it secondary to the physician's role. Response C represents an attempt on the part of the nurse to share control with the physician. The nurse rejects the physician's request for dominance but offers the alternative of assisting the physician, which does acknowledge the physician and his or her request. In essence the nurse is saying that the physician can have control, but not at the overall expense of the nurse, who retains control in this exchange. This may characterize a parallel relationship.

Each kind of relationship (complementary, symmetrical, and parallel) has advantages and disadvantages.

Complementary relationships are stable, efficient, and predictable because individuals in these kinds of relationships know where they stand and need not spend time negotiating who is in charge in every particular situation. On the negative side, complementary relationships are repressive because they inhibit the independence and creativity of the subordinate member in the relationship.

Symmetrical relationships are more equal. They promote mutual sharing of thoughts and feelings; both interactants are free to express their own values. However, symmetrical relationships may be inefficient and may promote needless competition. When making decisions, it can be time consuming to debate and discuss the implications of each person's position on every issue or decision. These discussions often create conflict since individuals in symmetrical relationships are often unwilling to compromise their own "one-up" positions.

Parallel relationships are ideal in many ways. In parallel relationships, individuals share control equally in some areas and distribute control to one another in other areas. Although not as stable as complementary relationships, and not as equal in all situations as symmetrical relationships, parallel relationships do function efficiently and fairly, allowing persons to share control with minimal conflict.

Sharing control in communication is complex and difficult, and there are no simple prescriptions for how it is best done. Being aware of professionals' and clients' needs for control is a first step in the process. This awareness, coupled with flexibility and willingness to adapt one's own needs for control to the needs of others, will result in better interpersonal communication and more productive professional-professional and professional-client relationships.

TRUST

Trust is another central variable in the human communication process. Trust involves accepting others without evaluating or judging them. It plays an essential part in establishing effective counseling relationships (Johnson & Noonan, 1972). Pearce (1974) points out in his review of the literature that trust exists when a person feels that another individual will behave in ways that are beneficial to the relationship, without attempting to control or direct it. For our discussion, *trust* is defined as an individual's expectation that he or she can rely on the communication behaviors of others. Trust gives relationships a special, unique, positive quality that sets them apart from other relationships.

To illustrate the uniqueness of trusting relationships, presented below are some selected responses that students made when asked to describe the individuals in their lives whom they trusted most. Consider which responses most closely parallel your own feelings about trust. Would you describe the individuals in your life whom you trust most in similar ways?

> He understands me for what I am and he isn't concerned with trying to make me something or someone I'm not. He gives me a feeling of security.

> When I talk to her, she doesn't judge me or my behavior. She knows my innermost feelings and doesn't make fun of them.

> He values my ideas and feelings. I can depend upon him at all times. Whatever I say, he understands it.

> When I talk with her, I usually feel as though she really cares about what I'm saying, plus, I've never had the problem of worrying about whether or not she's going to tell people the confidential things I tell her.

> We can talk about anything, and I know he won't lie to me.

> She seems to allow me to be me (both good and bad). When I tell her a
> bad side of me she doesn't make me feel bad about myself. I feel I can
> talk about anything with her.

These quotes from students indicate that trust is a highly desirable element in our relationships, because it allows us to show both our good and not-so-good sides in the presence of another human being. Although trust is a rather broad and vague concept, its general meaning is clear: We rely on other individuals or events that are outside of ourselves. Trust creates feelings that events are predictable and that people are basically sincere, competent, and accepting.

In health care settings, trust is particularly important to clients because clients often feel helpless, extremely vulnerable, and in need of support. The act of trusting health professionals gives clients a bridge to building relationships that lessen their feelings of depersonalization or vulnerability. Clients will also feel that they can depend on professionals to behave in predictable ways, and that they can rely on professionals' knowledge and integrity. For these reasons, trust appears to be an important variable to study in health care.

Conceptual Frameworks of Trust

Researchers have approached trust from three different orientations: game theory (Deutsch, 1958; Vinacke, 1969), credibility research (Giffin, 1967), and interpersonal trust research (Pearce, 1974; Wheeless, 1978). In the game theory literature, trust has been studied most often by having individuals play what is called the Prisoner's Dilemma game (Luce & Raiffa, 1957)[1] and observing participants' behaviors during the game. Prisoner's Dilemma is a two-person game in which individuals are asked to choose between two alternatives, both of which produce gains or losses for the individual and for the individual's partner. The key psychological element of the game is that mutual trust must exist between the players in order to solve the game, since independent individual behavior does not result in a reasonable solution to the game (Deutsch, 1960, p. 138). The theorists measure trust through the choices participants make in the game setting that let them maximize the potential gains for one another. In the game,

---

[1] Luce and Raiffa (1957) describe the Prisoner's Dilemma game as follows: "Two suspects are taken into custody and separated. The district attorney is certain they are guilty of a specific crime, but he does not have adequate evidence to convict them at a trial. He points out to each prisoner that each has two alternatives: to confess to the crime the police are sure they have done or not to confess. If they both do not confess then the district attorney states that he will book them on some very minor trumped-up charge . . . ; if they both confess, they will be prosecuted, but he will recommend less than the most severe sentence; but if one confesses and the other does not, then the confessor will receive lenient treatment for turning state's evidence whereas the latter will get the "book" slapped at him" (p. 95).

trust is the reliance that one individual places on another in a risky situation in which the individual has a lot to lose.

Game theory is useful because it provides researchers an easy method for establishing a variety of conditions under which trusting behavior can be observed. However, the overall value of this approach is limited because it is difficult to interpret and apply the outcomes of these games to trust in ongoing personal relationships.

A second way of conceptualizing trust emerges from the research that has been conducted on what is called *source credibility*. Studies of source credibility actually originated with Aristotle's *Rhetoric*. Aristotle argued that audiences would believe and trust speakers who exhibit intelligence, character, and good will (Cooper, 1932). Subsequent research by Hovland, Janis, and Kelly (1953) and McCroskey (1966) has empirically confirmed that the first two dimensions—intelligence and character—are indeed factors that contribute to a speaker's credibility. Trust research has focused specifically on the character dimension.

Character is related to how one person perceives the trustworthiness of another person (Wheeless & Grotz, 1975). From this perspective, then, trust is seen as the degree to which one individual perceives another to have certain positive characteristics. For example, by observing certain behaviors in some of our colleagues, such as the fact that they are sincere with clients or conscientious about professional responsibilities, we most likely develop a perception of these colleagues as credible and trustworthy. Put another way, we learn to trust certain individuals because we have seen them act in positive, consistent, and reliable ways.

This concept of trust has been measured by researchers using a series of word-choice scales that are based on measures developed by McCroskey (1966) and Berlo, Lemert, and Mertz (1969). On these scales, individuals describe trustworthy persons as being very benevolent, candid, respectful, considerate, faithful and reliable, to name a few qualities. In short, an individual is highly trusted if others see the individual as having a worthy character. Based on descriptions given by individuals in experimental situations, researchers are able to determine the degree to which individuals trust others.

Trust research has also been approached from an interpersonal perspective. This line of research, taken by Wheeless and Grotz (1975, 1977) and Northouse (1979), indicates that interpersonal trust actually occurs and can be measured at two levels: *general trust* (the trust an individual has of other people in a global sense), and *specific trust* (the trust an individual has of a particular person in a relationship). For example, you may consider yourself to be basically trusting because you openly accept people you meet (high general trust), while at the same time you may have a particular supervisor or colleague whom you at times distrust (low specific trust). Similarly, some paranoid clients may have a general mistrust of other persons, yet they are able to develop a specific trust in a particular mental health nurse or psychiatric social worker.

To measure *general* trust, researchers have employed the widely used Rotter Interpersonal Trust Scale (Rotter, 1967). To measure *specific* trust in the context of interpersonal communication, researchers have used the word-choice scales we mentioned two paragraphs earlier. Using both types of measures, researchers are able to compare and contrast individuals with regard to the general trust and specific trust they exhibit in interpersonal situations. Unlike the other research frameworks, which view trust more as a quality that a person does or does not have, the interpersonal trust perspective can also look at trust as a variable that may change when an individual is involved in specific relationships and specific situations.

Applications of Trust in Health Care

Two positive outcomes emerge when trust is present in interpersonal relationships. First, trust helps individuals to experience a sense of security and connectedness, to feel that they are not alone and that others care about them. Second, trust creates a supportive climate in relationships which reduces defensive communication: It makes individuals more open and honest about their attitudes, feelings, and values. In health care settings, the first outcome—security—is especially important to clients; the second outcome—a supportive climate—is important to both health professionals and clients.

Trust: The client's perspective

The nature of various health care situations can increase clients' needs to establish trusting relationships with professionals. Undergoing brain surgery, selecting a treatment regimen, receiving an intravenous medication, or having their chest X-rays read are just a few of a multitude of complex and disturbing situations in which clients need to depend on and trust health professionals. Cantor (1978), describes how important it is for cancer patients to establish a relationship with a skilled and competent oncologist: "Being able to trust those upon whom we must depend is essential. . . . We seek out the best in others and attach our hopes to their abilities" (p. 75). Clients are simply unable to do many of the things that health professionals do, and in many ways they are forced to depend on the competent skills of the professionals (Tagliacozzo & Mauksch, 1979). Being able to trust the professionals reduces some of the fear and uncertainty that is inherent in this forced dependence. Furthermore, clients have a need to be able to see professionals as competent, sincere, and caring individuals (Tagliacozzo & Mauksch, 1979). Being able to trust professionals produces in clients the sense of being connected to others and the feeling of not being alone.

Trust: The professional's perspective

Knowing that trust reduces uncertainty in clients and helps them to feel secure is important for professionals to understand. But in addition, professionals will want to be aware of ways in which they can help clients to develop that trust.

As we described in the preceding section on conceptual frameworks, clients trust professionals if they believe professionals are worthy (source credibility) and if they develop caring relationships with health professionals (interpersonal trust). Health professionals who want to establish trust with clients will try to build both their professional credibility as well as trusting interpersonal relationships. Too often these two kinds of trust are fostered separately from one another or not fostered at all. For example, the health professional may go to great lengths to convince the client of his or her expertise or credibility in technical matters, while totally disregarding the elements of a caring relationship that are necessary to develop interpersonal trust. The following example illustrates a situation in which neither credibility nor a caring atmosphere was present.

A young brain surgeon hurriedly walked into the room of a 75-year-old woman, and introduced himself as the neurosurgeon who had been asked by another physician to assess her neurological condition. The woman and her family had never heard of this neurosurgeon and were immediately skeptical about his competence because he was quite young. After quickly assessing the woman's physical status and giving her the results of the CAT scan and laboratory reports, the surgeon recommended that the woman be scheduled for surgery at 8:00 A.M. the next morning. The woman and her family were startled at this sudden suggestion for surgery, since another physician had previously diagnosed the woman as having had a stroke and had prescribed outpatient physical rehabilitation for the past three months. The woman and her family expressed their concern to the physician, stating that events were moving too fast and that they needed time to think and talk about the situation. The surgeon appeared dismayed at the woman's hesitation and the request for more time. He told her that he had two accident victims with severe head injuries waiting for him in the emergency room and he had no more time to talk with her. . . . The woman refused the surgery.

In the next few days the family members called different health professionals they knew to gather more information on the neurosurgeon. They learned that he was noted for his surgical skills but not for his interpersonal skills. Also, over the next few days, the neurosurgeon altered his approach to the woman and her family, spent a little more time discussing the pros and cons of surgery and building rapport. After learning about the surgeon's expertise and after building a limited rapport with the surgeon, the woman consented to surgery.

This example vividly illustrates the importance of trust in professional-client communication. The patient and her family find themselves in a situation in which they must depend on a health professional to perform a difficult operation. They do not understand the details behind the two different diagnoses they have received, and they are frightened. Naturally, they want to trust the surgeon and they know they need to trust him; yet his attitude and approach reduce his credibility in the minds of the patient and her family.

By the initial refusal of surgery, the message is sent to the surgeon "We don't trust you. . . . Show us that we can trust you." The surgeon responds to the patient and family by demonstrating an increased degree of concern. The additional time he spends helps the patient and family feel more a part of the treatment process and more secure with the surgeon. Also, as the family hears other health professionals' opinions of the surgeon's competence, his source credibility increases. In the end, the surgeon is trusted for both his competence and his supportive behavior, and the patient and her family agree to the surgery.

Building trust with clients is not an easy task for health professionals, especially because of the many demands on their time. Nonetheless, health professionals need to realize that their behavior toward others does influence, either positively or negatively, the development of trust. For example, health professionals who actively try to be knowledgeable, sincere, honest, predictable, and caring can enhance their source credibility with others. In a similar way, health professionals who try to nurture supportive relationships can encourage others' trust.

Up to this point, we have been discussing the importance of developing trust in relationships. Now we would like to assess which communication factors in professional-client and professional-professional relationships will foster trust.

Our primary source for this discussion will be a classic article by Gibb (1961) which divides different types of communication behaviors into only two categories: those communication behaviors that produce a *supportive climate* and those that produce a *defensive climate*. Those that produce a supportive climate could be trust-producing behaviors; the opposite behaviors, which result in a defensive climate, could be termed distrust-producing behaviors (see Table 2.1)

Trust is enhanced in health care relationships when professionals use supportive communication behaviors (e.g., description, problem orientation, spontaneity, etc.). Gibb's work implies that health professionals should try to avoid using communication behaviors that arouse defensiveness and distrust (e.g., evaluation, control, strategy, etc.). In the next section each trust-producing behavior is described and contrasted with its opposite distrust-producing behavior.

**TABLE 2.1   Categories for Communication Behaviors
That Produce Trust and Distrust**

DEFENSIVE CLIMATES	SUPPORTIVE CLIMATES
1. Evaluation	1. Description
2. Control	2. Problem orientation
3. Strategy	3. Spontaneity
4. Neutrality	4. Empathy
5. Superiority	5. Equality
6. Certainty	6. Provisionalism

Reprinted from J. R. Gibb, "Defensive Communication."
Journal of Communication, 1961, *11* (3), 143. Reprinted with
permission of the International Communication Association.

Evaluation versus description. Professionals whose communication is
evaluative in tone or content will increase defensiveness in others. "If by
expression, manner of speech, tone of voice, or verbal content the sender
seems to be evaluating or judging the listener, then the receiver goes on
guard" (Gibb, 1961, p. 143). Descriptive communication, on the other
hand, reduces defensiveness in the receiver and increases trust. It is being
free of moral or value judgments; it does not prescribe what the listener
ought to do differently. For example:

> EVALUATION: You haven't positioned this patient properly. You have
> to do it this way. (*Demonstrates.*)
>
> DESCRIPTION: I have found that patients experience less pain when
> they are turned on their unaffected side with two pillows placed be-
> tween their legs like this (*demonstrates*) and another pillow behind
> their back.

Control versus problem orientation. Professionals whose communication
attempts to control the receiver will create a reaction of distrust. When the
listener senses that the professional is trying to change his or her attitudes,
values, or behaviors through the communication, it implies that the listener
is inadequate, less informed, immature, or unable to make independent
decisions—and the listener will set up resistance. The opposite of this is
problem-oriented communication, which reduces resistance and builds
trust because it involves the listener in defining the problem and finding
solutions. A problem orientation "allows the receiver to set his/her own
goals, make his/her own decisions, and evaluate his/her own program—or
to share with the sender in doing so" (Gibb 1961, p. 145). For example:

> CONTROL: John, you know that desserts are not a part of your diabetic
> diet. You must cut them out of your diet completely or your diabetes
> will not stabilize at a manageable level.

PROBLEM ORIENTATION: John, I gather that you are very fond of desserts. Have you thought of any alternate ways to manage your craving for desserts that would fit into your diabetic diet?

Strategy versus spontaneity.   Listeners distrust communicators who appear to have hidden intentions or specific plans in their messages. Listeners prefer to have professionals communicate with them in uncomplicated ways that are marked by openness, honesty, and directness. Although spontaneity is not always common among health professionals, it is effective in reducing the defensive barriers put up by clients and by other health professionals. For example:

STRATEGY: Jean, you have such great skill in writing nursing care plans, would you mind writing up care plans on Mr. F. and Mr. M. in addition to those other patients?

SPONTANEITY: Jean, I really feel frustrated and pressed for time about writing those two care plans. Would you be willing to help me out and show me how to develop the nursing diagnoses?

Neutrality versus empathy.   When the tone and content of communication express neutrality, the listener tends to resist it. In essence, neutrality makes others feel as if they are not valued as unique persons. Clients resent the clinical, detached patient-as-object approach. On the other hand, empathic communication increases trust because it indicates that others value the listener enough to set their own thoughts and values aside and attempt to place themselves into the listener's personal world. For example:

NEUTRALITY: For patients like your husband who have had a CVA, we typically expect eight out of ten to survive the initial phase and about 30 to 60 percent of the patients to return to a productive work life. It is also likely that your husband will regain only 65 percent of the movement of his right arm.

EMPATHY: Mrs. B., even though this has been a difficult period for you and the family, Mr. B.'s condition seems to be improving now. I am hoping that with some intensive physical rehabilitation, he will be able to regain much of his arm movement, and be able to return to his office on a limited basis.

Superiority versus equality.   People whose communication gives the impression that they feel superior to the listener in some way will be met with a defensive response. Communicating superiority indicates an unwillingness to participate and share in a mutual problem-solving relationship. On the other hand, communicating equality suggests that the speaker is interested in others' perspectives and is willing to participate in planning that will involve mutual trust and respect. As we discussed before, the nature of health care settings actually works against equality between communicators. Nevertheless, attempts to reduce superiority will usually increase trust and have a positive impact on the development of relationships. For example:

> SUPERIORITY: I know you have worked with the family a long time Mrs. L., but my work toward a specialist degree gives me a broader perspective. Here are my ideas about how the family dynamics can be altered.
>
> EQUALITY: Your experience with the family is extremely important in helping me to understand the family relationships. Perhaps we could work together to find some ways to deal with their problems.

Certainty versus provisionalism.   When individuals communicate in a way that indicates absolute, unquestionable certainty, they often evoke distrust in the listener. If professionals imply that their way is always correct and their approach to a problem is the only approach, this belittles the clients' ideas. On the other hand, communication that sounds more provisional will create more trust in the client, because it implies willingness on the professional's part to share control in analyzing a problem. The client then has a chance to participate in the outcome of the interaction. For example:

> CERTAINTY: I give *my* mastectomy patients all the information that they need to know about their rehabilitation from breast surgery. Mrs. K. doesn't need this "touchy-feely" support group you are suggesting!
>
> PROVISIONALISM: You mentioned a support group for mastectomy patients for Mrs. K. Although I don't think she needs it, tell me what you think these groups offer to patients.

All the different types of communication behaviors that health professionals use will have a major impact on the development—or the lack of development—of trust between client and health professional, as well as on trust between professionals. Health care professionals cannot automatically assume that others will immediately trust them and grant them credibility just because they occupy a particular position. By attending to others' needs and communicating in ways that will create positive reactions, health professionals can foster trust and credibility.

SELF-DISCLOSURE

The fourth communication variable we have chosen to discuss in this chapter is self-disclosure. Self-disclosure is included because of its critical importance in facilitating open communication, which is essential in the development of healthy interpersonal relationships. The recognition of self-disclosure as a communication variable can be traced to Sidney M. Jourard's book, *The Transparent Self*, first published in 1964. A central tenet of Jourard's work is that people can attain health only insofar as they gain the courage to be themselves with others, that is, to self-disclose.

Since Jourard's book appeared, self-disclosure has become a popular concept. Many people regard it as a simple straightforward process: The more you are able to disclose about yourself, the healthier you are. Some researchers, however, have begun to question this assumption and have suggested that very high and very low levels of self-disclosure may not be healthy for the self-disclosing individual (Chaikin & Derlega, 1974a; Chelune et al., 1979). In the following discussion, we will take the position that there are appropriate levels of self-disclosure for different situations, and that one of the keys to building effective relationships is being sensitive to how much or how little self-disclosure should be offered to others.

The variable, self-disclosure, can be characterized as any message about the self that one person communicates to another (Cozby, 1973; Wheeless & Grotz, 1975; Wheeless, 1978). Some researchers have defined self-disclosure more specifically by describing it as "the communication of intimacy, or the act of revealing personal information to others" (Gilbert & Horenstein, 1975; Jourard & Jaffee, 1970). For our discussion, self-disclosure will be defined as a process whereby an individual communicates personal information, thoughts, and feelings to others.

Conceptual Frameworks of Self-Disclosure

Jourard's studies of self-disclosure (1964, 1968, 1971) emphasize that self-disclosure benefits individuals because it enables them to find meaning and direction for their lives. Through the process of sharing, individuals discover their true selves in relation to others. Jourard believes that individuals remain healthy as long as they are able to develop human relationships in which self-disclosure is possible. People become less healthy when they are estranged from other human beings and when the opportunities for self-disclosure are no longer possible: In effect, self-disclosure is directly linked to the healthy personality. Although he has reported some evidence that suggests self-disclosure is curvilinearly related to mental health (i.e., the benefits taper off at high and low levels) (Jourard, 1971, p. 234), Jourard's *theoretical* position emphasizes the positive relationship between self-disclosure and personality adjustment as illustrated in Figure 2.3 (D. A. Taylor, 1979).

Other researchers have approached self-disclosure more analytically, examining the *nature* of self-disclosing messages rather than the *benefits* of self-disclosure by itself (Altman & Taylor, 1973; Cozby, 1973; Gilbert & Horenstein, 1975; Pearce & Sharp, 1973; Wheeless & Grotz, 1976). These studies revealed that self-disclosure is composed of at least five separate di-

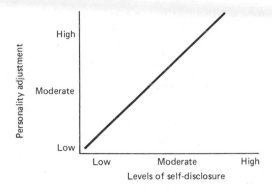

FIGURE 2.3   A positive relationship between self-disclosure and personality adjustment.

mensions or aspects: (1) intention, (2) amount, (3) valence, (4) honesty, and (5) depth.

1. The *intention* aspect of self-disclosure refers to a person's demonstrated willingness to disclose to others. Sometimes individuals disclose information that they had not really planned to share with someone else, such as an unintentional slip of the tongue. However, when individuals consciously choose to reveal their personal thoughts and feelings, they are engaged in intentional self-disclosure.
2. The *amount* aspect refers to the quantity of information a person communicates to others. Individuals who share a lot of information about themselves when talking with others are demonstrating greater amounts of self-disclosure. A client who tells you little about his or her feelings would exemplify a low degree of self-disclosure.
3. The *valence* aspect refers to the positive or negative content of the self-disclosure. If individuals tend to disclose good aspects about themselves, the valence would be labeled positively (+), whereas it would be labeled negatively (−) if the information provided about themselves was primarily unfavorable.
4. The *honesty* dimension refers to the accuracy of the disclosures that an individual makes to others. Self-disclosure may vary in the degree to which what is said accurately matches what an individual really thinks or feels. For example, certain individuals find it difficult to reveal their true experiences to others and may cloak some of their feelings, while others are comfortable "telling it like it is."
5. The *depth* dimension refers to the intimacy level of the content of disclosures. Information of a very personal nature is described as being of greater depth than less personal information.

In addition to studies of the nature of self-disclosing messages, other studies examine self-disclosure from a *situational* perspective, emphasizing variables that affect how appropriate self-disclosure may be in various situations (Chaikin & Derlega, 1974b; Cozby, 1973). In contrast to the position taken by Jourard and others, who assert that increased amounts of self-disclosure are related to increased levels of mental health, other researchers have stressed that self-disclosure is curvilinear (see Fig. 2.4) with extremely high or low levels of self-disclosure being related to adjustment problems in individuals (Chaikin & Derlega, 1974a; Cozby, 1973).

Chaikin and Derlega (1974a) contend that certain factors, such as the nature of interpersonal relationships themselves and different types of situational contexts, mediate or influence the relationship between self-disclosure and mental health. Although there has not been a great deal of research on the general rules governing appropriate self-disclosure, there are some indications that disclosing personal information at an inappropriate time or to the wrong persons may in fact reflect some kind of maladjustment (Chaikin & Derlega, 1974a; Wortman et al., 1976).

The situational approach to self-disclosure taken by Wenburg and Wilmot (1973) also acknowledges both the benefits and risks of self-disclosure. They maintain (1) that situational constraints cannot be ignored and (2) that self-disclosure should be *reasoned.* "In reasoned self-disclosure, one is concerned with the other person as well as himself/herself" (Wenburg & Wilmot, 1973, p. 227). In this perspective, the individual is encouraged to disclose only the amount and kind of information that he or she feels is appropriate to others and to the situation. Wenburg and Wilmot believe that it is legitimate for individuals to keep some things to themselves. Reasoned self-disclosure means the individual can be honest about his or her true feelings without being expected to disclose everything.

To assess self-disclosure, researchers have most frequently used Jourard's Self-Disclosure Questionnaire (Jourard & Lasakow, 1958),

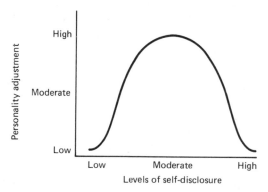

FIGURE 2.4 A curvilinear relationship between self-disclosure and personality adjustment.

consisting of 60 items that measure the extent to which individuals share specific kinds of information with significant others. It should be pointed out, however, that this instrument and subsequent shorter versions of it have been criticized by researchers who have found little evidence that the test is valid—that it actually measures what it claims it does (Cozby, 1973). More recently, Wheeless and Grotz (1976) have developed a new and valid measuring instrument, consisting of sixteen statements that measure the intention, amount, valence, honesty, and depth of self-disclosure.

Applications of Self-Disclosure in Health Care

In the preceding section, we discussed ways of thinking about or conceptualizing self-disclosure. Now we would like to look more closely at how self-disclosure applies to interpersonal relationships in health care settings. Those health care organizations that support open communication among professionals and clients will foster the positive outcomes that can result from self-disclosure. In health care, clients and professionals often approach the self-disclosure process from distinct perspectives, which we will discuss in the next two sections.

Self-disclosure: The client's perspective

Given the many positive outcomes of self-disclosure, why is there so little client self-disclosure in health care settings, and what makes the process of self-disclosure so difficult? Part of the answer lies in the feelings of vulnerability and uncertainty experienced by clients who may wish to share feelings with other clients or health team members. For example, clients often wonder if their reactions to illness and stress are normal. They worry that if they disclose their feelings about their illness, others will evaluate them and find them to be responding in weak, excessive, or strange ways.

Clients may also fear that their self-disclosure could disrupt relationships they have already established with health professionals (Tagliacozzo & Mauksch, 1979). For example, a client who is concerned about some aspects of the health services being provided may fear that a complaint or negative reaction could disrupt the relationship that he or she has with the health team member and could also have a negative impact on the kind of care he or she receives. The point is that clients, because they feel vulnerable, are careful about what they say to health professionals; therefore, they may refrain from self-disclosure because they fear negative repercussions in their care.

Clients' concerns about how others will respond to their self-disclosures are not totally unfounded. In a study of people's reactions to victims, Coates, Wortman, and Abbey (1979) note that when victims disclose their misery and their need for support, others often evaluate them as less well adjusted and less attractive than victims who do not disclose. Similarly, Wortman and Dunkel-Schetter (1979) noted that cancer patients often receive mixed messages or confusing feedback from others in response to the personal concerns that they voice. Perhaps it is not surprising, then, that disclosing feelings can be a difficult process for some patients. Clients may want to self-disclose and yet fear to do so because of the risks that make it so difficult.

One way for clients to resolve this dilemma is to assess the context of the situation and the nature of the relationship. It is unrealistic for professionals to expect clients to freely disclose information about their health or personal matters to anyone at anytime. Instead, it is important for clients to identify trustworthy people who may give them personal support and to have access to settings where there is enough privacy for self-disclosing communication. Clients need to be encouraged to participate actively in the process of choosing people and places for self-disclosure, so that the experience is comfortable and positive for them, rather than threatening and nonproductive.

Consider the following example in which a woman is encouraged by an acquaintance to self-disclose in a very public setting. As you read the example, assess the difficulties faced by the woman who is being asked to talk about a personal health-related matter.

Joanne was a 30-year-old woman who miscarried in her eighth month of pregnancy. One month after the loss of her baby, Joanne was asked to serve punch at a reception in a hospital dining room.

A former colleague and acquaintance of Joanne's came to the reception. Upon arriving at the reception, she went to the punchbowl where Joanne was serving and expressed her sympathy to Joanne. She told Joanne that she was sorry about the loss of her baby and then proceeded to ask questions such as, "What do the doctors feel the problem was that caused you to lose the baby?" and "This won't affect your ability to have children in the future, will it?" Joanne gave brief responses to the questions and excused herself from the punchbowl saying she had to use the bathroom. In the bathroom Joanne tried to gain back the composure which she had lost while choking back the sad feelings these questions rekindled.

Later, when discussing this incident, Joanne said that she wished that the woman had waited until she was not in the middle of serving punch or she wished the woman had visited her in her office. She felt very uncomfortable sharing such private information in such a public setting. Joanne also noted that she and this woman had never really talked about personal things before, even when they had worked together, and that it seemed quite unnatural to discuss those kinds of things now.

This case illustrates a situation in which neither a trusting relationship nor privacy was available and the person found self-disclosure almost impossible. Health care settings are notorious for the lack of privacy available to clients and their families. Large four-bed wards and semiprivate rooms make disclosure of personal information very difficult. Giving families information in front of other families in waiting rooms, or asking them to step into hallways to hear results of surgical procedures obviously inhibits self-disclosure. The clinic waiting room is another example of a public setting that could hinder not only clients' disclosures to professionals, but also professionals' disclosures to clients. If health professionals accept the importance of self-disclosure for clients, it is important for professionals to work toward creating contexts in health care settings in which self-disclosure can be fostered, and then to nurture trusting relationships in which client disclosure can be facilitated.

Another aspect to take into consideration is that clients vary in their preference for self-disclosure (Bradac, Tardy, & Hosman, 1980). You may know some people who are comfortable sharing personal information with many people without any hesitation. You may also know people who are comfortable disclosing information to only one or two close family members and, even then, do so with great difficulty and restraint. Because of this variability in individuals, health professionals need to assess clients' readiness and preferences for self-disclosure. Expecting immediate self-disclosure from clients who seldom self-disclose to anyone or who have not yet developed a comfortable rapport with us may be an unrealistic expectation (Klotowski, 1980). Only as we take into consideration the preferences of the other person, the nature of our relationships, and the settings of the interactions will we be able to assist clients in showing *reasoned* self-disclosure.

Self-disclosure: The professional's perspective

Most health professionals see self-disclosure as important for clients. As professionals they are faced with the problem of creating contexts in which clients feel free to self-disclose, building relationships that foster self-disclosure in these situations, and doing both without failing to meet their other professional obligations. At the same time, however, professionals need to find ways to self-disclose and ventilate their own feelings. Even though there is not a long tradition to support professional self-disclosure in the health care fields, there is evidence that it is important for professionals (Jourard, 1964). A closer examination of the professional's perspective may provide some insight into why self-disclosure is a difficult aspect of the communication process for professionals in health care.

In a study of self-disclosure at a large public urban hospital, Johnson

(1980) noted three explanations that were commonly given by staff nurses who were asked whether they self-disclosed to patients or whether they encouraged patients to self-disclose to staff. First, nurses in this study indicated that they did not have sufficient time to listen to clients once the clients started to talk about personal matters and feelings. Second, nurses indicated that other nursing care activities were given higher priority than self-disclosure. Last, nurses pointed out that they did not have the skills to handle self-disclosure from clients and they could do little to change clients' personal problems. The first two explanations are understandable in light of the nature of health care systems that stress the importance of technical tasks over interpersonal processes. But the third explanation, the health professionals' discomfort with patients' disclosures, needs further consideration.

Some health professionals feel they do not have the skill or do not feel comfortable enough to elicit client self-disclosure. In the following example, an oncologist describes his interactions with cancer patients and the approach that he takes toward their self-disclosure.

> I know that patients who have cancer have much going on inside themselves about the meaning of life, death, and their cancer experience. I value these feelings. . . . But I don't feel prepared to respond to them, so I don't encourage patients to talk about their feelings. Allowing patients to talk about the existential anxiety they feel is important, but I don't really deal with this aspect.

The physician acknowledges patients' needs to air their feelings, yet he expresses personal concern about how he should handle patients' self-disclosures. This illustration is not an isolated case, but may represent the response of many health professionals to patients' self-disclosure. Health professionals can recognize the importance of self-disclosure for clients and yet find it hard to feel comfortable with it or know how to react. Apart from the constraints of lack of time and the many tasks that must be done, why do professionals often feel this way? What are the possible explanations for their problem?

Perhaps one explanation for the discomfort that some professionals feel in the presence of client self-disclosure is that their education does not stress the importance of psychosocial factors in the health care process. Physicians, for example, have in-depth preparation in the physical sciences, such as chemistry, physiology and biochemistry, but they have little academic preparation in social sciences such as psychology, social psychology, and sociology.

Another reason why health professionals may be hesitant to respond to clients' disclosures is that their education stresses that there is a "right way" to respond to each patient's condition. For example, the presence of symptom A (lung congestion) in the patient requires the correct reaction B (encouraging coughing and deep breathing) on the part of the professional. However, not all patient problems can be addressed in such a straightforward cause-and-effect manner. When patients and their family members share psychosocial concerns (such as feelings of anger, sadness, and frustration about their health), professionals are confronted with a problem for which they have no *exact* treatment. Many times there is no "right way" to respond to client self-disclosure. There is more ambiguity and uncertainty in psychosocial areas of treatment; therefore, sorting out appropriate responses to clients seems less than clear-cut and more difficult for professionals.

Finally, concerns about their own ability to remain objective and to remain composed in their responses to client self-disclosure may inhibit professionals from eliciting open expression of feelings from clients. Some professionals fear that being in touch with clients' feelings can be an obstacle to good treatment. Yet, as the following example from a cancer patient's unpublished journal so clearly suggests, patients *do* want health professionals to help them in the self-disclosure process.

> The emotional support I received during my experience with cancer was limited. I wanted to talk to someone who could put the medical facts in the proper perspective for me. My need for support was most overwhelming when I started receiving radiation treatments. Yet this is when I had the least support.
>
> I felt hostile, desperate, frightened, and totally alone. I needed answers to my questions about the "machines." The technicians later told me they did not talk much to me because they were not supposed to talk with patients and they thought leaving me alone was the best thing! I think they were as frightened of me as I was of them.
>
> I don't know why people were afraid to talk with me about my cancer. I'm the one who had the disease, not them, I'm the one who had to walk away from the clinic and live with it.
>
> It seemed like there was no place for me to release my daily anxieties. At 29 years old, I felt that I did not belong in the waiting room with the "old" people with "cancer." Even if I wanted to talk to them I couldn't because it was blatantly discouraged by the sign on the wall which read: *Please do not talk about your problems with other patients.* What help we might have been to each other! It would have outweighed any harm. Certainly a cancer patient did not make that sign and hang it on the wall.

In essence, this patient is expressing her desire to be heard by health professionals. Her remarks suggest that clients do not want health professionals to be insulated; they want professionals to help them in the self-disclosure process and to communicate with them about personal and health-related subjects.

Up to this point in our discussion we have been focusing on possible explanations for why health professionals find it difficult to promote client self-disclosure. Another aspect that deserves consideration is the approach health professionals themselves take toward self-disclosing to clients and to other professionals. Several questions are commonly raised in this regard: For example, should health professionals engage in self-disclosure at all? Is it appropriate for them to self-disclose to clients? What is the role of self-disclosing communication in professional-professional relationships?

Based on our preceding discussion of conceptual frameworks for self-disclosure, these questions would be answered affirmatively. It is helpful when health professionals share their personal feelings with other professionals and to some extent with clients. All the positive outcomes of self-disclosure, so strongly espoused by Jourard and others, are available to professionals just as they are to clients. So, too, the rules for appropriate self-disclosure apply to professionals as they do to clients. Too much or too little self-disclosure is maladaptive for professionals just as it is for any individual.

In communication between professionals and clients, the focus of the interaction needs to remain on the client. Fostering patient disclosure does not require that professional disclosure be inhibited—in fact, to be fully effective, self-disclosure needs some element of reciprocity. However, reciprocal disclosure does require that professional self-disclosure be appropriately expressed. It does *not* mean that the professional "tells all" to the client or switches the focus of the interaction onto the needs of the professional—only that the professional uses self-disclosure to facilitate empathic understanding. Therefore, reciprocity of disclosure calls for sharing honest feelings and observations with clients, as in the following statements:

> The situation you're telling me about sounds really frightening. I probably would have felt the same way you did.

> I'm glad that you told me about that. It gives me a better understanding of what you are going through. I really sense you have deep inner strength that was untapped before this crisis.

> I know you're angry about the missing laboratory report. I'm also very mad and frustrated at the way this thing has worked out.

> I can understand your hesitancy to see a marriage counselor. A few years ago I was in a similar crisis and found my talks with a mental health professional very helpful. . . . You may want to give the idea a little more thought.

In these situations the focus of the interaction remains on the client, even though the professional is sharing some of his or her own feelings and perceptions.

Even in the area of treatment decisions, sharing concerns and questions can create a participatory relationship between the professional and the client. The following example illustrates this type of reciprocal self-disclosure.

A 55-year-old man who had had surgery for an obstructed bowel exhibited symptoms including nausea, distended abdomen, and moderately severe pain. Three days after surgery, the following brief conversation took place between the man and the surgeon.

PATIENT: I'm still feeling bad. My pain isn't going away and I don't feel any better than I did before surgery. What do you think is the matter? (*Puzzled look on his face.*)

SURGEON: I just don't know; I'm concerned too. I know the bowel has been reattached properly, so that couldn't be causing these problems. I can't figure it out. (*Sitting with a frown on his face, arms closed in front of his chest, one hand supporting his chin.*)

PATIENT: Well, I'm glad to know that you think the bowel attachment is OK. . . . Anything I can do to get rid of some of this bloated feeling? (*Looking at physician.*)

SURGEON: We might increase your exercise a little to help with the peristalsis. I'll check back with you tonight. We'll work this one out. (*Touches patient's shoulder as he leaves.*)

The following day the symptoms subsided and the patient went on to a complete recovery. Later, in recalling his postsurgery complications the patient graphically described how the surgeon, while pacing at the foot of the patient's bed, had expressed his bewilderment with the complications. He said that although he was concerned that the surgeon didn't know exactly what was wrong, he felt assured by the physician's open, honest approach and willingness to involve him in the problem-solving process.

In disclosing his concerns about the postsurgery problems, the surgeon allowed the patient to perceive him as fallible. This disclosure encouraged the patient to become actively involved in his care and also let him see a very human side of the physician. To honestly express his frustrations and concerns about the patient's progress in this way was appropriate professional-client self-disclosure, and it had a positive impact on their relationship.

In addition to the importance of professionals using disclosure with clients, it is also important for professionals to feel that they can self-disclose to other professionals. When professionals engage in self-disclosure with other professionals, they can express their feelings and talk about things that concern them with others who are likely to understand and be supportive. In professional-professional relationships, health care workers can be their true selves. Facades and roles can be discarded, thus enabling deeper disclosure. Although it is more common for professionals to share feelings and concerns with their own colleagues (nurses with nurses, social workers with social workers, and administrators with administrators), it is also important for interdisciplinary sharing to take place. A common problem facing health professionals is the lack of understanding of the unique problems faced by professionals in different disciplines (see Chapter 3). Through interdisciplinary communication and self-disclosure, nurses can increase their sensitivity to social workers, and physicians can increase their sensitivity to nurses, to name only a few possibilities. Through appropriate self-disclosure, health care professionals can begin to relax some of their defensive postures, and exchange some of their true concerns and feelings. The result may well be increased cooperation and understanding among the staff, and higher quality care for their clients.

CONFIRMATION

Confirmation, the final human communication variable we have selected to discuss, overlaps in some ways with the variables we have already presented (empathy, control, trust, and self-disclosure). Confirmation involves dimensions of showing empathy, sharing control, exhibiting trust, and disclosing personal thoughts and feelings to others. However, confirmation is also a distinct variable that plays a unique role in health communication. Confirmation occurs when individuals respond to others in ways that indicate to others that they are acknowledged and understood. Confirmation is a means of communicating that focuses on the ways individuals experience the world and ascribe meaning to events. It is a relatively new concept which is starting to receive more emphasis in health care (Heineken, 1982). In the following sections we will try to make the meaning of confirmation clearer and more concrete by discussing how researchers have defined confirmation. In addition, we will examine how health professionals can apply theoretical information about confirmation to improve their communication.

The writings of existentialists, such as Martin Buber, Viktor Frankl, and R. D. Laing, stress the importance of confirmation. According to Buber (1957), all individuals wish to be confirmed and accepted for what they are and what they can become. Societies in which confirmation flourishes are the most human. In addition, Buber believes that every person in society is able to fulfill this wish *in others* by confirming them as unique human beings (p. 102). Approaching confirmation from a different perspective, Viktor Frankl (1963), in a moving account of how he and others survived Auschwitz and the Nazi concentration camps, describes the importance of being able to ascribe meaning to one's *own* existence, whether it be through doing a deed, through experiencing the love of another human being, or through suffering (p. 176). For Frankl, the essence of life revolves around our ability to find meaning through actively choosing the way in which we respond to life's circumstances. The meaning we establish for our lives—and our actions and responses—all become more meaningful when they are acknowledged and *validated* by others. In a quite different context, R. D. Laing, a psychiatrist interested in the consequences of *dis*confirming communication on patients, has written about confirmation from his clinical observations. He has focused on finding ways to prevent people from disconfirming others. Laing (1967) describes the opposite of confirmation as being those "attempts to constrain the other's freedom, to force him to act in the way we desire, but with ultimate lack of concern, with indifference to the other's own existence or destiny" (p. 36).

In our discussion, confirmation will refer to specific kinds of communicative responses that one individual makes to another. *Confirming responses* acknowledge and validate the other person's perspective. They are responses that enable someone else to value himself or herself more fully as a human being (Sieburg & Larson, 1971). Engel (1980) has suggested that confirming responses include acceptance of the other individual's self-definition despite the fact that this definition may be very different from one's own definition of the other. On the other hand, *disconfirming responses* express indifference to and denial of the presence and experiences of another. They are responses that cause another person to place less value on himself or herself as a human being (Sieburg & Larson, 1971). In other words, disconfirming responses imply that we perceive others as being incapable of creating a sense of who they are on their own (Werner-Beland, 1980, p. 180).

Conceptual Frameworks of Confirmation

As we discussed in Chapter 1, every communication event occurs on two levels: content and relationship. Confirmation can be thought of as occurring on the *relationship* level. Individuals define who they are through other's responses to them (Sieburg, 1975). Thus it is satisfying if others respond in ways that affirm the receiver's own experience, and it is painful if others respond in a disconfirming manner that negates the receiver's self-experience.

Confirming and disconfirming responses were first identified in studies by Sieburg (1969) and Sieburg and Larson (1971). Sieburg's initial work included a factor analytic study of a list of "ways of responding" and peoples' preferences for these ways of responding in their interactions with others. Two major factors that described the communication responses emerged from her analysis: The first factor, identified as *confirming responses,* included items labeled direct responses, agreement, clarification, supportive responses, and expression of positive feelings. The second factor, identified as *disconfirming responses*, included imperviousness, interruption, irrelevant responses, tangential responses, and unclear responses.

Receiving confirming responses can validate an individual's experience in three ways (Sieburg, 1979, pp. 9–10): (1) Confirming responses decrease a person's fears of depersonalization by acknowledging that person's presence; they confirm the receiver's feeling, "I exist." For example, health professionals who show confirmation to clients are communicating to clients the obvious but extremely important message that the professional is aware of the presence of the client as a unique human being. (2) Confirming responses relieve the individual's fears of being blamed or rejected, by validating the individual's own way of experiencing events. Individuals learn to feel that their own perspective is legitimate and that it is all right for them to be who they are. (3) Confirming responses reduce feelings of loneliness, alienation, and abandonment by creating in the receiver the undeniable feeling that he or she is engaged in a human relationship with another person. In essence, the confirming response is saying to the receiver, "I see you, you are OK, and you and I have established a relationship."

Applications of Confirmation in Health Care

Throughout this book it has been stressed that health professionals have a responsibility to be sensitive to the circumstances of clients and to assist clients in finding ways to participate in their own treatment. Of all the variables discussed in this chapter, confirmation is probably the most important in this process.

Confirmation: the client's perspective

As previously mentioned, when health professionals' communication is confirming, it helps clients in a variety of ways. First, through communicating in confirming ways, health professionals provide recognition of clients as unique persons with real problems. Clients often feel like inanimate objects, as if they were objects rather than people. A vivid illustration of this is provided in the following example of a nurse who was a patient in a rehabilitation hospital.

> One day, as I was sitting on the toilet, a volunteer brought a group of visitors through the bathroom. The volunteer threw back the curtain that served as the door of the toilet stall, exposing both me and my wheelchair (the latter of which was slightly more socially acceptable at that moment). Then the volunteer proudly announced to the group of visitors, "This is one of our quadriplegics!" I literally felt as though I was nothing, and as far as meaning anything, I did not. I might just as well have been a resident on Monkey Island at the zoo. In order to reconfirm that I was indeed somebody, I shouted a few phrases that would have make a longshoreman blush. The volunteer and the visitors

retreated while uttering comments about what an ungrateful, uncouth wretch I was. Well at least "ungrateful and uncouth" constitutes an identity of sorts and one which at that moment I preferred to no identity at all.[2]

In the above situation, the nurse loudly voiced a desire to be treated as a person and not as an object to be studied. Clients are vulnerable and, unfortunately, easily viewed only as cases—the "gallbladder in room 518," "the triple bypass in the stepdown unit," or the "C-section in 306"—which negates their humanness. Although these labels are not intended to be harmful in any way, they are examples of the subtle ways health professionals disconfirm clients. Health professionals have a responsibility to recognize clients as *people* with unique, innate human needs.

Second, by confirming communication, health professionals assure clients that their responses to illness and their concerns are normal, and that they will not be rejected for the feelings they experience.

Clients in health care settings find themselves in a strange environment, and they are often expected to do things they would not normally have to do in their home settings such as wear identifying wristbands, urinate in plastic cups, and expose their bodies to the scrutiny of numerous people. Not only do these new situations and relationships produce stress, but they also can result in clients' developing feelings of being different. It is not unusual for clients to wonder if they are coping adequately with these changes and if their responses are appropriate.

For example, the woman who is experiencing acute grief over the loss of her husband may sometimes hear the voice of her deceased husband and wonder whether she is going crazy. An informed health professional who understands the grieving process can confirm her response as being perfectly normal. In another situation, while clients are waiting for laboratory results, X-ray readings, or pathology reports that sometimes take a long time to return, they may react to the uncertainty of the situation by conjuring up their own reasons for the delays. For example, a client may think, "They must have found something bad that they don't want to tell me about." Or, "It must mean that something really unusual is going on." Clients will interpret the events around them in their own unique way and probably much differently from the way in which we health professionals would interpret the same event. A health professional can give a confirming response to clients' reactions in these uncertain situations. Confirmation does not have to mean that health professionals *agree* with clients—just that it is all right for clients to respond in their own way.

---

[2]Jean A. Werner-Beland, *Grief Responses to Long-Term Illness and Disability*, 1980, p. 181. Reprinted with permission of Reston Publishing Co., a Prentice-Hall Co., 11480 Sunset Hills Road, Reston, Va. 22090.

Third, we have observed that confirmation is also important in providing clients in health care settings with a sense of connectedness. In hospitals, clients can feel disconnected, not only from family and work, but even from the health professionals who are caring for them. These feelings are illustrated in the following comments a patient made to one of the authors about her intense feelings of alienation while undergoing a series of exploratory surgeries.

> I wish I knew what was happening. No one seems to know what's going on around here. Are they going to have to operate on me again? What did the last biopsy show? Why are they doing more X-rays? Will the same person operate if they choose to do more surgery? Who is coordinating all of this? I feel like no one is in charge of what's happening to me. No one cares a bit. It's like I'm a cabbage sitting here in a field; I'm left out and no one even knows it.

This client was describing deep feelings of fear that things were happening to her and that the health professionals around her did not seem to be concerned. She wanted and needed information and confirmation. Information concerning her X-rays, biopsies, and surgeries would have helped to lessen her fears of being a meaningless object (a cabbage in a field) that no one cared about. Acknowledging her circumstances (the lack of coordination) through confirming responses would have reduced her feelings of alienation and helped her to feel involved with health professionals in her own treatment.

Confirmation: The professional's perspective

Confirmation is essential for clients, but it is also important for nurses and other health professionals. Perhaps one of the reasons for this is that health professionals themselves experience so little confirmation from clients and other health professionals. Time pressures, rotating shifts, and staff shortages make it difficult for professionals to share in meaningful communication with others. In this environment it is not surprising that nurses and other health professionals often feel as if they are just one of many cogs in a wheel.

Just as clients have a need to be treated personally, professionals also have a need to be seen by others as fully human and able to make unique professional contributions to the health care process. Health professionals dislike being treated as insignificant persons. For example, a psychiatric nurse who develops a treatment plan for a depressed client does not like to hear that the psychologist working with the patient has cancelled the treatment plan because it did not originate with him or her. The psychologist's invalidating the treatment plan disconfirms the psychiatric nurse as an independent professional who is competent to make assessments and formulate treatment plans. Similarly, a medical social worker who arranges a discharge planning meeting with an entire staff to discuss procedures for placing patients in nursing homes does not want to learn at the start of the meeting that the attending physician on the unit is not going to be present. In this example, the physician's absence communicates that the social worker's professional actions (to call a planning meeting) are without value and significance. These examples by no means exhaust the impersonal and disconfirming ways in which professionals treat each other.

Furthermore, health professionals, like clients, also have a need to feel accepted and worthwhile. Although they seldom say it out loud, many professionals have a strong desire to be viewed as an integral member of the health care team. They want to participate, make contributions, and be involved. Regardless of the level of status of the health care team member, each member desires to have his or her professional contributions accepted or recognized by others. Nurses, social workers, health educators, chaplains, physicians, pharmacists, physical therapists, occupational therapists, and others, each have unique contributions that they want to offer the health care team and that they think deserve feedback from others on the team. During meetings and conversations professionals have a chance to listen to and acknowledge each other's ideas. By confirming communication, professionals expand the potential for mutual acceptance and shared respect.

Health professionals can feel just as separated from their co-workers as alienated clients feel separated from professionals and from their families. Health care settings sometimes demand that each professional work isolated from others in order to fulfill professional responsibilities. As we discuss in Chapter 3, the tasks to be performed by professionals can become so numerous and so complex that professionals seem to have little or no time for personal interaction. Nonetheless, professionals want and need to be related to others. Being confirmed by other professionals satisfies health professionals' desire to be humanly connected to the helping process.

Unfortunately, however, a chain reaction can occur, which begins when health professionals who feel disconfirmed lack the emotional energy to become involved with clients, whom they then treat as objects (see Fig. 2.5). Clients who are themselves experiencing emotional isolation will increase their own disconfirming responses toward the staff. Health professionals interpret these responses as further evidence that they are misunderstood and not appreciated. This chain of reciprocal events can continue until the client is discharged or until one of the persons in the interaction actively seeks to alter this cycle that has evolved.

Interrupting this disconfirming cycle is not easy because system pressures often perpetuate its occurrence. Although changing system pressures is not always possible, learning to alter interpersonal communication patterns is possible. A change toward showing more confirmation of others is

DISCONFIRMING INTERACTION CYCLE

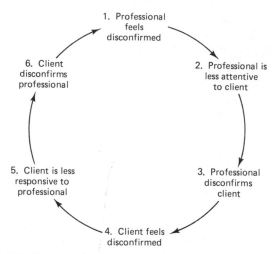

FIGURE 2.5 The cyclical process of disconfirming communication showing the negative effect it has on communication between professionals and clients.

not a cure-all for health communication problems, but confirmation can benefit professionals as well as clients. In the succeeding discussion we will describe negative communication behaviors that perpetuate the cycle as well as positive communication behaviors that will alter the cycle. Sieburg (1969) has identified 12 basic categories of confirming as well as disconfirming responses in interpersonal communication (see Table 2.2 and Table 2.3). Ask yourself which of these responses you generally use with your colleagues and clients. Are you aware of disconfirming responses that you may use when feeling tired or stressed? Are you aware of disconfirming responses that others (clients and colleagues) make to you? Are there disconfirming responses that you too frequently show toward others that you would like to change?

These confirming and disconfirming responses can affect our communication with other professionals as well as our communication with clients. It is not unusual for professionals to slip into old ways of interacting that disconfirm other professionals and clients without noticing the effects this has on others. Altering common communication patterns involves practicing new modes of communication that are confirming, and then adjusting our responses to be consistent with the feedback we receive from others.

The conversations provided in Tables 2.4 and 2.5 illustrate the difference between disconfirming and confirming responses. In the first conversation (Table 2.4), the nurse unintentionally disconfirms the client and

TABLE 2.2   Confirming Responses

Confirming responses are those that make another person value herself or himself more as an individual. They acknowledge the other's existence as a unique person.

The following responses are characterized as confirming:

1. *Direct acknowledgment.*   To respond directly to what the other person communicated. To attend directly to another.

2. *Agreement about content.*   To reinforce or support what the other person is talking about. Examples: "Yes, that is an important area." "At least now I can see your side of the issue."

3. *Supportive response.*   To express understanding, reassurance, or to try to make the other person feel better. Examples: "I think I know what you mean." "With your attitude, I know you'll do well." "I'm impressed with the progress you are making."

4. *Clarification.*   To attempt to make the content of another's message or the other's present or past feelings more understandable. This may include asking for further information or encouraging the other person to express in greater detail how he or she feels. Examples (content): "Tell me more about your reasoning for that point." "I'm not sure I understand; could you explain it further?" Examples (feelings): "Could you describe for me how you feel about that person?" In attempting to clarify the other person's feelings, the emphasis is on description, not on interpreting the feelings.

5. *Expression of positive feelings.*   To respond to another person with affirming uncritical feelings. Examples: "I'm glad you told me that." "What you said makes me want to look further into this."

Adapted from E. Sieburg, "Dysfunctional Communication and Interpersonal Responsiveness in Small Groups." Doctoral dissertation, University of Denver, 1969. *Dissertation Abstracts International,* 1969, *30,* 2622A (University Microfilm No. 69-21, 156).

leaves the client feeling that his concerns are rather stupid. In the second conversation (Table 2.5), because the nurse is more confirming, the client is able to express his underlying concerns and will probably be able to solve his problems more productively.

Tables 2.6 and 2.7 illustrate how confirmation can significantly affect professional-professional interaction. In the first conversation (Table 2.6), the night supervisor fails to acknowledge the pressures being experienced by the staff nurse and hence reacts to the nurse with impervious, irrelevant, tangential, and impersonal disconfirming responses. The end result of the conversation is distant communication, more similar to monologue than dialogue. In the second conversation (Table 2.7) the night supervisor utilizing confirming responses is able to have a more meaningful interaction with the staff nurse, and identifies strong feelings and concerns of the nurse. The scenario in the first interaction perpetuates a disconfirming cyclical interaction, while in the second encounter, the night supervisor alters the interaction, and both people feel confirmed.

Effective communication in health care depends on health professionals who will continually assess their interactions with clients and peers. Conscious attempts to utilize confirming communication responses that are based on the underlying belief in the uniqueness of people and the unique-

TABLE 2.3   Disconfirming Responses

Disconfirming responses deny the other person's existence. These responses are inappropriate or irrelevant to what the other person has communicated. They make the other person value herself or himself less as an individual.

Disconfirming responses may be characterized as follows:

1. *Impervious.*   To ignore or disregard the other person's attempt to communicate by making no verbal or nonverbal acknowledgment of what they have communicated.
2. *Interruptive.*   To cut the speaker off before she or he has a chance to finish a statement or fully elaborate on a point.
3. *Irrelevant.*   To respond in an unrelated way to what another person has communicated. This can be done by introducing a new topic or shifting to a previous topic without warning.
4. *Tangential.*   To acknowledge what the other has said, but to immediately take the conversation in another direction. Examples: "Yes, I know you're having pains in your stomach, but I'm concerned that you're not getting enough exercise." "Yes, I see the problem, but I'm sure it will go away. Let me tell you how another one of my friends got around this problem."
5. *Impersonal.*   To respond in the third person in an intellectualized tone. This type of response often contains many cliches and euphemisms. Examples: "The problem with working double shifts is that one is always tired and prone to make many mistakes." "In debating that particular position, you people need more evidence."
6. *Incoherent.*   To respond in incomplete sentences or long, rambling speeches. This response is often difficult to follow because it contains much retracing and rephrasing which adds nothing to the content of the message.
7. *Incongruous.*   To act in a different way from what you say. It is sending two messages (verbal and nonverbal) that are not consistent. Examples: "No, you're not bothering me." (*Stated in a high voice with shaky hands.*)

Adapted from E. Sieburg, Dysfunctional Communication and Interpersonal Responsiveness in Small Groups." Doctoral dissertation, University of Denver, 1969. *Dissertation Abstracts International,* 1969, *30,* 2622A (University Microfilm No. 69-21, 156).

TABLE 2.4   Example of Disconfirming Interaction between Professional and Client

INTERACTANTS	DISCONFIRMING INTERACTION	KIND OF RESPONSE
MALE PATIENT:	You know, I'm kind of worried about this minor knee surgery . . . Seems a little silly doesn't it, compared to all those other guys who have to have back surgery and heart surgery.	
NURSE:	There is nothing for you to worry about. . . The surgery is fairly easy and won't take too long. (*Straightening up the room.*)	Impervious Irrelevant
MALE PATIENT:	I guess you're right. It's kind of crazy of me to worry. I've got to stop overreacting to things I guess. (*Nervous laugh to self.*)	
NURSE:	Why don't you try to watch a little TV? Watching TV helps keep one's mind off other things. (*Walks out of room.*)	Irrelevant Impersonal

TABLE 2.5 Example of Confirming Interaction between Professional and Client

INTERACTANTS	CONFIRMING INTERACTION	KIND OF RESPONSE
MALE PATIENT:	You know, I'm kind of worried about this minor knee surgery. . . . Seems a little silly doesn't it, compared to all those other guys who have to have back surgery and heart surgery.	
NURSE:	No, I can understand that you might be worried. What are you especially concerned about?	Direct acknowledgment Clarification
MALE PATIENT:	Well, I kind of wonder how I'm going to get around at home. My wife hasn't been too well, and she depends on me to do a lot of things for her. Kind of crazy of me to be so worried about this surgery, isn't it?	
NURSE:	No, I think it's very understandable to wonder what effect the surgery is going to have on your life especially with your wife depending on you the way she does.	Direct acknowledgment Supportive

TABLE 2.6 Example of Disconfirming Interaction between Two Professionals

INTERACTANTS	DISCONFIRMING INTERACTION	KIND OF RESPONSE
STAFF NURSE:	We're really busy here tonight. We're short of staff and E.R. has sent up three new patients to be admitted. I'm feeling hassled and in need of some help.	
NIGHT SUPERVISOR:	You wouldn't believe it but things are that way throughout the hospital. You should have been here last night.	Impervious Irrelevant
STAFF NURSE:	It couldn't have been much worse than tonight. It seems like it's impossible to do everything. It's really a problem.	
NIGHT SUPERVISOR:	I know, but it's always going to be this way when the census is up. One just has to stay with it and do what one can do.	Tangential Impersonal

TABLE 2.7   Example of Confirming Interaction between Two Professionals

INTERACTANTS	CONFIRMING INTERACTION	KIND OF RESPONSE
STAFF NURSE:	We're really busy here tonight. We're short of staff and E.R. has sent up three new patients to be admitted. I'm feeling hassled and in need of some help.	
NIGHT SUPERVISOR:	I can see you're under pressure here. This place is really busy. As far as additional staff to help out, I don't know what to tell you. All the float-staff have already been assigned.	Direct acknowledgment Agreement about content
STAFF NURSE:	On nights like this, trying to fulfill *all* my responsibilities really makes me feel up-tight. I want everything to get done but I just can't do it all by myself.	
NIGHT SUPERVISOR:	I understand your situation. You're trying to do *everything* but it's impossible. I'm glad you've made me aware of this. I'll try to get more staff up here to relieve some of this pressure, if I can.	Supportive response Expression of positive feelings

ness of their responses to situations provide the means for clients and professionals to experience connectedness with others and for them to experience minimal alienation and rejection.

SUMMARY

In this chapter, conceptual frameworks of five selected communication variables were presented and the effects of these variables on the communication of clients and professionals in health care settings were discussed. Our intention has been to demonstrate how the application of these variables—empathy, control, trust, self-disclosure, and confirmation—can enhance health communication.

Empathy is the process of observing the world from another person's point of view. It is a complex variable that occurs within the source, within the receiver, and within messages. Through empathy clients are helped to feel that they are understood, accepted, and that they have a sense of control over their circumstances. For professionals, empathy improves the accuracy of communication and reduces misunderstanding.

Control is an intrinsic part of human interaction. There are two kinds of control: personal and relational. When individuals sense that they can influence the circumstances surrounding their lives, they have personal control. In health care, clients have intense needs for personal control. Relational control is the process whereby individuals share influence with other individuals within relationships. Three kinds of relationships can be established through different approaches to relational control: complementary, symmetrical, and parallel. A willingness to adapt one's own needs for control to the needs of others is the key to building productive relationships. Effective professional-professional and professional-client relationships are usually based on shared control.

Trust is present in relationships when individuals feel that they can rely on others. Being able to trust health professionals as competent and caring helps clients face the fears and uncertainties of illness. In professional-professional and professional-client relationships, building trust requires that individuals' communication be descriptive rather than evaluative, problem oriented rather than control oriented, spontaneous rather than strategic, empathic rather than neutral, equal rather than superior, and provisional rather than certain.

Self-disclosure is a process in which an individual communicates personal information, thoughts, and feelings to others. If exhibited appropriately, self-disclosure has many benefits for clients and professionals: If there is too much or too little disclosure, or if it is given in inappropriate circumstances, it can be maladaptive. In health care settings, many factors make it difficult for both clients and professionals to self-disclose. Nevertheless, it is important for health care organizations to foster reasoned self-disclosure in client-professional and professional-professional relationships.

Confirmation refers to the communication that enables others to value themselves more fully as unique human beings. By communicating in confirming ways, health professionals help clients to cope with feelings of depersonalization, rejection, and alienation. Confirming responses show to others direct acknowledgment, agreement about content, supportiveness, clarification, and expression of positive feelings. Disconfirming responses are impervious, interruptive, irrelevant, tangential, impersonal, incoherent, and incongruous. Professionals need confirmation from other professionals just as much as clients need confirmation from professionals.

Each of these five variables describes a different component in the highly complex process of health communication. By observing these variables from both the client's perspective and the professional's point of view, the communication that takes place in health care settings can be enhanced.

REFERENCES

Altman, I., & Taylor, D. A. *Social penetration: The development of interpersonal relationships.* New York: Holt, Rinehart & Winston, 1973.
Arakelian, M. An assessment and nursing application of the concept of locus of control. *Advances in Nursing Science,* 1980, *3*(1), 25–42.

Barrett-Lennard, G. T. The empathy cycle: Refinement of a nuclear concept. *Journal of Counseling Psychology*, 1981, *28*(2), 91–100.

Bateson, G. *Naven* (2nd ed.). Stanford, Calif.: Stanford University Press, 1958.

Bergin, A. E., & Strupp, H. H. *Changing frontiers in the science of psychotherapy.* Chicago: Aldine-Atherton, Inc., 1972.

Berlo, D. K., Lemert, J. B., & Mertz, R. J. Dimensions for evaluating the acceptability of message sources. *Public Opinion Quarterly*, 1969, *33*, 563–579.

Blum, R. H. *The management of the doctor-patient relationship.* New York: McGraw-Hill Book Company, 1960.

Bradac, J. J., Tardy, C. H., & Hosman, L. A. Disclosure styles and a hint at their genesis. *Human Communication Research*, 1980, *6*(3), 228–238.

Buber, M. Distance and relation. *Psychiatry*, 1957, *20*, 97–104.

Cantor, R. C. *And a time to live: Toward emotional well-being during the crisis of cancer.* New York: Harper & Row, Publishers, Inc., 1978.

Carkhuff, R. *Helping and human relations* (2 vols). New York: Holt, Rinehart, & Winston, 1969.

Chaikin, A. L., & Derlega, V. J. Liking for the norm-breaker in self-disclosure. *Journal of Personality*, 1974a, *42*, 117–129.

Chaikin, A. L. & Derlega, V. J. Variables affecting the appropriateness of self-disclosure. *Journal of Consulting and Clinical Psychology*, 1974b, *42*, 588–593.

Chanowitz, B., & Langer, E. Knowing more (or less) than you can show: Understanding control through the mindlessness-mindfulness distinction. In J. Garber & M. Seligman (Eds.), *Human Helplessness.* New York: Academic Press, 1980, 97–129.

Chelune, G. J., et al. *Self-disclosure: Origins, patterns, and implications of openness in interpersonal relationships.* San Francisco: Jossey-Bass, Inc., Publishers, 1979.

Cline, V. B., & Richards, J. M., Jr. Accuracy of interpersonal perception—A trait? *Journal of Abnormal Psychology*, 1960, *60*, 1–7.

Coates, D., Wortman, C. B., & Abbey, A. Reactions to victims. In I. H. Frieze, D. Bar-tal, and J. S. Carroll (Eds.), *New Approaches to Social Problems.* San Francisco: Jossey-Bass, Inc., Publishers, 1979.

Cooper, L. *The rhetoric of Aristotle.* New York: Appleton-Century-Crofts, 1932.

Cozby, P. C. Self-disclosure: A literature review. *Psychological Bulletin*, 1973, *79*(2), 73–91.

Cronkhite, G. *Communication and awareness.* Menlo Park, Calif.: Cummings Publishing Company, 1976.

Dance, F. E. X., & Larson, C. E. *Speech communication: Concepts and behavior.* New York: Holt, Rinehart & Winston, 1972.

Deutsch, M. Trust and suspicion. *Journal of Conflict Resolution*, 1958, *2*, 265–279.

Deutsch, M. Trust, trustworthiness, and the F Scale. *Journal of Abnormal and Social Psychology*, 1960, *61*(1), 138–140.

Dymond, R. F. A preliminary investigation of the relation of insight and empathy. *Journal of Consulting Psychology*, 1948, *12*, 228–233.

Dymond, R. F. Personality and empathy. *Journal of Consulting Psychology*, 1950, *14*, 343–350.

Egbert, L. D., Battit, G. E., Welch, C. E., & Bartlett, M. K. Reduction of postoperative pain by encouragement and instruction of patients: A study of doctor-patient rapport. *New England Journal of Medicine*, 1964, *270*, 825–827.

Engel, N. S. Confirmation and validation: The caring that is professional nursing. *Image*, 1980, *12*(3), 53–56.

Forsyth, G. L. Analysis of the concept of empathy: Illustration of an approach. *Advances in Nursing Science*, 1980, *2*(2), 33–42.

Frankl, V. *Man's search for meaning: An introduction to logotherapy.* New York: Simon & Schuster, Inc., 1963. (Originally published 1959)

Freud, S. *Group psychology and the analysis of the ego,* trans. J. Strachey. London: Hogarth Press, 1948.

Friedman, H. S., & DiMatteo, M. R. Health care as an interpersonal process. *Journal of Social Issues,* 1979, *35*(1), 1–11.

Gagan, J. Methodological notes on empathy. *Advances in Nursing Science,* 1983, *5*(2), 65–72.

Gage, N. L., & Cronbach, L. J. Conceptual and perceptual problems in interpersonal perception. *Psychological Review,* 1955, *62,* 411–423.

Gazda, G. M., et al. *Human relations development.* Boston: Allyn & Bacon, Inc., 1973.

Gibb, J. R. Defensive communication. *The Journal of Communication,* 1961, *11,* 141–148.

Giffin, K. The contribution of studies of source credibility to a theory of interpersonal trust in the communication process. *Psychological Bulletin,* 1967, *68,* 104–120.

Gilbert, S. J., & Horenstein, D. The communication of self-disclosure: Level versus valence. *Human Communication Research,* 1975, *1*(4), 316–321.

Haley, J. Marriage therapy. *Archives of General Psychiatry,* 1963, *8,* 213–224.

Hammond, D. C., Hepworth, D., & Smith, V. *Improving therapeutic communication.* San Francisco: Jossey-Bass, Inc., Publishers, 1977.

Heineken, J. R. Disconfirmation in dysfunctional communication. *Nursing Research,* 1982, *31,* 211–213.

Hobart, C. W., & Fahlberg, N. The measurement of empathy. *American Journal of Sociology,* 1965, *70,* 595–603.

Hovland, C. I., Janis, I. L., & Kelly, H. H. *Communication and persuasion.* New Haven, Conn.: Yale University Press, 1953.

Jackson, D. D. Family interaction, family homeostasis and some implications for conjoint family psychotherapy. In J. Masserman (Ed.), *Individual and familial dynamics.* New York: Grune & Stratton, Inc., 1959, 122–141.

Johnson, D. W., & Noonan, M. P. Effects of acceptance and reciprocation of self-disclosures on the development of trust. *Journal of Counseling Psychology,* 1972, *19*(5), 411–416.

Johnson, M. N. Self-disclosure: A variable in the nurse-client relationship. *Journal of Psychiatric Nursing and Mental Health Services,* 1980, *18,* 17–20.

Jourard, S. M. *The transparent self.* Princeton, N.J.: Van Nostrand Reinhold Company, 1964.

Jourard, S. M. *Disclosing man to himself.* Princeton, N.J.: Van Nostrand Reinhold Company, 1968.

Jourard, S. M. *The transparent self* (2nd ed.). New York: Van Nostrand Reinhold Company, 1971.

Jourard, S. M., & Jaffee, P. E. Influence of an interviewer's behavior on the self-disclosure behavior of interviewees. *Journal of Counseling Psychology,* 1970, *17,* 252–257.

Jourard, S., & Lasakow, P. Some factors in self-disclosure. *Journal of Abnormal and Social Psychology,* 1958, *51,* 91–98.

Kalisch, B. J. Strategies for developing nurse empathy. *Nursing Outlook,* 1971, *19,* 714–718.

Kalisch, B. J. What is empathy? *American Journal of Nursing,* 1973, *73*(9), 1548–1552.

Klotkowski, D. Self-disclosure: Implications for mental health. *Perspectives in Psychiatric Care,* 1980, *18*(3), 112–115.

Krantz, D. S., & Schulz, R. A model of life crisis, control, and health outcomes: Cardiac rehabilitation and relocation of the elderly. In A. Baum & J. Singer (Eds.), *Advances in Environmental Psychology, Vol. 2, Applications of Personal Control,* Hillsdale, N.J.: Erlbaum, 1980, 131–148.

Laing, R. D. *The politics of experience.* New York: Pantheon Books, Inc., 1967.

Laing, R. D., Phillipson, H., & Lee, A. R. *Interpersonal perception: A theory and a method of research.* New York: Harper & Row, Publishers, Inc., 1966.

Lambert, M. J., DeJulio, S. S., & Stein, D. M. Therapist interpersonal skills: Process, outcome, methodological considerations and recommendations for future research. *Psychological Bulletin,* 1978, *85*(3), 467–489.

LaMonica, E. L. Construct validity of an empathy instrument. *Research in Nursing and Health,* 1981, *4*(4), 389–400.

Lewis, F. Research questions and answers: Health locus of control. *Oncology Nursing Forum,* 1982(a), *9*(3), 108–109.

Lewis, F. Experienced personal control and quality of life in late-stage cancer patients. *Nursing Research,* 1982(b), *31*(2), 113–119.

Lipps, T. *Leitfaden der psychologie.* Leipzig: Engelmann, 1909.

Lowery, B. J. Misconceptions and limitations of locus of control and the I-E Scale. *Nursing Research,* 1981, *30*(5), 294–298.

Luce, R. D., & Raiffa, H. *Games and decisions: Introduction and critical survey.* New York: John Wiley & Sons, Inc., 1957.

McCroskey, J. C. Scales for the measurement of ethos. *Speech Monographs,* 1966, *33,* 65–72.

McIntosh, J. Processes of communication, information seeking and control associated with cancer: A selective review of the literature. *Social Science and Medicine,* 1974, *8,* 167–187.

Mehrabian, A., & Epstein, N. A measure of emotional empathy. *Journal of Personality,* 1972, *40,* 525–543.

Millar, F. E., & Rogers, L. E. A relational approach to interpersonal communication. In G. R. Miller (Ed.), *Explorations in interpersonal communications.* Beverly Hills, Calif.: Sage Publications Inc., 1976, 87–103.

Miller, G. R., & Steinberg, M. *Between people: A new analysis on interpersonal communication.* Chicago: Science Research Associates, 1975.

Mortensen, C. D. *Communication: The study of human interaction.* New York: McGraw-Hill Book Company, 1972.

Morton, T. L., Alexander, J. F., & Altman, I. Communication and relationship definition. In G. R. Miller (Ed.), *Explorations in interpersonal communications.* Beverly Hills, Calif.: Sage Publications, Inc., 1976, 105–125.

Northouse, P. G. Interpersonal trust and empathy in nurse-nurse relationships. *Nursing Research,* 1979, *28*(6), 365–368.

Northouse, P. G. An analysis of the concurrent validity of three types of empathy measures. Paper presented at the meeting of the Central States Speech Association, Chicago, April 1981. (ERIC Document Reproduction Service No. ED 204 828)

Parks, M. R. Relational communication: Theory and research. *Human Communication Research,* 1977, *3*(4), 372–381.

Pearce, W. B. Trust in interpersonal communication. *Speech Monographs,* 1974, *41,* 236–244.

Pearce, W. B., & Sharp, S. M. Self-disclosing communication. *Journal of Communication.* 1973, *23,* 409–425.

Rogers, C. R. *Client-centered therapy.* Boston: Houghton Mifflin Company, 1951.

Rogers, C. R. The necessary and sufficient conditions of therapeutic personality change. *Journal of Consulting Psychology,* 1957, *21,* 95–103.

Rogers, C. R. A process conception of psychotherapy. *American Psychologist,* 1958, *13,* 142–149.

Rogers, C. R. A theory of therapy, personality, and interpersonal relationships, as developed in the client-centered framework. In S. Koch (Ed.), *Psychology: A study of a science,* Vol 3. *Formulations of the person and the social context.* New York: McGraw-Hill Book Company, 1959, 184–256.

Rogers, C. R. Characteristics of a helping relationship. In C. R. Rogers, *On becoming a person.* Boston: Houghton Mifflin Company, 1961, 39–58.

Rogers, C. R. Empathic: An unappreciated way of being. *The Counseling Psychologist,* 1975, *5*(2), 2–10.

Rogers, L. E., & Farace, R. V. Analysis of relational communication in dyads: New measurement procedures. *Human Communication Research,* 1975, *1*(3), 222–239.

Rotter, J. B. *Social learning and clinical psychology.* Englewood Cliffs, N.J.: Prentice-Hall, Inc., 1954.

Rotter, J. B. Generalized expectancies for internal versus external control of reinforcement. *Psychological Monographs,* 1966, *50*(1). (Whole No. 609)

Rotter, J. B. A new scale for the measurement of interpersonal trust. *Journal of Personality,* 1967, *35,* 651–665.

Rotter, J. B. Some problems and misconceptions related to the construct of internal versus external control of reinforcement. *Journal of Consulting Clinical Psychology,* 1975, *43,* 56–67.

Schulman, B. A. Active patient orientation and outcomes in hypertensive treatment. *Medical Care,* 1979, *17*(3), 267–280.

Seligman, M. E. P. *Helplessness.* San Francisco: W. H. Freeman & Company Publishers, 1975.

Shillinger, F. Locus of control: Implications for clinical nursing practice. *Image: The Journal of Nursing Scholarship,* 1983, *15*(2), 58–63.

Sieburg, E. Dysfunctional communication and interpersonal responsiveness in small groups (Doctoral dissertation, University of Denver, 1969). *Dissertation Abstracts International,* 1969, *30,* 2622A. (University Microfilms No. 69-21, 156)

Sieburg, E. Interpersonal confirmation: A paradigm for conceptualization and measurement. San Diego: United States International University, 1975. (ERIC Document Reproduction Service No. ED 098 634)

Sieburg, E., & Larson, C. E. Dimensions of interpersonal response. Paper presented at the International Communication Association Annual Conference, Phoenix, Arizona, 1971.

Tagliacozzo, D. L., & Mauksch, H. O. The patient's view of the patient's role. In E. G. Jaco (Ed.), *Patients, physicians, and illness* (3rd Ed.). New York: The Free Press, 1979.

Taylor, D. A. Motivational bases. In G. J. Chelune, *Self-disclosure: Origins, patterns, and implications of openness in interpersonal relationships.* San Francisco: Jossey-Bass, Inc., Publishers, 1979.

Taylor, S. E. Hospital patient behavior: Reactance, helplessness, or control? *The Journal of Social Issues,* 1979, *35*(1), 156–184.

Thompson, S. C. Will it hurt less if I can control it? A complex answer to a simple question. *Psychological Bulletin,* 1981, *90*(1), 89–101.

Truax, C. B., & Mitchell, K. M. Research on certain therapist interpersonal skills in relation to process and outcome. In A. E. Bergin & S. L. Garfield (Eds.), *Handbook of Psychotherapy and Behavior Change: An Empirical Evaluation.* New York: John Wiley & Sons, 1971.

Vaccarino, J. M. Malpractice: The problem in perspective. *The Journal of the American Medical Association,* 1977, *238,* 861–863.

Vinacke, W. E. Variables in experimental games: Toward a field theory. *Psychological Bulletin,* 1969, *71,* 293–318.

Wallston, B. S., Wallston, K. A., & DeVellis, R. Locus of control and health: A review of the literature. *Health Education Monograph,* 1978, *6*(2), 107–117.

Wallston, B. S., Wallston, K. A., Kaplan, G. D., & Maides, S. A. Development and validation of the health locus of control (HLC) scale. *Journal of Consulting Clinical Psychology,* 1976, *44,* 580–585.

Watzlawick, P., Beavin, J., & Jackson, D. D. *Pragmatics of human communication.* New York: W. W. Norton & Co., Inc., 1967.

Wenburg, J. R., & Wilmot, W. W. *The personal communication process.* New York: John Wiley & Sons Inc., 1973.

Werner-Beland, J. *Grief responses to long-term illness and disability.* Reston, Va: Reston Publishing, 1980.

Wheeless, L. R. A follow-up study of the relationships among trust, disclosure, and interpersonal solidarity. *Human Communication Research,* 1978, *4*(2), 143–157.

Wheeless, L. R., & Grotz, J. Self-disclosure and trust: Conceptualization, measurement, and inter-relationships. Paper presented at the annual convention of the International Communication Association, Chicago, April 1975.

Wheeless, L. R., & Grotz, J. Conceptualization and measurement of reported self-disclosure. *Human Communication Research,* 1976, *2*(4), 238–346.

Wheeless, L. R., & Grotz, J. The measurement of trust and its relationship to self-disclosure. *Human Communication Research,* 1977, *3*(3), 250–257.

Wilmot, W. W. *Dyadic communication: A transactional perspective* (2nd ed.). Reading, Mass.: Addison-Wesley Publishing Co., Inc., 1979.

Wortman, C. B. Causal attributions and personal control. In J. H. Harvey, W. J. Ickes, & R. F. Kidd (Eds.), *New Directions in Attribution Research.* Hillsdale, N.J.: Erlbaum, 1976, 23–51.

Wortman, C. B., Adesman, P., Herman, E., & Greenberg, R. Self-disclosure: An attributional perspective. *Journal of Personality and Social Psychology,* 1976, *33,* 256–266.

Wortman, C. B., & Brehm, J. W. Responses to uncontrollable outcomes: An integration of reactance theory and the learned helplessness model. In L. Berkowitz (Ed.), *Advances in Experimental Social Psychology,* Vol. 8. New York: Academic Press, 1975.

Wortman, C. B., & Dunkel-Schetter, C. Interpersonal relationships and cancer: A theoretical analysis. *Journal of Social Issues,* 1979, *35*(1), 120–155.

3 Communication in Health Care Relationships

In order to facilitate interdisciplinary education and practice, a climate of shared communication and interactional opportunities based on respect and concern for one another should be nurtured. . . . Status differences, power controls, distorted role expectations, and other views can seriously influence interdisciplinary goal efforts. —Leininger, 1971

Numerous kinds of relationships exist in health care settings. These include physician-patient, nurse-social worker, dietitian–family member, administrator-clinician, to name just a few. Communication that occurs within these relationships is affected by the roles each person plays within the relationship and by the expectations that they hold of one another. Some roles are clearly established and generally accepted within an organization, while others are ambiguous.

Presently in the health care system the traditional roles of physician, nurse, and patient, for example, are being challenged and are undergoing considerable change. As a result, the stereotyped rules that previously governed these roles and relationships are no longer valid. For example, it is no longer true that the physician gives the order, the nurse carries it out, and the patient accepts it. Changing roles have increased role ambiguity, stress in relationships, and communication difficulties among participants (Hardy, 1978).

In keeping with the health communication model presented in Chapter 1, the present chapter includes discussions of the four major types of relationships in health care settings: (1) professional-patient, (2) professional-professional, (3) professional-family, and (4) patient-family. We will discuss the nature of these relationships and identify potential barriers to effective communication within each type of relationship.

PROFESSIONAL-PATIENT RELATIONSHIPS

The relationship between the person who provides health care and the person who receives the care has been identified as one of the most crucial components of the entire health care delivery process (Rodin & Janis, 1979). The professional-patient relationship has been cited as a major factor in patients' failure to follow treatment regimens (Stone, 1979), in patients' dissatisfaction with the health care system (DiMatteo, 1979), and in their increased resort to malpractice suits (Taylor, 1979).

The nature of each professional-patient relationship is influenced by the personal and professional characteristics that both patient and professional bring to the relationship. Characteristics such as an individual's age, sex, ethnic background, personality, and values all impact on the nature of professional-patient communication (Davitz & Davitz, 1980; Hooper et al., 1982). Professionals' characteristics also have an impact on health communication. The professional's specialty, education, socialization, and aspirations all affect the way in which the professional establishes relationships with patients.

In addition to the unique personal and professional characteristics that influence professional-patient relationships, several other specific factors affect this relationship. Four of these factors that are potential barriers to effective professional-patient communication will be considered in detail: (1) role uncertainty, (2) responsibility conflicts, (3) power differences, and (4) unshared meanings. While there are many other factors that could be identified, these four have been selected because of the central role they play in explaining obstacles to effective professional-patient communication. Figure 3.1 amplifies the segment of the health communication model that portrays the professional-patient interaction and presents the four potential communication barriers.

Role Uncertainty

Kasl (1975) states that one of the key factors affecting communication between the professional and patient involves the expectations that persons hold about their roles in the relationship. To develop an effective relationship, there has to be a fairly high degree of agreement about what the individuals expect of each other, and it also helps if both "sides" are able to revise their expectations. Although it is easy to assume that patients know what is expected of them and what they can expect from health profession-

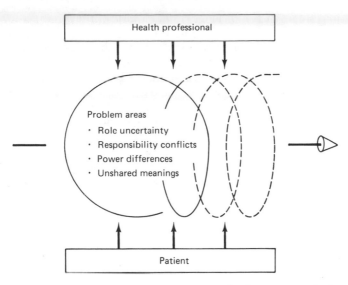

FIGURE 3.1 Potential barriers to effective communication in professional-patient relationships.

als, on closer inspection it appears that the roles of patient and health professional are not clearly defined.

Patients are often uncertain about what "being a patient" requires. Patients typically enter the health care system as loners who are unfamiliar with the physical structure, the organization, and the numerous people with whom they will be dealing (Lorber, 1975). Patients often shed, or at least lose sight of, the familiar roles they occupied before entering the health care agency. Roles of husband, wife, father, mother, employer, employee, sports enthusiast, gardener, and so on are overshadowed by the new role of patient. Although patients may receive brief introductions to their hospital roommates or a quick tour of their immediate surroundings, they are still left on their own to figure out how they fit into the maze of people and places.

Patients who are uncertain about their role sometimes worry that they are asking for too much time from staff or that they are not functioning independently enough. For example, patients may evaluate their own requests for help and assistance by comparing the severity of their own illness to that of other patients, assuming that the more severe the illness, the more appropriate it is to request help from staff members (Tagliacozzo & Mauksch, 1979). Role uncertainty makes it hard for patients to know how to act, and their communication with health professionals may contain considerable hesitation and ambivalence as illustrated in the following case situation of a woman with viral pneumonia.

I waited as long as I could before calling the doctor. I know how busy he is and I didn't want to bother him. I was *very* hesitant to make the call. When I got to his office I saw a whole lot of other people who looked worse off than I and I started to think that maybe I was making a lot out of nothing, and that maybe I should have waited a couple more days before contacting him. I was glad when the nurse took my temperature and it was 102 degrees. Usually what happens is that I have a temperature at home and by the time I get to the doctor's office it's normal—then I really feel foolish, and wish that I hadn't bothered him.

Patients' uncertainty about their role is compounded by the fact that they have to interact with a variety of health providers. Considering that a hospitalized patient may be in contact with as many as 30 different people within one day, it is not surprising that the patient has some confusion about what is expected of him or her (Brown, 1963; Taylor, 1979). The comments of a psychiatric patient below indicate how patients try to juggle the expectations of a team of people.

So, what are the things the staff expect? Well, if you are talking about the ward staff, they want you to make life easy for them and to not be unreasonable about the hospital rules. You know, do what you are told and not make demands on them. And of course, be considerate and thankful. . . .

Now if you are talking about what the therapist wants, that's a different story. Complete trust in her ability to solve all of my problems in three or four hours of spilling my guts was what she was after. . . .

It's hard to say what the expectations of the doctor were. I guess he had more to do than stand around talking to patients. My contacts with him were too indirect to ever learn what he wanted of me. When I wanted special permission to go to town or something, I would go through the nurse to get it. I suppose doc did the same if he wanted something from me (Templin, 1982, p. 108).

Having to respond to many different demands from many different providers makes the role of patient problematic. It is not unusual for a patient to be told that he or she can stay in bed for another day by the physician, yet be told to become more active by the nurse (Tagliacozzo & Mauksch, 1979). Contradictory communication from members of the health team increases the patient's uncertainty about his or her role. Not wanting to anger one professional or the other, the patient is often in a double bind as to which person's directives to follow. Sorting out lines of authority or determining which of several conflicting messages is correct presents a complex situation for the patient (Taylor, 1979).

Although patients are uncertain about their own roles, they are even more uncertain about the roles of health professionals. The trend away from traditional professional uniforms, such as a cap with a black ribbon for the registered nurse and a long white lab coat for the physician, and toward street clothes and name tags (with small print) eliminates specific ways of identifying different professionals. Ambiguous introductions further complicate matters. For example, "I am Dr. Jones," does not tell patients whether they are dealing with a medical student, an intern, a resident, or a staff physician, much less the type of medical or surgical specialty of that individual. Similarly the introduction, "I am the person who will be working with you today," does not tell the patient whether the person is an aide, an L.P.N., an R.N., a clinical nurse specialist, a respiratory therapist, or an occupational therapist. Health professionals often overlook the fact that the patient is unsure of who they are and what can be expected of them. This uncertainty about *what* to expect from *which* professional can make the patient hesitant to talk with the provider.

One of our students made an interesting observation about role expectation. She said,

> On hotel doors they tell you what they expect—the price, check-in time, and check-out time. Maybe we need that in health care. We could tell people what they can expect of us and what we will expect of them.

The point she makes is important; patients want and deserve to know what they can expect from others in health care settings. Although the movement toward informing patients of their own rights has done a great deal in letting patients know the specific rights that they have within a health care agency (such as the right to refuse treatment or the right to obtain a second opinion), these guidelines seldom indicate what specific kind of care they can expect from which type of professional. The only professional whose role is discussed in the Patient's Bill of Rights is the physician. None of the roles of the many other professionals who will be providing care are addressed in this document.

Just as patients are often uncertain about professionals' roles, the health professionals themselves are often uncertain or ambiguous about *both* their own professional role and the role of the patient. As we will discuss in the section on professional-professional relationships, the new and expanding roles of health professionals blur traditional responsibilities and increase professionals' uncertainty about their roles (Hardy, 1978). In addition, with the trend toward increased patient participation, some professionals are uncertain about how active or passive a role patients want to assume. With the changes in health care, considerably more role negotiation now needs to take place between patients and professionals (Haug, 1979).

What happens when patients and professionals are uncertain about one another's roles?

1. Patients may hesitate to raise health concerns because they are uncertain about which of the many professionals is the appropriate one to approach with a problem.
2. Professionals may interpret the lack of initiation on the patient's part to mean that the patient has no concerns, or else that the patient's concerns are only *minimally* important.
3. Patients may express only *physical* concerns, excluding emotional concerns, because physical concerns seem more legitimate when asking for a professional's time.
4. Uncertainty about roles and expectations can cause the patient and professional to deal with one another in traditional or stereotyped ways, and to use only a few of one another's resources. For example, patients who think the nurse only passes medication will not seek out the nurse for his or her expertise in health matters. If dietitians are seen only as menu distributors, patients will not ask them about other dietary concerns. Each of these problems occurs as a result of role uncertainty.

Considering the potential problems that can occur in the communication patterns of the patient and professional, it becomes apparent that clarifying expectations, negotiating perceived and actual roles, and dealing with one another in a personalized and individualized manner are essential to effective professional-patient relationships.

Responsibility Conflicts

A second barrier that can emerge in professional-patient relationships is conflict over the issue of responsibility. For example, who is responsible for managing the patient's illness—the patient or the health professional? How much patient participation is optimal in promoting desired health outcomes? What happens when the patient and professional do not agree on areas of responsibility and desired levels of involvement in care? With the growing trend toward holistic health care and increased patient responsibility, these questions are being debated more among health professionals and consumers. How these issues are negotiated can have considerable impact on the patient-professional relationship and on desired health outcomes (Schulman & Swain, 1980).

Responsibility conflicts and the problems they can create in professional-patient relationships have been addressed by Brickman and his associates (1982) in their work on models of responsibility in health care. They named their theoretical framework "models of helping and coping" because they believe that how professionals "help" and how patients "cope" are based on their often unspoken beliefs about responsibility (see Fig. 3.2). Problems can occur, they contend, when a professional and pa-

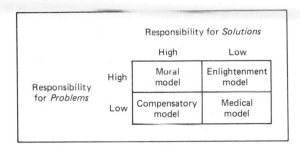

FIGURE 3.2 Four models of helping and coping. (Adapted from P. Brickman, V. Rabinowitz, J. Kuruza, Jr., D. Coates, E. Cohn, and L. Kidder, "Models of Helping and Coping." *American Psychologist*, 1982, 37 (4), p. 370.)

tient are operating from different models that do not fit with one another. The models differ in how much responsibility (high or low) the patient bears for causing health problems, and how much responsibility the patient has for finding solutions to his or her problems. The four models are described below.

The *moral model* of helping and coping views people as highly responsible for creating their own problems and therefore also highly responsible for changing their situation. For example, a person who believes in the assumptions of the moral model would argue that obese people cause their obesity by overeating and are consequently responsible for correcting their weight problems by mustering up enough willpower to stop overindulging.

The *compensatory model* characterizes people as having little responsibility for causing their problems, but having a higher level of responsibility for altering their health problems. For example, a cancer patient would not be held responsible for *causing* his or her cancer, but would be expected to assume an active role in *solving* the problems associated with the cancer by attending self-help groups such as Make Today Count or cancer education groups such as I Can Cope.

The *medical model,* the third model of helping and coping, has generally been associated with practitioners in the medical profession. However, this model can also characterize nurses, social workers, or others who ascribe little responsibility to the patient. According to the medical model, patients are neither responsible for causing their problems nor responsible for finding solutions to them. For example, the person who develops an intestinal abscess of unknown origin and who has the abscess excised by an expert surgeon would not be held responsible for the onset of the problem or for providing a solution.

The *enlightenment model* is the final combination of levels of responsibility. Patients, according to this model, are held highly responsible for causing their problems but are not as responsible for solving their problems. Responsibility for solving problems is placed into the hands of a powerful "other," such as a religious figure or community group who will provide the solution or "enlighten" people about the real nature of their problems. Alcoholics Anonymous has been identified as a group based on this model of helping and coping (Brickman et al., 1982). Recovering alcoholics are expected to give testimony to their responsibility for having caused their drinking problems rather than blaming problems on outside circumstances. Since responsibility for resolving the drinking problem is viewed as resting outside of the power of the alcoholic, the alcoholic must maintain close ties with a community of supporters, such as Alcoholics Anonymous, whose encouragement and support will help the recovering alcoholic stay on the nondrinking path. Advocatès of other groups, that are usually outside of the traditional health care setting, have also been linked to the beliefs of the enlightenment model. Early practitioners in the natural childbirth movement and "folk healers" of cancer patients have also been identified as basing their practice on the assumptions of the enlightment model (Cronenwett & Brickman, 1983; Northouse & Wortman, 1983).

Each of the four models of helping and coping has particular strengths and limitations. Brickman and his associates (1982) note that the *moral model* with its high emphasis on responsibility is probably most beneficial to those who have the intellectual or behavioral resources to take charge of their lives. The moral model, however, places more blame on patients for causing health problems or for not changing negative health states. The *compensatory model* may be helpful in mobilizing people to work through their problems without being blamed for them. Yet there is a question about how long people can continue to stay motivated to work through problems they have not caused. The *medical model* is criticized for the dependency that it frequently encourages in patients. However, on the positive side, if people are not regarded as responsible for causing or solving their problems, they may feel more justified and willing to seek out health services. Finally, the *enlightenment model* is advantageous because it helps to mobilize a group of supporters for the ill person. On the other hand, this model can lead to abuse of power, illustrated in the classic cases of Jim Jones and Charles Manson whose control over others had negative consequences. Also, like the moral model, the enlightenment model tends to blame the person for causing his or her illness.

Many questions about these four models or ways of viewing responsibility cannot be answered easily. Which of these four models generally guides professional practice with patients? Do professionals change the type of model that they use when working with one type of patient versus another, with old versus young patients, or with physically ill patients versus mentally ill patients? When working with a patient who might be described as passive, unmotivated, or noncompliant, could the professional be operating from a moral model while the patient is operating from a medical model? How do the issues of *responsibility* and of varying preferences for involvement affect the relationship between the patient and the professional?

Obviously, the optimal situation is one in which there is a perfect match between the amount of responsibility desired by the patient and the amount encouraged by the professional. Situations in which the patient and professional differ on issues of responsibility are more problematic and require more assessment and negotiation.

Communication assists patients and professionals to work through these issues of responsibility. First, without direct communication, patients and health professionals may be unaware that they are operating from different models of responsibility—a factor that could block the development of a collaborative relationship. Brickman contends that many of the problems that occur between the help giver and help receiver are due to the fact that the two people's models are "out of sync" with one another (1982). Second, the language that each person uses to describe active involvement can influence perceptions about responsibility for care. For example, the health professional who states that the patient is *responsible* for health outcomes sends a quite different message to the client than one who says the patient *participates* in the health care outcome. Third, communication is an essential means of assessing patients' preferences for involvement in care. Cassileth and his associates (1980) encourage clinicians to attend closely to the patients' verbal requests and nonverbal cues regarding the degree of involvement they prefer. Although we know very little about what happens when patients are pushed to become more involved in their care when they prefer less involvement, or when patients are prevented from participating when they wish to be more involved, it seems likely that either situation blocks the development of a collaborative role between professional and patient.

Up to now, we have been talking about patients' *preferences* for participating in care and models of perceived responsibility. Orem (1980), a nurse theorist, emphasizes also assessing patients' *abilities* to participate in care. She notes that patients' abilities to engage in self-care vary considerably. For example, a severely depressed patient, a cardiac patient, and a diabetic patient may differ tremendously in their ability to engage in self-care. Both Orem's and Brickman's perspectives are similar in that each highlights the importance of individualizing approaches to patient care depending on patients' abilities (Orem) or preferences for responsibility (Brickman).

Power Differences

It is no surprise that health professionals are generally perceived as the "powerful" and patients as the "powerless." Nor is it unusual that the professional-patient relationship has been characterized as asymmetrical, with the balance of power tipping in favor of the practitioner (Anderson & Helm, 1979). What is surprising, however, is that this unequal relationship is so difficult to change in today's health care system and that it still remains a barrier to effective professional-patient relationships.

Sources of the *practitioner's power* are diverse. Practitioners have access to all five sources of power identified by French and Raven (1959) (see Chapter 7). Health professionals' knowledge and perceived authority in health matters make their claim to expert and legitimate sources of power obvious to consumers. Equally important, but more subtly exercised, is the health professional's use of reward and coercive power. For example, some patients fear that professionals will provide inadequate care if patients do not follow the prescribed pattern of behavior. In addition, as Kalisch (1975) noted, the health professional's power base remains strong because of the patient's faith in professionals and because patients believe that professionals have nearly mystical powers. Also, people who can "fix bodies" are held in very high esteem by patients who are worried about life and death issues (DiMatteo & Friedman, 1982).

Patients have fewer sources of power than health professionals. Health professionals seldom see the patient as an "expert," even though the patient is the person most familiar with the onset, symptoms, and duration of the distress that he or she is experiencing. Similarly, patients are accorded little legitimate power although they pay high fees for the services they receive from health professionals. Coercive power *is* available to patients in the form of malpractice suits, aggressive behavior, or negative evaluations, but patients seldom use this power because of the time and cost involved (malpractice) and because of their fears of retaliation or inadequate treatment if their power tactics fail (Kalisch, 1975; Kritek, 1981). Patients will, at times, resort to reward power in the form of "good" patient behavior or praise for the professional's skills. However, as Kritek (1981) suggests, this does not result in any sustained source of power for the patients.

Leary's model of human interaction presented in Chapter 1 is useful for understanding what happens in health care settings when power imbalances occur. According to Leary (1955), communication occurs along dominant-submissive and love-hate dimensions; when one person uses specific communication behaviors, this elicits specific behaviors in another person. Traditionally (see Fig. 3.3), the professional has been dominant because of the power attributed to the role of expert and because patients have wanted professionals to act in a dominant manner (Krause, 1977). In terms of Leary's model, patients have participated in the health communication process from a submissive position. This submissiveness elicits dominant responses from health professionals. So, too, health professionals have communicated in dominant ways toward patients and this has elicited submissiveness from patients. Although there are a few instances in which

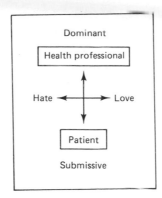

FIGURE 3.3 Traditional patient-professional relationships.

patients act dominant and professionals act submissive, it is far more common in health care settings for the professional to assume a position of power in an asymmetrical professional-patient relationship.

What happens to relationships in which there is an uneven balance of power? One major problem is that the more powerful person assumes more authority than warranted. The psychiatrist Thomas Szasz (1970) writes about this problem in strong language:

> Power is power. It does not really matter—especially to the victim—who wields it. Pope or prince, politician or physician, each can oppress, persecute, and kill those subject to his power. Politicians wage war against enemies, and in the process sacrifice their own people. Physicians wage war against diseases, and in the process often degrade, injure, or even kill persons who voluntarily surrender to them as patients or who, as in Pediatrics and Institutional Psychiatry, are surrendered to them by their families and the state (p. 193).

Another problem pointed out by Kalisch (1975) is that the authority of the professional can spill over into making decisions for patients in areas in which patients are capable of making their own decisions. Similarly, Krause notes in his book *Power and Illness* (1977) that professionals (in this case he talks about physicians) "tend to extend their rightful area of expertise far outside the direct delivery of services to an individual" (p. 233). The submissive persons, in this case the patients, are not given the opportunity to use their potential resources to cope with their circumstances; they stay locked into a rigid role of dependency even though the initial health crises may subside.

To promote effective patient-professional relationships, power needs to be shared more equally between patients and professionals. While there will continue to be differences in the professional's and the patient's education, knowledge, and economic background, the opportunity for shared power will allow patients to maintain control over their lives and the decisions affecting their bodies (DiMatteo & Friedman, 1982). Kalisch (1975) advocates a more balanced relationship to increase the likelihood that patients will agree to follow treatment regimens. Lastly, shared power will lead to more balanced and effective relationships that do not violate patients' rights or induce patient dependency.

Unshared Meanings

The final barrier to effective professional-patient communication that will be considered here is the issue of unshared meanings—differences in perceptions between the professional and the patient. As we discussed in Chapter 1, it is difficult for effective communication to occur without a common set of meanings between a source and a receiver.

Berger and Luckman, in their classic work, *Social Construction of Reality* (1967), explain why we often miss or fail to share the same meanings with other people. They believe that what we perceive to be "real" depends on our unique interpretation of events *and* on our different interactions with others—hence our reality is socially constructed. Each person, therefore, carries around a reality that is real to her or him, but not necessarily shared with a second person.

> I know, of course, that the others have a perspective on this common world that is not identical with mine. My "here" is their "there." My "now" does not fully overlap with theirs. My projects differ from and may even conflict with theirs; all the same, I know that I live with them in a common world (Berger & Luckman, 1967, p. 23).

According to Berger and Luckman, conversation is the most important factor that enables us to maintain our shared perceptions of reality with others as well as to modify our perceptions. Furthermore, they believe that conversation between people must be *continued* and *consistent* to be effective.

The professional and the patient often do not see eye to eye on the same issue due in part to the different perceptual fields from which they are viewing their realities. Danziger (1981) suggests that the professional may be preoccupied with work concerns while the patient is mainly concerned with his or her well-being. Similarly, Mechanic (1982) suggests that health professionals such as physicians tend to focus on a narrow range of factors when diagnosing disease while patients consider a broader range of factors including their social functioning as well as their overall state of mind.

Although there are many factors that contribute to unshared meanings between professional and patient, two specific sources that will be discussed here are (1) the jargon used by health professionals and (2) their different interpretations of the same words. The problems that medical jargon creates in communication are well known to health professionals. Words such as *decubitus ulcer, incontinence,* and *alopecia,* are often too technical for some patients to understand. They can actually prevent patients from being aware of their health problems or of the side effects of treatments (DiMatteo & Friedman, 1982). Professionals are often educated to use technical terminology so they will be able to communicate more precisely with other professionals. However, when these same words are used in professional-patient interactions, the opposite can occur—communication can be blocked. Although many professionals use medical jargon unintentionally and simply out of habit, overuse of medical jargon can be a way of indirectly withholding information from patients (DiMatteo & Friedman, 1982).

Although jargon is a prime cause of unshared meaning, the problems that arise when professionals and patients have different interpretations or attach different meanings to common words also needs to be considered. The problem is humorously illustrated by the following interaction between a patient and physician.

> I'd been asked to see an elderly man suffering from a urinary tract infection. I asked him if his urine burned, "Well, to tell the truth Doc," he replied earnestly, "I haven't really tried to light it" (Ruderman, 1966, p. 8).

It is difficult for professionals to help patients solve their problems, needs, and concerns when each person has a different frame of reference.

In our own work with cancer patients, we discovered that several specific words cause problems. *Prognosis,* for example, is a very emotionally charged word to cancer patients; they often think it means *the chances that I won't make it* or *death.* To practitioners, however, this word is much less negative; it often refers to how long the patient will *live* or *chances of surviving.* Other words like *side effects, weight loss,* and *cure* often carry very different meanings for different individuals.

To illustrate the potential problems that unshared meanings can create, consider the following situation which occurred between a patient and health professional.

> A patient, recently diagnosed as having cancer, was just told that she had a "good prognosis." The patient, still feeling threatened and fearful about having a disease like cancer, focused on the word *prognosis* and was struck by the fact that she never thought of life in terms of a shortened life-span. The patient overlooked the adjective *good* and responded to the message "good prognosis" with worry and concern.
>
> The staff member was unaware of how the patient was interpreting the words *good prognosis* and did not understand why the patient re-

sponded to this good news with anxiety and apprehension. The staff member started to question why the patient was pessimistic and not coping better with her illness.

Obviously, if the staff member continued to miss the interpretation that the patient had given to the word *prognosis,* the staff member would not be able to assist this patient in working through problems related to her diagnosis.

There are numerous other situations in which meanings are missed and communication becomes ineffective between individuals. You may be aware of words or events that are commonly missed in your own practice. To an orthopedic social worker the term *nursing home* probably conjures up a different meaning than it does for the 80-year-old previously independent patient who is being transferred to a nursing home. To a nurse, the word *hospital* may elicit a different meaning than it does from a Spanish-speaking family member in the nurse's community health practice. *Locked ward* means one thing to a psychotic adolescent and something different to a psychologist. The words *God's will* may be interpreted in one way by a 10-year-old leukemic patient, in a different way by his parents, and in a still different way by the hospital chaplain. *Meanings are in people not in words.*

Communication is important in facilitating shared meanings between individuals. As Berger and Luckman (1967) noted, we can only understand one another's reality through conversation. Communication is the vehicle through which professionals can develop an understanding of the anxieties and problems experienced by patients. To help patients cope with their situation, health care workers require an understanding of how patients perceive their world. For illustration, a recent study compares the perceptions of cancer patients and the perceptions of nurses about what cancer patients want to learn. Cancer patients and nurses ranked a group of learning needs very differently: Patients said "minimizing side effects of therapy" was a number one learning need, while nurses ranked "dealing with feelings" as the top learning need of the patients (Lauer, Murphy, & Powers, 1982). Obviously, professionals who assume that they know what patients want, rather than assessing patients' actual needs, will miss important areas and be less effective in helping patients. Learning to share common frames of reference is an essential component in effective professional-patient relationships (Mechanic, 1978).

Haney (1979) has summarized six commonsense ways that professionals can be more aware of previously missed meanings (see Table 3.1). Accurate assessment and understanding of the meaning of words and events are an important aspect of communication. Shared meanings do not develop effortlessly. On the contrary, shared meanings develop from an interactional process that takes time, commitment, and a conscious effort. Going through this process, however, will continue to be essential to effective professional-patient interactions.

TABLE 3.1   Sharing Meaning

1. *Be aware of the multiple meanings of words.*   The same word can have more than one meaning. The word *responsibility* may mean "take control" to one patient, while it means "take blame" to another patient.

2. *Be person-minded, not word-minded.*   Frequently ask yourself, "This is what it means to me; what does it mean to him or her?"

3. *Paraphrase frequently.*   Put the other persons' statements in your own words. Restate what they have said to you in similar but different language.

4. *Be approachable.*   Create a personal atmosphere that will invite or encourage the other person to ask questions if he or she does not understand your message.

5. *Use multiple methods of communicating.*   Try to use a variety of ways to get your message across to another person. For example, if teaching a psychiatric patient about medications, use pictures and written instructions as well as verbal communication.

6. *Be aware of the contexts (verbal and situational).*   Verbal context: How was the particular word used in the sentence? Situational context: What was happening in the environment during the interaction with the patient?

Based on W. Haney, *Communication and Interpersonal Relations,* 4th ed. Homewood, Ill.: Richard D. Irwin, Inc., 1979, pp. 284–321. Copyright © 1979, Richard D. Irwin, Inc.

To summarize, there are four problem areas that we believe are disruptors to professional-patient communication: (1) role uncertainty, (2) responsibility conflicts, (3) power differences, and (4) unshared meanings. As noted earlier in Figure 3.1, these are potential problem areas that can occur in any type of professional-patient relationship.

PROFESSIONAL-PROFESSIONAL RELATIONSHIPS

Researchers have found that a spirit of collegiality among health professionals is essential to the delivery of quality health care services (Feiger & Schmitt, 1979). Health professionals need to collaborate and cooperate with one another in order to help patients resolve complex health care problems (Williams & Williams, 1982). Ironically, this spirit of collegiality and collaboration has not always been present among health care professionals. Although improvements have been made in the past few years, areas of contention and misunderstanding still exist (Mauksch, 1981) and interfere with professionals' communication with one another.

Focusing on the segment of the health communication model that depicts interprofessional relationships (see Fig. 3.4), this section will address three problem areas that have an impact on professional-professional relationships: (1) role stress, (2) insufficient interdisciplinary understanding, and (3) autonomy struggles. The disruptive effect of professional-professional conflicts is important because ultimately it will affect the quality of patient care.

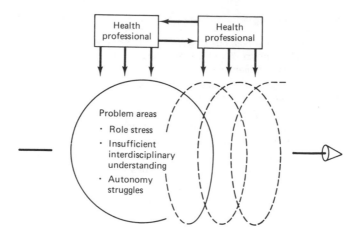

FIGURE   3.4 Potential   barriers   to   effective   communication   in professional-professional relationships.

Role Stress

Facing sick and suffering people every day is no easy task. Health professionals' work constantly places them in contact with patients who are struggling with life crises and who are trying to overcome serious emotional or physical illness. For example, physicians often need to tell patients about life-threatening diagnoses; social workers need to deal with the resulting family chaos; and nurses need to help patients maintain their courage to live through each day (DiMatteo & Friedman, 1982). In acute care institutions the nature of health care work demands decision making on matters that affect life and death. In community settings, health care work can involve locating scarce resources for patients' long-term health problems. In both settings the nature of the health care work contributes to the job stress experienced by persons in health care fields.

Yet, the role stress experienced by health professionals is due only in part to the nature of their work. Another major source of work stress and strain is related to problems in carrying out professional roles. Hardy (1978) has identified many types of role stress. We will discuss two types of role stress—role conflict and role overload—as a way to illustrate how they can eventually lead to problems in professional-professional relationships.

A considerable amount of research has been done on *role conflict*, especially as it relates to health professionals who are socialized to fit one role, and yet are expected to fulfill a different role in the work setting. Kramer's book, *Reality Shock* (1974), has helped to illuminate the stress created by the gap between education and service. Kramer, studying the stresses experienced by new graduate nurses, coined the term *reality shock* for the shocklike symptoms experienced by nurses who suddenly realize that their education has not adequately prepared them for the work setting. Kramer notes that new graduates learn that their ideals and aspirations are seldom the same as the values that receive praise on the job. Role conflict occurs as new graduates experience the discrepancy between these two very different value systems.

Seasoned professionals also experience role conflict. Fourcher and Howard (1981) report that health professionals experience a conflict between what they have labeled *personal rationality* and *organizational rationality*. Personal rationality describes a "work experience that is organized in relatively unique and immediately creative ways by the individual worker" (p. 299). In contrast, organizational rationality refers to a "work experience that is organized in a relatively pre-established way to suit the systemic requirements of a larger organization" (p. 299).

Role conflict between organizational rationality and personal rationality is often expressed by health professionals. Devereux (1981) notes that nurses experience frustration about the numerous nonnursing tasks imposed upon them (organizational rationality); these tasks interfere with their ability to give anything more than routine nursing care. The comments of a psychiatric staff nurse illustrate the frustration and role conflict:

> I remember the weekend vividly. Most of my time was spent giving medications, charting medication, checking orders, correcting pharmacy errors, playing ward clerk, and assessing dietary needs. I did not do *true* nursing care. That is, I spent only a little time with each client, so I couldn't assess their individual needs or plan specific care to meet those needs. Many clients' concerns went unmet. I resorted to bringing clients into the nursing station to do one-to-one interactions, so that I could simultaneously supervise the unit, put out crisis fires, and try to tend to their needs.

This psychiatric nurse believed that organizational rationality, such as demands to get functional tasks completed, interfered with personal rationality, or her ability to carry out individualized nursing care. Role conflict arose as she tried to meet these opposing demands in a limited period of time.

Other health professionals are also plagued by role conflicts originating from the organizational versus personal rationality dichotomy in their daily work settings. Borland (1981), for example, discusses stress and burnout among social workers. He cites discharge planning as a typical problem in which institutional efficiency often demands that the social worker quickly place a client into a community setting that may not be completely suited to meet the individual's needs. Hurried discharges into less than optimal settings can lead to the client's later rehospitalization. Balancing the professional's desire for better discharge planning with the system's demands for efficiency leads to considerable role stress among these health care providers.

Role conflict occurs when health professionals try to balance these two different perspectives within their work setting. Health professionals often become frustrated as they realize that agencies are set up to reward organizational rationality rather than personal rationality—or reward it only after organizational priorities are accomplished (Fourcher & Howard, 1981).

Role overload is a second factor affecting the role stress experienced by professionals. Due to the nature of health care settings, the health professional is often required to react like an amoeba—constantly expanding or changing to meet the increased demands on his or her time. Emergencies frequently arise in which health professionals need to take on more responsibilities than they can reasonably manage within a given period of time. In addition, health professionals often are expected to wear many hats and to negotiate with numerous other departments or agencies.

Role overload often occurs when a health professional's workload consists mostly of referrals made by others. For example, the number of referrals made to a psychiatric nurse specialist or a clinical social worker may vary considerably from one week to another. One social worker's comments illustrate the role overload that she experienced due to an increased number of referrals.

> I was supposed to have 12 patients in my caseload, but for some reason a lot of patients came in with family problems and were referred to me. Within a couple of days the number of patients and families in my caseload jumped to 20. I tried to see as many of them as I could, but I wasn't able to see as many as I know I *should* have seen. I tried to give some of my cases to another social worker, but she was overloaded herself and was not familiar with the agencies to which my patients needed referrals. I felt in a real bind: if I kept all of the cases, the patients would not get adequate care; if I transferred them to other caseworkers, they would be more overloaded and ticked off at me for not managing the patients myself.

The social worker is frustrated by the role overload that she is experiencing. The mental energy that she is expending to try to resolve the situation also adds to her job stress.

Assuming that role stress (e.g., role conflict and role overload) is common among health professionals, what effect does role stress have on the interpersonal relationships among health care providers? We believe that role stress is often the underlying source of professional-professional tensions. Role stress leaves the professional in a vulnerable position, more easily stressed by minor conflicts with co-workers. The social worker mentioned previously also described the following situation:

> At 4:30 P.M. I got a telephone call from the physician working with the
> K. family. He wanted to discharge Mrs. K. as soon as possible and he
> wondered if I had the nursing home placement worked out. I suddenly
> felt my anger rising—I don't know why, it was a legitimate question on
> his part. I snapped back to him that I had a million other things that I
> had to do that were more important, so I did not have one spare minute
> to see her. He didn't sound too pleased about the situation. . . . I don't
> know if he realizes it but he took the brunt of my feelings about a
> missed lunch break, my physical exhaustion, and my general frustra-
> tion.

In this situation, the social worker felt tense and irritable as a result of her
role stress. As the social worker's tension increased, it eventually spilled
over into her interaction with the physician. With less role stress, the social
worker would probably have been able to handle the physician's inquiry
with less exasperation.

The example above also illustrates how the role overload from one
professional can eventually interfere with the role functioning of another
health professional, causing increased conflict between them. This is especially common among health professionals who need to function
interdependently to meet patients' needs (see Chapter 8). In the case
above, the social worker and physician had interdependent roles. The physician's desire to discharge the patient was blocked by the social worker who
was too busy with other role responsibilities. The social worker's role overload and subsequent inability to carry out her portion of an interdependent
task became the underlying source of the conflict between these two
professionals.

In a similar way nurses working in hospital settings are interdependent on other nurses who work different shifts. Nurses who are unable to
meet role demands during a day shift may leave these tasks undone, and
the work spills over into the work responsibilities of the nurses working the
evening shift. Interpersonal conflicts emerge between nurses on different
shifts as they struggle to cope with the role overload. What makes this problem particularly difficult to deal with is that the participants attribute their
professional problems to inefficiency or lack of follow-through on the part
of the other professionals, rather than attributing it to the role stress that is
the underlying cause of the problem.

A second effect of role stress is that professionals may withdraw from
one another as a means of coping with role conflicts and role overloads
(Hardy, 1978; Kahn et al., 1964). As role stress increases, the health professional may shift priorities from process or relationship-building functions
to task functions. The professional under stress may become unwilling to
invest energy in maintaining professional relationships (Hardy, 1978) and
instead direct all energies into getting the job done. For example, a nurse
feeling very stretched by role demands may resolve role overload by

skipping an interdisciplinary team meeting and by focusing solely on task accomplishment (e.g., passing medications). This nurse's absence from the meeting removes one opportunity for important professional-professional relationship building and also limits the nurse's input into important patient care decisions.

Obviously the effect of role conflict and overload will eventually have an impact on the patient. Professionals who are physically and mentally exhausted by these role stresses will have less energy remaining to attend to patients' needs.

A number of programs have been developed to help professionals cope with role stress. Kramer and Schmalenberg suggest in *Path to Biculturalism* (1977) programs that can be implemented in hospitals to help nurses bridge the gap between the subculture of idealistic education and the subculture of new work settings. Ways to manage stress (Maslach, 1979) and ways to change the health care system (Jacox, 1982) have both been proposed as means to lessen role stress and strain. Our purpose is not to describe these programs, but rather to point out how role stress underlies and contributes to problems in professional-professional relationships and eventually to problems in professional-patient relationships.

Insufficient Interdisciplinary Understanding

We would expect health care providers, of all people, to understand the many professional roles in health care settings. Amazingly, this is not the case. Leininger (1971) reported that problems in health care are related "to a lack of understanding and appreciation for the actual and potential contributions of the different disciplines" (p. 78). Although some progress has been made in understanding one another's role, much confusion about the unique expertise of each professional still remains (Leininger, 1978; Weiss, 1983). This lack of understanding has been cited as a cause of "role confusion and territorial disputes among the various disciplines" (Williams & Williams, 1982, p. 17).

Why do health professionals know so little about one another's roles? Professional education that takes place in virtual isolation from other health disciplines is a major cause of this problem. Leininger (1971) notes that a health professional can spend between two and eight years in an educational program and yet get little exposure to the roles and skills of the other professionals. However, as soon as these new graduates enter health care settings, they are suddenly expected to collaborate with one another in a collegial manner—without any understanding about the other professionals' roles (Leininger, 1971). Examining the specific problems between the disciplines of nursing and medicine, Kalisch and Kalisch (1977) report that the distinctly separate educational experience of these two professional groups leads to a lack of insight into one another's roles and responsibilities. Milne (1980) studied students in various health disciplines and found that they have only a very rough idea of one another's professional roles. She also noted that students tend to hold a broader view of their own professional role and a more restricted view of other professionals' roles.

In addition to specialized education, the characteristics of health care settings create a second factor that contributes to a lack of awareness of the various professional roles. Levine and Kliebhan (1981) contend that many health care personnel work in locations that are physically distant from one another. This complicates the communication among health care providers such as occupational therapists, physicians, and physical therapists. In addition, the rapid tempo in health care settings and the busy schedules of professionals leave little time for professionals to sit down and learn more about one another's role responsibilities (Devereux 1981).

How does lack of knowledge of one another's roles contribute to the problems in professional-professional relationships? First of all, health professionals may make demands on other professionals that are not compatible with others' perceptions of their own responsibilities. These discrepancies in role expectations can lead to professional-professional conflicts. Nurses, for example, are often frustrated that other professionals expect them to carry out nonnursing tasks (Byrne 1982). One nurse shared her frustrations with us about being asked to do nonnursing tasks:

> One day when a ward clerk was not assigned to the unit, I remember the phone constantly ringing and interrupting my plans for nursing care. The physician who entered the unit station never answered the phone. Yet during this very busy time he asked me to write down a couple of verbal orders for him. Noting no overt sign of hand paralysis in the physician, I cheerfully responded that I would write his physician notations if he would write my nursing notes for me. . . . Why should I interrupt my professional responsibilities to be unit control clerk or stenographer?

Here the physician erroneously assumes a nurse's role includes answering the phone, keeping the unit in order, and transcribing orders (nonnursing tasks). As the staff nurse's comments show, tensions and misunderstandings can occur when health professionals relate to each other in stereotyped ways or are unaware of one another's *real* areas of responsibility.

Second, a lack of understanding of professional roles also leads to underutilizing others' professional expertise. For example, if pharmacists are stereotyped as pill dispensers, they will not be utilized by other professionals as educational consultants to the interdisciplinary team or to individual patients. If chaplains are viewed only as people who provide early morning communion, they will not be used as valuable resource people who can help staff members learn how to help patients with existential concerns, such as anxiety or finding meaning in life.

A third problem created by a lack of interdisciplinary understanding is an increase in territorial disputes among health professionals. In recent years, health professionals' roles have expanded considerably (Leininger, 1978), leading to confusion as to which professional has expertise in a particular area. Lister (1980), reporting on a survey of 13 types of health professionals, found numerous areas in which health professionals' roles overlapped or conflicted with one another. Lister noted that role overlap occurred especially in those areas that were outside of the more traditional role of a particular discipline. In a more recent study, Weiss (1983) reported that when subjects in her study (nurses, physicians, and consumers) were asked to place 417 health-related behaviors into the domain of the physician, nurse, or both, the respondents placed 82 percent of the items into the area considered common to both groups. In other words, the respondents reported a large amount of overlap between the role of the nurse and the role of the physician.

When health professionals have considerable role overlap, it is not unusual for one professional to think that the other person is trying to take over his or her power and responsibilities. This can result in unproductive competition. For example, Kalisch and Kalisch (1977) identified role overlap as a common problem between pediatric nurse practitioners and physicians. They reported, for example, on a situation in which the American Academy of Pediatrics withdrew from previous plans to collaborate with pediatric nurse practitioners, because the AAP feared too much competition from the practitioners in similar areas of patient care. Role overlap and the lack of understanding of one another's areas of expertise lead to interprofessional conflict.

Several innovative approaches have been proposed to deal with the lack of awareness of one another's professional roles. Probably one of the most innovative (yet least practical in terms of wide usage by others) was reported in the *American Medical News*. A physician worked alongside of intensive care nurses for one week in order to get a first hand understanding of the nurses' work experiences. He said

> Although everyone talks about the high level of stress among intensive care nurses, I realized that despite all of my medical training, I really had little idea of what a nurse's day-to-day experience was really like. . . .

> Physically, the work is exhausting, I can't remember ever being as tired, even during my days as an intern or resident. . . .

> And I didn't even have the usual patient care responsibilites since I was always working with one of the nurses rather than having the full load the way a nurse actually would. . . .

> I think more physicians would be more receptive to the nursing staff if they observed first hand as I did. The doctors are so busy with their

own responsibilities that they may not stop to think how valuable the nursing staff is in improving patient care. . . . [1]

Although few health professionals would be willing to take one week to work alongside another health professional, the value of such an activity is unmistakably clear.

Hoping to achieve similar interprofessional understanding, other approaches such as sharing common core courses during educational experiences (Leininger, 1971), increased contact with one another during the clinical rotations (Weinberger, Green, & Mamlin, 1980; Williams & Williams, 1982), and interdisciplinary seminars (Balassone, 1981) have been proposed to increase role knowledge among professionals.

Other innovative approaches hold considerable promise. Interdisciplinary conferences have been rather common in mental health settings but less common in other acute care settings. Interdisciplinary rounds have also been utilized. Unlike traditional rounds in which only one professional speaks and everyone else listens, in these interdisciplinary rounds each professional contributes to the process based on his or her own area of expertise. These rounds have been found to increase communication and collaboration among professionals (Devereux, 1981). Finally, joint progress notes, which encourage professionals to read each other's observations regarding the patient's health status, have been used in some health care settings to promote interprofessional communication (Devereux, 1981).

Leininger (1971) advocated recognizing one another's area of expertise, while at the same time realistically accepting that there will be areas of overlap or common knowledge among the health disciplines. She portrays these interrelationships schematically as shown in Figure 3.5. Health professionals' well-defined areas of expertise are indicated as well as areas of overlap with other disciplines (gray areas). Similarly, Schindler, Berren, and Beigel (1981) contend that health professionals need to continue an open dialogue on competencies they *share* with other disciplines, as well as competencies that health professionals think are *unique* to their area of expertise. As health professionals continue to increase their familiarity with one another's roles, they will be able to make better use of one another's expertise and be less threatened by areas of role overlap. Increased interdisciplinary understanding will enhance professional-professional relationships.

Autonomy Struggles

A final problem that threatens harmony in professional-professional relationships is the issue of autonomy—the freedom to be self-governing or self-directing. The importance of autonomy is underscored by Conway

[1]Excerpts from *American Medical News*, Staver, 1983, 13.

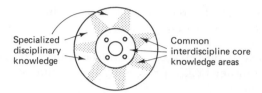

(1978), who states that the capacity to exercise autonomy is crucial in order for professionals to fulfill their professional roles. However, not all health professionals perceive the same degree of autonomy in their practice—a discrepancy that has caused considerable tension among the various disciplines (Fagin, 1981; Hamburg, 1981).

The degree of autonomy experienced by a health professional depends on three factors:

1. The permissible scope of practice for that group contained in state licensing laws;
2. The ability of that group to secure access to necessary health facilities, such as hospitals; and
3. The ability of that group to obtain reimbursement from private and governmental third party payers (Latanich and Schultheiss, 1982, p. 421).

Looking more closely at these three factors, it is evident that the various health disciplines differ considerably on these criteria for autonomy.

To illustrate, the medical profession generally scores well on all three criteria. Physicians have considerable latitude in their actions in professional practice; they have ready access to admit and discharge patients from health care settings, and can easily obtain third party reimbursement for the services they render to patients.

Other health professionals do not compare as favorably on these three criteria. Nurse practitioners, for example, complain that restrictive state licensing laws limit their ability to practice at the level for which they have been educationally prepared to practice (Latanich & Schultheiss, 1982). Social workers, nurses, and physical therapists often are limited in their access to health organizations. While nurse midwives and psychologists continue to contest their perceived professional rights to obtain hospital privileges, their ability to fully exercise this second criterion for autonomy remains limited. The third criterion, reimbursement for third-party payments, is also less available to other professionals at this time. While gains have been made by some professionals, such as reimbursement by CHAMPUS (insurers for the armed forces) for nurse midwife services (Diers, 1982), many restrictions still remain for other professionals in this area. If we compare the medical profession to the other health professions, we see that major differences exist with regard to professional autonomy.

How has the medical profession been able to establish a high degree of autonomy in health care? In addition to their strong political influence, which they have established through lobbying and forming strong professional organizations, physicians have been socialized into assuming a highly autonomous role (Conway, 1978; Weiss, 1983). Others have observed that physicians have developed the traditional notion that "members of the health care team worked for them, rather than with them" (Allen, Jackson, & Younger, 1980, p. 838).

This viewpoint helps to cement the physicians' highly autonomous view of themselves. In addition, in their medical training, physicians are often taught to retain the central responsibility for patient care, a factor that could make them hesitant to share responsibility with other health professionals (Keenan, Aiken, & Cluff, 1981; Weinberger, Green, & Mamlin, 1980).

Finally, the hierarchical nature of health care has contributed to the highly autonomous nature of medical practice. Kalisch and Kalisch (1982) note that dominance of the medical profession has persisted despite the fact that physicians make up less than 10 percent of the health care personnel. Figure 3.6 depicts the hierarchical nature of personnel in health care institutions. In this model the physician maintains the top position on the pyramid, with other professionals viewed as having less power, less authority, and consequently less autonomy over their practice.

Leary's transactional model of dominance and submission (as discussed in Chapter 1) is relevant to our discussion of factors influencing the dominance of physicians in some health care settings. While characteristics of the medical profession have been influential in making physicians domi-

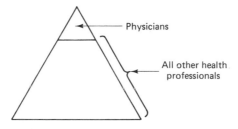

FIGURE   3.6 Hierarchical nature of health care. (Adapted from M. Leininger, "This I Believe . . . about Interdisciplinary Health Education for the Future." Copyright © 1971, American Journal of Nursing Company. Reproduced with permission from *Nursing Outlook,* December, vol. 19, no. 12, p. 789.)

nant throughout history, characteristics of the other health professions have played a role in maintaining their submissive position. Kalisch and Kalisch contend that professions such as nursing with large female memberships have been deferent (due to their socialization as women) to the predominantly male medical profession. Other factors such as unassertive approaches in the doctor-nurse game or unequal ways of addressing other professionals (e.g., *Dr.* Physician versus *Firstname* health professional) continue to perpetuate submissive roles (Mauksch, 1983).

How do discrepancies in professional autonomy affect professional-professional relationships? The dominant profession tends to underestimate the professionalism or competence of other professionals. In other words, the members of the dominant profession tend to rate themselves higher in such areas as autonomy of judgment or evaluative skills than they would rate other health professionals (Silva, Clark, & Raymond, 1981).

Discrepancy in degrees of autonomy among the professionals can also lead to interpersonal tension, especially if one group of professionals perceives overt or covert maneuvers by other professionals to exert their dominance over them. Discussing tensions between nurse practitioners and physicians, Ford (1982) gives the following report:

> The nurse practitioner has been a particular target in interprofessional conflicts with medicine, especially in the delivery of primary care. The scenario is played out in many ways: the withdrawal of support of the American Medical Association from the National Joint Practice Commission; the efforts of physicians in New Jersey to prevent school nurse practitioners from practicing, and the hospital administrators' strategy to bus nurses to the State Nurses Association to rescind the previously accepted position supporting the entry-into-practice resolutions; [and] the attempts of Arkansas physicians to control the delivery of health care to rural and deprived populations by establishing restraints on nurse practitioners working collaboratively with a physician in a rural and deprived area (p. 244).

Dominance of one professional group can lead to erroneous assumptions about control over other professions or to an exaggerated sphere of influence.

Finally, the dominance of one profession can interfere with the flow of communication between the higher- and lower-status professionals. Wessen (1958) found that in a hierarchical hospital organization, hospital personnel tended to interact only with members of their *own* group; as the social distance between the various occupational groups increased, their interactions with one another decreased. Wessen found that rigid status roles and limited intergroup communication can be disruptive to professional relationships.

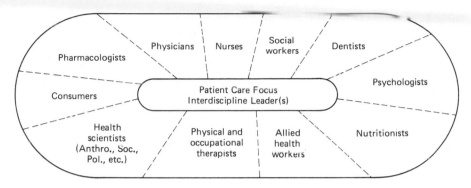

FIGURE 3.7 Interdisciplinary health team model. (Reprinted from M. Leininger, "This I believe . . . about Interdisciplinary Health Education for the Future." Copyright © 1971, American Journal of Nursing Company. Reproduced with permission from *Nursing Outlook,* December, vol. 19, no. 12, p. 789.)

Leininger proposes a model for interdisciplinary collegiality to replace the hierarchical system (see Fig. 3.7). The oval model of interdisciplinary teamwork recognizes the professional contributions and autonomy of many health professionals. Although this model or similar models are often assumed to be already in place in many health care settings, actually a lot of negotiation about issues of professional autonomy is still going on. Obviously, real changes in the legal and political spheres are needed in order for all professionals to function appropriately in the roles for which they have been educated. However, recognition of these issues and their impact on professional-professional relationships will promote an understanding of present communication problems among health professionals.

In summary, this section of Chapter 3 has addressed three potential barriers to communication among health professionals: (1) role stress, (2) insufficient interdisciplinary understanding, and (3) autonomy struggles. In order to solve complex patient problems, health professionals need to invest energy into collaborative efforts with one another, utilizing each professional's unique expertise, so that territorial problems and role stress do not interfere with patient care.

PROFESSIONAL-FAMILY RELATIONSHIPS

In contrast to the vast amount of literature describing professional-patient relationships and professional-professional relationships, there is relatively little literature describing relationships between health professionals and family members (Litman, 1979). This lack of systematic study of professional-family interaction is symptomatic of the lack of importance that health professionals have traditionally attributed to this relationship in health care. The emphasis in health care has generally been on the provider-patient relationship with all other relationships assigned lesser importance.

During recent years, however, health professionals have become increasingly aware that family members play an important role in promoting positive health outcomes for the ill person (Kaplan et al., 1973). Research on social support networks has helped to highlight the role of significant others in mediating various life stresses (Eckenrode & Gore, 1981) and serious illnesses (DiMatteo & Hays, 1981). Family members, for example, have been identified as the "first line of defense to support one of its members who faces a crisis" (Giacquinta, 1977, p. 1585). Family members and other significant individuals affect patients' compliance with treatment regimens (Litman, 1979), their ability to cope with illness (DiMatteo & Hays, 1981), and their successful convalesence after hospitalization (Stern & Pascale, 1979).

For family members to maintain their supportive role in health care, they need to have effective communication with health professionals. Family members have traditionally faced two problems: (1) they often feel excluded from the treatment process, and (2) their access to information about the patient's status is limited or "managed." These two problems are shown on the segment of the health communication model illustrated in Figure 3.8.

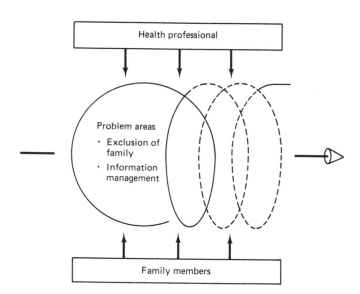

FIGURE   3.8 Potential barriers to effective communication in professional-family member relationships.

Exclusion of Family Members

Serving as the primary support person for the patient produces considerable stress for family members (Klien, Dean & Bogdonoff, 1967; Stern & Pascale, 1979). In spite of the stress that family members experience, they generally receive *little* support from professionals. Hampe's study of the needs of grieving spouses (1975) revealed that only 15 percent of the spouses felt that they had received support from health professionals. However, subjects in this study reported that nurses did meet the needs of their ill spouses. These subjects (family members) acknowledged that, although ideally they would have liked more support from health professionals, they also realized that staff members were "too busy" to be concerned with family members' difficulties. Reporting similar responses, Breu and Dracup (1978) noted that spouses of cardiac patients were reluctant to "bother" the hospital staff and as a result tended not to voice their concerns. Family members of critically ill patients often believe that the professional's responsibility is toward the patient, especially when the professional appears to have so little time (Molter, 1979). Similarly, family members of psychiatric patients have reported that the hospital and personnel existed for the patient, and were not a resource for them (Leavitt, 1975).

In light of the stress experienced by family members, why have health professionals directed so little attention to their needs? From a transactional perspective we believe *both* family members and staff have contributed to the problem. Family members at times act in ways that hinder professionals from learning about their needs. Typically, family members have been hesitant to ask for help (Leavitt, 1975), thinking that they do not have a legitimate right to take up professionals' time because they are not really "sick" (in the sense of being physically ill). Also, family members have feared that if they use the professional's time, valuable resources would be diverted away from the primary needs of the ill family member. Studies have indicated that family members rank the needs of patients higher than their own needs (Freihofer & Felton, 1976). Intuitively, this seems reasonable. But it also means that family members and their needs are thrust into a position of secondary importance. In trying to place the ill patient's needs first, family members give messages to health professionals that their own needs are not important when in fact this is not the case. Family members have real needs just as the sick person has needs, as illustrated in the following example.

> Mrs. F., a 72-year-old woman, was hospitalized for transient periods of confusion and disorientation. Prior to her hospitalization she had been living independently in her own home. During her hospitalization it became apparent that she could no longer manage by herself at home.

When Mrs. F. was approached about an alternative living situation, she adamantly stated that she would not go to a nursing home since "those were places where they put people to be forgotten and to die." Mrs. F. said that she would much rather move in with her son.

Mrs. F.'s son Robert was 50 years old and operated a small microcomputer business. He lived alone and spent many hours working at the office. Robert felt considerable conflict about his mother's situation. On the one hand, he felt he should have his mother move in with him—he had a large house, adequate income, and no other family responsibilities. He was also receiving a great deal of pressure about the situation from out of town relatives. On the other hand, he felt that the added responsibility of his mother living at his house would be emotionally exhausting. She was a very religious woman and could be quite domineering at times. He was also convinced that his work schedule and life style would change drastically if she started living in his house.

Robert felt that there was no one with whom he could discuss his ambivalence and guilt. He was hesitant to talk these worries over with the staff. He was afraid that they would think he was self-centered and that he did not care for his mother. When it became clear that his mother would have to leave the hospital within the week, he finally shared his worries with one of the evening nurses. When the health care team became aware of his feelings a family conference was scheduled to discuss discharge plans.

Health professionals have also contributed to the problems faced by family members. Until recently, health professionals have been relatively unaware of the effects of illness on the family unit (Northouse, 1984). Professionals have also been unattentive to family members' needs for information or have left the responsibility for obtaining information up to the family members. Bond (1982), for example, studied the communication between nurses and family members and found that in all but one instance the family members reported that they had initiated the interaction with the professional. Furthermore, the attitudes of professionals toward family members have not always been positive. At times staff members have considered family members a nuisance, as getting in the way of patient care (Litz, 1957) or as a source of the patient's problem, especially in psychiatric settings (Leavitt, 1975). Sometimes health professionals simply rank family members' needs lower than the patient's because they realize their own resources are limited and that nearly all resources need to be directed toward the ill patient.

With the emergence of family systems theory (Bowen, 1971; Minuchin, 1974), it is becoming more apparent that the "healthy" family member versus "sick" family member dichotomy is more of a myth than a reality. According to family theorists, the stress of illness reverberates throughout the entire family system (Minuchin, 1974). Although objective signs of illness are more obvious in the "sick" person, the mental anguish is often high in all family members who are affected in one way or another by the illness.

There is increasing evidence that family members are an integral part of the overall treatment process. As family members experience more stress, they will be less effective in providing ongoing support to the ill family member (Neuhring & Barr, 1980). Rigid boundary lines between who is sick and who is "only a family member" are limiting because they lessen family members' access to care or support. Family members who feel they have no "rights" to professionals' time will hesitate to initiate interactions or to express concerns to staff members. On the other hand, professionals who are unaware of family members' needs will not actively try to support the whole family system.

Overall, an overstressed, undersupported family network will have a negative effect on patient care goals. Yet if more attention is given to the needs of family members and friends, they will be able to join forces with staff to support the patient and achieve health care goals.

Information Management

Information management is a second problem that surfaces in professional-family relationships. Information management between health care providers and family members often takes one of two forms, which we have labeled *privileged* communication, and *filtered* communication. Privileged communication occurs when family members are given information that has not been made available to the patient (see Fig. 3.9). Filtered communication, in contrast, is "secondhand" information that family members obtain after it has been filtered indirectly through the patient or someone else.

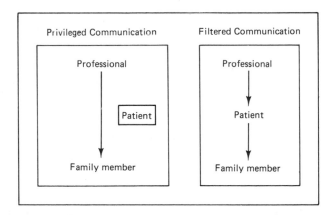

FIGURE 3.9 Common channels of communication utilized in information management.

Privileged communication was more common in earlier years when health professionals did not disclose information or diagnoses to patients. Okun (1961), for example, reported that 90 percent of the physicians in his study did not tell cancer patients their diagnoses. In some of these situations family members were given this privileged information so that they could get financial or business matters arranged prior to the death of the patient (Okun, 1961). Although more recent studies indicate that the majority of physicians now tell patients their diagnoses (Novack et al., 1979), remnants of this practice still remain (Gould & Toghill, 1981). For example, it is not unusual when family members are either told the diagnosis sooner than the patient or in more detail than is given to the patient. Comments from the daughter of a cancer patient illustrate this problem.

> Dad was admitted to the hospital for a growth in his lung. It turned out to be cancer, but the doctor decided not to tell Dad for a few days. The doctor did tell Mom and me about the cancer but wanted Dad to regain his strength before he got the bad news. It was hard for us—especially Mom—to know Dad had cancer when he didn't know. Mom became a nervous wreck. She finally called the family doctor for a nerve pill. A few days later they told Dad. It wasn't easy, but at least we all knew about it.

Another type of privileged information takes the form of family members' knowing more detailed information than is given to the patient. This situation is illustrated in the comments of a patient's wife:

> The doctor was at the nursing station when he called me aside and said, "Your husband has cancer and it's hopeless." I was shocked and didn't know what to say. I asked him if there was a place where we could go and talk about it and he said, "There's really nothing more to talk about." I asked him to tell my husband and he said that he would. When he told my husband about the cancer he soft-pedaled my husband's prognosis. He did not use the word *hopeless* which he had used with me.

These two situations illustrate how privileged information can create problems for family members. Privileged information is often given on the assumption that family members are "healthy" while patients are "sick" and less able to take the truth. Although some family members may encourage these practices by asking professionals not to tell the patient a particular type of information or to give them more specific details than are given to the patient, information management of this type can eventually lead to problems in professional-family and in patient-family communication.

Family members not only have problems of dealing with privileged communication but also with interpreting filtered communication, which is relayed to them by the patient or other nonprofessionals (see Fig. 3.9). The family members of hospitalized patients often receive only filtered information because they usually are not in the hospital during the times in which health professionals give reports to patients. Similarly, family members of outpatients remain in the waiting room during examinations and receive only secondhand information. In nursing homes the same problem occurs. Family members are frequently not present for status reports on patients and therefore have to rely heavily on the patients or other residents for feedback on the patient's status.

Problems that arise from filtered information are analogous to the problems that arose from the telephone game that many of us played as children. As you may recall, during the telephone game the first person whispers a message to the second person and so on down the line until the last person announces the message. As children we would laugh with amusement that the message changed so drastically from the first person to the last person. In the same way, but without the amusement, family members often receive information that is incorrect—especially if the patient who is transferring the information is hard of hearing, has transient periods of confusion, or is highly anxious and unable to attend closely to detailed information. Receiving information in a roundabout way prevents family members from asking for clarification, correcting misassumptions, and developing a rapport with health professionals. All in all, filtered communication is a problem because it is one-way communication that does not allow for direct feedback between family members and the professionals.

The need for direct communication is expressed by the woman in the following example.

> I told my mother that I wanted to talk with the doctor after her examination. At the end of the examination Mother told him that I wanted to hear from him about what he thought was wrong. He told her, "I don't need to talk to your daughter, I'd just tell her the same thing that I told you." Mother was insistent that he talk to me—I guess she knew how worried I was—but when he saw me he acted sort of put out and briskly glossed over her problems. I felt like I was needlessly taking his time.

This example illustrates the problems that confront family members in their attempts to communicate directly with the health professional, rather than rely on filtered information. Family members' requests for information that has already been given to the patient may be brushed off as unnecessary by professionals or seen as needlessly taking up professionals' time.

It is true that communicating with family members or significant others involves professionals' time, but giving direct communication to family members can assist them to cope better and more realistically. Welch

(1981), in a study of the families of cancer patients, reported that a majority of the spouses in the study "strongly agreed" with the statement that if a doctor or nurse were to talk with them and provide explanations about treatments, these events would be easier to "cope with" (p. 367). The point is that family members often have a strong need for information. If professionals can help family members to satisfy their needs, family members will be strengthened and better able to help the ill family member.

Some attempts have been made to attend to the needs of family members and to enhance their relationships with health professionals. Among these approaches have been family support groups, joint patient-family educational groups, family conferences, and family involvement in interdisciplinary team meetings. Interventions such as these can give professionals the opportunity to assess family needs and to provide a forum for more direct and open communication as illustrated in the following case study.

> Mr. Mason had a stroke and was admitted to an acute care hospital. The family was very concerned about Mr. Mason and felt frustrated by the lack of information that they were able to obtain from staff members about his condition.
>
> Three weeks later, Mr. Mason was transferred to a rehabilitation center. The family was amazed at the sharp contrast between the two settings. In the rehabilitation setting, family members were viewed by staff members as important participants in the patient's recovery. In addition, family members were also viewed as having their own emotional concerns and needs for information.
>
> The staff held weekly progress conferences on Mr. Mason's condition. The meetings were attended by Mr. Mason's primary nurse, physician, social worker, occupational therapist, and physical therapist. Mr. Mason and his wife and children were also encouraged to attend the weekly conferences. At these sessions, each professional described their own assessment of Mr. Mason's progress and offered their own recommendations for treatment. Mr. Mason and his family were encouraged to ask questions or share comments throughout these conferences.
>
> The family members found the conferences extremely helpful. Mrs. Mason said, "It really helped me to understand how my husband was progressing and gave me an opportunity to talk directly with some of the staff members whom I seldom saw during visiting hours. I also had the feeling that my comments were important to them—even helpful."

In summary, in this section two barriers to effective professional-family relationships were identified: (1) Family members often feel excluded from health care, and (2) they have difficulty with information management (privileged or filtered communication). By recognizing the needs of family members health professionals will assist family members to feel involved, supported, and less isolated from the health care environment. By attempting to provide direct communication to family members without violating patients' rights to privacy, health professionals will have more accurate communication with family members, and they can also assist family members to cope with the stress involved in maintaining their supportive role to the patient.

More and more, patients are leaving acute care settings earlier and are moving out into settings in the community (family homes, nursing homes, extended care facilities, and hospices) where family members are being asked to assume active roles in the patient's care. Recognizing this trend, health professionals can direct more attention to professional-family relationships.

PATIENT-FAMILY RELATIONSHIPS

The fourth set of relationships that we believe are central to the communication process in health care settings are the relationships between patients and their families. When the traditional focus of health care has been on the sick individual, health professionals have frequently overlooked the many ways in which patients affect family members and family members affect patients (Litman, 1979). This two-way interaction affects patients' and family members' ability to cope with health crises and influences their interactions with other members of the health care team (Pratt, 1976).

Family systems theorist Salvador Minuchin (1974) contends that the family is an open system, and that changes in one part of the system are accompanied by compensatory changes in another part of the system. The onset of a stress such as serious illness can disrupt the family system and force each family member to make adaptive changes. Family goals, income level, role relations, communication patterns, and family lifestyles can all be disrupted by the onset of an illness (Bell, 1966; Litman, 1979; Minuchin, 1974). Two major problems that affect the relationship between patients and family members are (1) the disruption of family members' roles and (2) the closed patterns of communication used by family members (see Fig. 3.10).

Disruption of Family Member Roles

Some families are able to adapt to change, but other families find change difficult and disruptive. Ackerman (1966) believes that disruption in families is primarily due to problems of role adaptation. Problems with role adaptation can occur in two extremes: (1) uncontrolled role fluidity, in which family roles become too loose and undefined, and (2) constrictive role rigidity, in which family roles become too rigid and narrowly defined (Ackerman, 1966; Jones, 1980). Each of these patterns will be discussed in the next section.

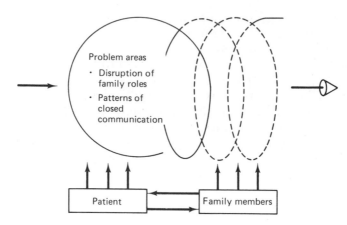

FIGURE 3.10 Potential barriers to effective communication in patient-family member relationships.

Family members normally assume various roles within the family. Each member knows what needs to be done and who will be responsible to do it (Parad & Caplan, 1965). However, with the onset of serious illness, old roles and patterns of relating to one another in the family undergo drastic alteration, leaving family members uncertain as to who will do what to maintain family functioning. As roles become fluid, individuals become unsure of their own role as well as others' roles. There is no control over how they are supposed to act. This uncontrolled *role fluidity* creates confusion and then stress in the family system as illustrated in the following example:

> Helen, a 34-year-old woman, fractured her femur during a motorcycle accident and was hospitalized for several weeks. Her husband, Keith, and four young school-aged boys were totally unprepared for the abrupt shift in their home life. Keith tried to keep their home life running smoothly in Helen's absence by making weekly chore lists for the boys and by using the help of family and friends. In spite of these attempts, considerable chaos still occurred in the family, especially around mealtimes and bedtimes. These were the specific times when Helen normally oversaw the activities in the home.

The amount of confusion and role change accompanying an illness may depend on a number of factors. Litman (1979) found that more prolonged and complicated illnesses have a greater impact on family role relations than acute temporary illnesses. Temporary illnesses are easier to cope with because family members realize that the disruption will be short-lived and that they will soon be returning to their traditional family roles (Bell, 1966). In addition, the amount of role fluidity is also affected by which family member becomes ill. If the wife-mother becomes ill, this disrupts the family more than if the father falls ill (Litman, 1979). Also, illness in a child will influence family functioning differently than illness in a parent (Bell, 1966). Taken together, these various factors influence the amount of role confusion experienced by family members.

The other role pattern that can be disruptive to families is *role rigidity*. Role rigidity occurs when individuals are inflexible or are unable to change their roles to meet the demands of a new situation. Role rigidity can lead to constricted roles among family members and limit their adaptive potentials (Ackerman, 1966; Jones, 1980). A form of role rigidity is typified by a pattern in which one family member assumes an overfunctioning role and another family member assumes an underfunctioning role. Either pattern can be detrimental to family functioning (Helm, 1979).

In families where the stress of illness is present, the overfunctioning role is frequently assumed by the spouse or significant other who does not have the illness, while the underfunctioning role has often been assumed by the ill family member. Bell (1966) observed that when a husband or wife becomes ill, the other spouse often takes on new responsibilities in addition to previous ones. The following example illustrates how these roles can develop and interfere over time with family relationships.

> Mr. W., a 52-year-old man, developed severe back problems after an automobile accident. He underwent several back surgeries and was unable to return to his previous job. Also, due to his back injury, he was told to stop doing heavy lifting and yard work. After Mr. W.'s accident, his wife took on a full-time job to help defray the medical costs and to maintain the family income. She also took on many of the household and yard tasks that he previously did while continuing tasks such as cooking, laundry, and shopping.
>
> After several months, Mr. W. was told that he could return to work and resume some of his previous activities. He was not able to find a new job, primarily because employers were hesitant to hire a man of his age with back problems. Over the next few months he became more and more depressed. He did not resume the yard work, something he enjoyed previously, because he was afraid he would reinjure his back. He spent most of his day watching TV.
>
> Mrs. W. was frustrated that her husband helped so little around the house and "wasted so much time" just watching TV. She was hesitant, however, to make demands on him because of his despondency at not being able to find a job and his anger about facing a life of chronic pain. She continued in her many activities but found herself becoming increasingly tense and irritable around her husband.

The circumstances surrounding the accident and Mr. W.'s surgeries led to Mrs. W. taking an *over*functioning role and Mr. W. an *under*functioning role. Over a short period of time this could assist the family through the crisis; however, over a long period of time, especially when the original health problem subsides, this form of role functioning can lead to interpersonal conflicts between the family members.

How do these overfunctioning and underfunctioning roles get perpetuated in families during a health crisis? Both the patient and the family member can contribute to the development of these role patterns. For example, the anxiety that some patients experience while recovering from an illness such as heart disease can cause them to feel apprehensive about assuming an active role (Wishnie, Hackett & Cassem, 1971). Family members of these patients, on the other hand, may worry that the patient will have another heart attack and may discourage the patient from assuming more responsibilities (Wishnie, Hackett & Cassem, 1971). To compensate for the patient, family members take on overfunctioning roles. In addition, new roles may be perpetuated because individuals find them to be more satisfying than their roles before the illness. Finally, the directives from health professionals can perpetuate role overfunctioning and role underfunctioning: Vague instructions (e.g., "use in moderation" or "a few times a day") may contribute to underfunctioning roles (Wishnie, Hackett & Cassem, 1971), and instructions such as "do as much as you can" may add to overfunctioning roles.

Although role disruption and brief periods of overfunctioning and underfunctioning are likely, Pratt (1976) encourages families to maintain role flexibility. According to Pratt, family members need freedom to shape their roles rather than assuming rigid roles or having rigid roles dictated to them. Health professionals can assist families through the turmoil of role disruption by providing empathic understanding and by assisting them in working through difficult role changes. Also, professionals can avoid locking families into rigid roles by assessing each family on an individual basis. For example, not all families have the caretaking capacities or emotional resources to participate with a hospice team and to provide care for a dying family member in the home setting. For these families a hospice in an institutional setting may fit better with the patient's and family's needs and resources. Although many families show great resiliency in the face of stressful illnesses, other families will need additional assistance from professionals to cope with family disruption due to role changes.

Closed Communication Patterns

A second potential barrier to effective patient-family relationships occurs in the area of family communication. During stress, family communication can either become closed or communication can remain open with interactions continuing throughout the period of stress (Hill, 1958). Closed patterns of communication are often less constructive for family members.

Closed communication hinders effective relationship building among family members at a time when supportive relationships are needed the most.

Family members' tendencies to engage in closed communication have been reported by several researchers. Vachon and her associates (1977) reported on the communication between cancer patients and their spouses during the final stages of illness; they found that only 29 percent of these couples "discussed the possibility of the husband dying of his illness" (p. 1152). Of those couples who did not discuss death, 61 percent said that they consciously avoided the topic, not wanting to upset their partner. Stern and Pascale (1979) also reported decreased communication between cardiac patients and their spouses. Some people refused to even participate in the study because they believed that the "less said about it [the heart attack] the better" (p. 84). Jamison, Wellisch, and Pasnau (1978) reported that little discussion of mastectomy-related concerns occurred between mastectomy patients and their husbands. Eighty-nine percent described their discussion of mastectomy concerns as "little or none" prior to surgery; 87 percent said they had "little or none" during the hospitalization; and 50 percent rated their communication after the hospitalization in this same range. While a majority of patients in a more recent study of mastectomy patients said that they generally could discuss concerns with family members, a segment of the group were adamant that they would not discuss concerns with family members as they did not want to upset them (Northouse, 1981).

Given the fact that patterns of communication are sometimes closed, what factors contribute to closed communication? How do closed communication patterns get perpetuated? Two factors that can foster closed communication among family members are (1) family rules and (2) family protectiveness.

Family communication theorists develop the concept of *family rules* (Jackson, 1965; Satir, 1972). Family rules are a set of unwritten guidelines that indicate how family members will and "ought" to behave toward one another. These implicit ground rules for the family's operations are usually based on the family's values. When family members violate family rules or when family rules are ambiguous problems can surface. To open up family communication family rules need to be altered.

Satir (1972) lists a rule inventory that family members can use to determine what rules are operating in their family (see Table 3.2). Not all families operate under family rules that give family members permission to comment on feelings or thoughts. For example, some families have the rule that "angry feelings are not discussed." In other families, the rule "sad feelings are not shared with Dad" may be followed by family members. Although some of these rules may be effective when families are experiencing little stress or disruption, rules can block effective family

TABLE 3.2   Rule Inventory

1.   What are your rules?
2.   What are they accomplishing for you now?
3.   What changes do you now see you need to make?
4.   Which of your current rules fit?
5.   Which have to be discarded?
6.   What new ones do you have to make?

Adapted from V. Satir, *Peoplemaking*. Palo Alto, Calif.:
Science and Behavior Books, Inc., 1972, p. 111.

communication when families face major stresses such as serious illness. Satir states that some families operate on the basis of outdated family rules. For example, the old notion of "what is not expressed will not be felt" is typical of a family rule that specialists in nonverbal communication tell us is no longer correct (see Chapter 4).

Satir believes that a first step for some families is just to become aware of the unwritten, unspoken family rules that exert a powerful influence on their family communication. Once they are able to define the rules, family members may better understand the difficulties that they experience in communicating with particular family members or in discussing a specific topic. Satir notes that some families may need to update old and no longer useful family rules so that family communication can be more supportive of family members' needs.

In addition to family rules that hinder open communication, the *protectiveness of family members* toward one another can also lead to closed communication. Family theorist Murray Bowen (1976) states that family communication can become constricted when one member faces a life-threatening illness. Family members try to protect themselves as well as others from the anxiety they are experiencing. Stern and Pascale (1979) report that spouses of cardiac patients not only limit their discussion about medical problems but also about their concurrent family stress. They report that family members often become "preoccupied with their husband's health, feeling that a 'wrong move' or 'bad move' on their part would produce another infarct" (p. 84). As a result, these spouses often reported trying to solve family problems by themselves, a task that at times was overwhelming. Families of psychiatric patients also worry about the amount of stress an ill family member can tolerate and at times limit the person from involvement in family decision making. For example, the wife of a man who was hospitalized for depression decided not to tell him about the financial problems that she and the children were facing at home. She said, "He's just starting to feel better, more hopeful; if he finds out about the money problems he may start going downhill again."

Some family members think that they are protecting the patient when in fact they are also really trying to protect themselves from facing painful experiences. Hearing and accepting information about a family member's deteriorating health can be especially difficult for family members and something that family members may not be willing to acknowledge. The following excerpt from the play *The Shadowbox*[2] illustrates the unwillingness of the wife of a cancer patient to accept and communicate openly about her husband's failing health. The wife (Maggie) is trying to get her husband (Joe) to leave the hospice setting and to return home with her. Joe wants Maggie to accept the reality of his illness.

MAGGIE: Come home, that's all. Come home.

JOE: I can't, Maggie. You know I can't.

MAGGIE: No, I don't know. I don't.

JOE: I can't.

MAGGIE: You can. Don't believe what they tell you. What do they know? We've been through worse than this. You look fine. I can see it.

JOE: No, Maggie.

MAGGIE: You get stronger every day.

JOE: It gets worse.

MAGGIE: No. I can see it.

JOE: Everyday, it gets worse.

MAGGIE: We'll go home, tomorrow. I got another ticket. We can get a plane tomorrow.

JOE: Don't do this, Maggie.

MAGGIE: I put a new chair in the apartment. You'll like it. It's red. You always said we should have a big red chair. I got it for you. It's a surprise.

JOE: No! It won't work.

MAGGIE: We'll get dressed up. I'll get my hair done. We'll go out someplace. What do we need? A little time, that's all.

JOE: It's not going to change anything.

MAGGIE: No. It's too fast. Too fast. What'll I do? I can't remember tomorrow. It's no good. We'll look around. Maybe we can find a little place. Something we like.

JOE: No. This is all. This is all we got.

MAGGIE: No. Something farther out. Not big. Just a little place we like. All right, a farm, if you want. I don't care. Tomorrow!

JOE: (*Angry and frustrated*): Tomorrow is nothing, Maggie! Nothing! It's not going to change. You don't snap your fingers and it disappears. You don't buy a ticket and it goes away. It's here. Now.

MAGGIE: No.

JOE: Look at me, Maggie.

MAGGIE: No.

[2]Excerpt from *The Shadow Box* by Michael Cristofer, copyright 1979 by the author. Used by permission of Drama Book Publishers, New York.

Whether closed family communication is due to unspoken family rules or protectiveness on the part of family members, problems can arise in family communication as a result of these patterns. Closed communication can lead to unnecessary estrangement in relationships (Karpel, 1980). Persons confronting illness are often already experiencing some aloneness and isolation in their relationships with others. Concealment and closed communication perpetuate these feelings of separateness from others. In addition, closed communication can lead to distortions of information and erroneous assumptions (Karpel, 1980). Finally, when family members attempt to protect one another, they limit their ability to support one another and assist each other to work through emotional pain.

Pratt (1976), in an extensive study of families, found that regular and varied communication among family members was linked to sound health practices among family members. Open communication not only assisted them in reducing stresses associated with illness, but also in negotiating with others within the health care system. Pratt believes that open communication does not have to be intrusive; it can respect the autonomy of individual family members within the complex family setting.

Although the importance of open communication among family members has been emphasized in this section, it is important to add that for some families closed patterns of communication may be more comfortable and adaptive. In other words, for some families it may be unrealistic and undesirable to try to quickly change longstanding patterns of family communication. It may also be unrealistic to expect that their patterns of communication during a crisis will be better than their communication during stable, pre-illness times. Assessment is essential. What are the typical patterns of communication in the family? Are these patterns helpful during a health crisis? What alterations, if any, would family members like to make? Answers to questions such as these will give professionals an indication of the ways in which they can assist family members.

In summary, in this section two barriers to patient-family relationships were identified: (1) disruptions in family member roles and (2) closed patterns of family communication. Health care workers can assist families to cope with the stress of role disruption and to maintain open channels of communication. While many families are able to cope well with the stress of illness and are brought closer together during the stress (Litman, 1979), other families will need the help and assistance of health professionals. Providing empathic understanding of role disruption, encouraging role flexibility, refraining from overloading an already overfunctioning family member, and communicating with family members in a way that will enhance their supportive communication with one another will facilitate patient-family relationships and also relationships with members of the health care team.

SUMMARY

Four major types of relationships that exist in health care are professional-patient, professional-professional, professional-family, and patient-family relationships. In each type of relationship there are factors that have the potential for hindering effective communication.

Four factors that can affect the quality of professional-patient relationships are role uncertainty, responsibility conflicts, power differences, and unshared meanings. Role uncertainty hinders patients' understanding of their own role as well as the role of the many health care providers with whom they will be working. Responsibility conflicts may arise when professionals and patients do not adhere to the same models of responsibility (moral, compensatory, medical, or enlightenment). Power differences are problematic in this relationship since professionals have traditionally held more power and influence than have patients. Finally, the differing perceptions or unshared meanings that professionals and patients have about various words may block effective professional-patient communication.

Three factors that affect professional-professional relationships are role stress, insufficient interdisciplinary understanding, and autonomy struggles. Due to the nature of health care settings, professionals experience considerable role stress. This role stress can lead to interpersonal tensions among health professionals as they attempt to cope with role conflict or it can lead to withdrawal from one another as they attempt to cope with role overload. Insufficient interdisciplinary understanding can cause professionals to underutilize one another's unique areas of expertise or to become embroiled in "turf" negotiations. Finally, friction due to autonomy struggles can lead to professional-professional competition and decreased collaboration.

The professional-family relationship is one that until recently has not received much attention in health care. A potential problem in this relationship is exclusion of family members from health care. Family members have felt uninvolved in health care and often have not made their needs known to professionals. Professionals, on the other hand, have not always been attuned to the special needs of family members, or to the importance of a collaborative relationship with family members. Information management is another problem area for professionals and family members. Family members have often received privileged or filtered communication, with both patterns creating potential problems for family members.

In patient-family relationships, coping with the disruption of family roles is a major problem for both patients and family members. In the face of such disruption, too much role fluidity may lead to confusion, while too much role rigidity may inhibit appropriate adaptation to the circumstances of the illness. Closed communication is another problematic area for pa-

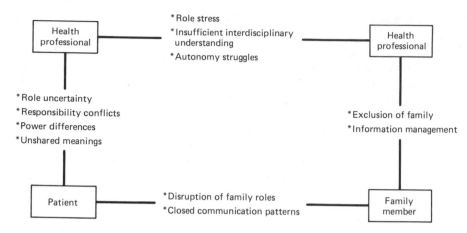

FIGURE 3.11   Potential barriers to effective communication among participants in health care settings.

tients and family. Closed communication, whether due to family rules or a desire of family members to protect one another, can limit supportive communication among family members during the stress of illness.

The four major relationships and potential barriers to effective health communication are summarized in Figure 3.11. As noted throughout the chapter, problems in one set of relationships, for example, professional-professional, can lead to problems in another set, such as professional-patient relationships. Ways to alter these potential problem areas were discussed throughout the chapter.

REFERENCES

Ackerman, N. *Treating the troubled family.* New York: Basic Books, Inc., Publishers, 1966.

Allen, M., Jackson, D., & Younger, S. Closing the communication gap between physicians and nurses in the intensive care unit setting. *Heart and Lung.* 1980, *9*(5), 836–840.

Anderson, W. T., & Helm, D. The physician-patient encounter: A process of reality negotiation. In E. G. Jaco (Ed). *Patients, physicians, and illness.* New York: The Free Press, 1979.

Balassone, P. Territorial issues in an interdisciplinary experience. *Nursing Outlook,* 1981, *29*(4), 229–232.

Bell, R. The impact of illness on family roles. In J. Folta and E. Deck (Eds.), *A sociological framework for patient care.* New York: John Wiley & Sons, Inc., 1966.

Berger, P. & Luckman, T. *The social construction of reality.* New York: Anchor Books, 1967.

Bond, S. Communicating with families of cancer patients: 2. The nurses. *Nursing Times,* 1982, *78*(24), 1027–1029.

Borland, J. Burnout among workers and administrators. *Health and Social Work,* 1981, *6*(1), 73–78.

Bowen, M. The use of family theory in clinical practice. In J. Haley (Ed.), *Changing families: A family therapy reader.* New York: Grune & Stratton, Inc., 1971.

Bowen, M. Family reaction to death. In P. Guerin (Ed.), *Family Therapy.* New York: Gardner Press, 1976.

Breu, C., & Dracup, K. Helping spouses of critically ill patients. *American Journal of Nursing,* 1978, *78*(1), 50–53.

Brickman, P., Rabinowitz, V., Karuza, Jr., J., Coates, D., Cohn, E., & Kidder, L. Models of helping and coping. *American Psychologist,* 1982, *37*(4), 368–384.

Brown, E. Meeting patient's psychosocial needs in the general hospital. *The Annals of the American Academy of Political and Social Science,* 1963, *346*, 117–122.

Bryne, M. Non-nursing functions: The nurses state their case. *American Journal of Nursing,* 1982, *82*(7), 1089–1092.

Cassileth, B., Zupkis, R., Sutton-Smith, K., & March, V. Information and participation preferences among cancer patients. *Annals of Internal Medicine,* 1980, *92*(6), 832–836.

Conway, M. Organizations, professional autonomy and roles. In M. Hardy & M. Conway (Eds.), *Role theory.* New York: Appleton-Century-Crofts, 1978.

Cristofer, M. *The shadowbox.* New York: Avon Books, 1977.

Cronenwett, L. & Brickman, P. Models of helping and coping in childbirth. *Nursing Research,* 1983, *32*(2), 84–88.

Danziger, S. The uses of expertise in doctor-patient encounters during pregnancy. In P. Conrad and R. Kern (Eds.), *The sociology of health illness.* New York: St. Martin's Press, Inc., 1981.

Davitz, L., & Davitz, J. *Nurses' responses to patients' suffering.* New York: Springer Publishing Co., 1980.

Devereux, P. Essential elements of nurse-physician collaboration, *Journal of Nursing Administration,* 1981, *11*(5), 19–23.

Diers, D. Future of nurse-midwives in American health care. In L. Aiken (Ed.), *Nursing in the 1980's.* Philadelphia: J. B. Lippincott Company, 1982.

DiMatteo, M. A social psychological analysis of physician-patient rapport: Toward a science of the art of medicine. *Journal of Social Issues,* 1979, *35*(1), 12–33.

DiMatteo, M., & Friedman, H. *Social psychology and medicine.* Cambridge, Mass.: Oelgeschlager, Gunn & Hain, 1982.

DiMatteo, M., & Hays, R. Social support and serious illness. In B. Gottlieb (Ed.), *Social networks and social support.* Beverly Hills, Calif.: Sage Publications, Inc., 1981.

Eckenrode, J., & Gore, S. Stressful events and social supports: The significance of context. In B. Gottleib (Ed.), *Social networks and social support.* Beverly Hills, Calif.: Sage Publications, Inc., 1981.

Fagin, C. Nursing education. In T. Keenan, L. Aiken, & L. Cluff, *Nurses and doctors: Their education and practice.* Cambridge, Mass.: Oelgeschlager, Gunn & Hain, 1981.

Feiger, S., & Schmitt, M. Collegiality in interdisciplinary health teams: Its measurement and its effects. *Social Science and Medicine,* 1979, *13A*(2), 217–229.

Ford, L., Nurse practitioners: History of a new idea and predictions for the future. In L. Aiken (Ed.), *Nursing in the 1980's.* Philadelphia: J. B. Lippincott Company, 1982.

Fourcher, L., & Howard, M. Nursing and the "managerial demiurge." *Social Science and Medicine,* 1981, *15A,* 299–306.

Freihofer, P., & Felton, G. Nursing behaviors in bereavement: An exploratory study. *Nursing Research,* 1976, *25*(5), 332–337.

French, R. P., & Raven, R. The bases of social power. In D. Cartwright (Ed.), *Studies in social power*. Ann Arbor, Mich.: Institute of Social Research, 1959.

Giacquinta, B. Helping families face the crisis of cancer. *American Journal of Nursing*, 1977, *77*(10), 1585–1588.

Gould, H. & Toghill, P. How should we talk about acute leukemia to adult patients and their families? *British Medical Journal*, 1981, *282*, 210–212.

Hamburg, D. Toward increasing collaboration among health professionals. In T. Keenan, L. Aiken, & L. Cluff, (Eds.), *Nurses and doctors: Their education and practice*. Cambridge, Mass.: Oelgeschlager, Gunn & Hain, 1981.

Hampe, S. O. Needs of the grieving spouse in a hospital setting. *Nursing Research*, 1975, *24*(2), 113–120.

Haney, W. *Communication and interpersonal relations*. Homewood, Ill.: Richard D. Irwin, Inc., 1979.

Hardy, M. Role stress and role strain. In M. Hardy & M. Conway (Eds.), *Role theory*. New York: Appleton-Century-Crofts, 1978.

Haug, M. The erosion of professional authority: A cross cultural inquiry in the case of the physician. In G. Turner and J. Mapa (Eds.), *Humanizing hospital care*. Toronto: McGraw-Hill Ryerson, 1979.

Helm, P. Family therapy. In G. Stuart and S. Sundeen (Eds.), *Principles and practice of psychiatric nursing*. St. Louis: The C. V. Mosby Company, 1979.

Hill, R. Generic Features of Families Under stress. *Social Casework*, 1958, *39*(2–3), 139–149.

Hooper, E., Comstock, L. M., Goodwin, J., & Goodwin J. S. Patient characteristics that influence physician behavior. *Medical Care*, 1982, *20*(6), 630–638.

Jackson, D. D. The study of the family. *Family process*, 1965, *4*, 1–20.

Jacox, A. Role restructuring in hospital nursing. In L. Aiken (Ed.), *Nursing in the 1980's*, Philadelphia: J. B. Lippincott Company, 1982.

Jamison, K., Wellisch, D., Pasnau, R. Psychosocial aspects of mastectomy: I. The women's perspective. *American Journal of Psychiatry*, 1978, *135*(4), 432–436.

Jones, S. *Family therapy*. Bowie, Md.: Robert Brady Co., 1980.

Kahn, R., Wolfe, D., Quinn, R., & Snock, J. *Organizational stress: Studies in role conflict and ambigiuty*. New York: John Wiley & Sons, Inc., 1964.

Kalisch, B. Of half gods and mortals: Aesculapian authority. *Nursing Outlook*, 1975, *23*(1), 22–28.

Kalisch, B., & Kalisch, P. An analysis of the sources of physician-nurse conflict. *Journal of Nursing Administration*, 1977, *7*,(1), 51–57.

Kalisch, B., & Kalisch, P. *Politics of nursing*, Philadelphia: J. B. Lippincott Company, 1982.

Kaplan, D., Smith, A., Grobstein, R., & Fischman, S. Family mediation of stress. *Social Work*, 1973, *18*(7), 60–69.

Karpel, M. Family secrets. *Family Process*, 1980, *19*(3), 295–306.

Kasl, S. Issues in patient adherence to health care regimens. *Journal of Human Stress*, 1975, *1*(3), 5–17.

Keenan, T., Aiken, L., & Cluff, L. *Nurses and doctors: Their education and practice*. Cambridge, Mass.: Oelgeschlager, Gunn & Hain, 1981.

Klein, R., Dean, A., & Bogdonoff, M. The impact of illness on the spouse. *Journal of Chronic Diseases*. 1967, *20*,(4), 241–248.

Kramer, M. *Reality shock*. St. Louis: The C. V. Mosby Company, 1974.

Kramer, M., & Schmalenberg, C. *Path to biculturalism*. Wakefield, Mass.: Contemporary Publishing, 1977.

Krause, E. *Power and illness*. New York: Elsevier, 1977.

Kritek, P. B. Patient power and powerlessness. *Supervisor Nurse*, 1981, *12*(6), 26–34.

Latanich, T. & Schultheiss, P. Competition and health manpower issues. In L. Aiken (Ed.), *Nursing in the 1980's.* Philadelphia: J. B. Lippincott Company, 1982.

Lauer, P., Murphy, S., & Powers, M. Learning needs of cancer patients: A comparison of nurse and patient perceptions. *Nursing Research,* 1982, *31*(1), 11–16.

Leary, T. The theory and measurement methodology of interpersonal communication. *Psychiatry,* 1955, *18* 147–161.

Leavitt, M. The discharge crisis: The experience of families of psychiatric patients. *Nursing Research,* 1975, *24*(1), 33–40.

Leininger, M. This I believe . . . about interdisciplinary health education for the future. *Nursing Outlook,* 1971, *19*(12), 787–791.

Leininger, M. Professional, political, and ethnocentric role behaviors and their influence in multidisciplinary health education. In M. Hardy & M. Conway (Eds.), *Role theory,* New York: Appleton-Century-Crofts, 1978.

Levine, M. S. & Kliebhan, L. Communication between physicians and physical and occupational therapists: A neurodevelopmentally based perception. *Pediatrics,* 1981, *68*(2), 208–214.

Lister, L. Role expectations of social workers and other health professionals. *Health and Social Work,* 1980, *5*(2), 41–49.

Litman, T. The family in health and health care: A social behavioral overview. In E. G. Jaco (Ed.), *Patients, physicians and illness.* New York: The Free Press, 1979.

Litz, T. and others. Patient-family-hospital interrelationships. In M. Greenblatt (Ed.), *The patient and the mental hospital.* Glencoe, Ill.: The Free Press, 1957.

Lorber, J. Good patients and problem patients: Conformity and deviance in a general hospital. *Journal of Health and Social Behavior,* 1975, *16*,(6), 213–225.

Maslach, C. The burnout syndrome and patient care. In C. Garfield (ed.), *Stress and survival.* St. Louis: The C. V. Mosby Company, 1979.

Mauksch, I. Nurse-physician collaboration: A changing relationship. *Journal of Nursing Administration,* 1981, *11*(6), 35–38.

Mauksch, I. An analysis of some critical contemporary issues in nursing. *Journal of Continuing Education in Nursing,* 1983, *14*(1), 4–6.

Mechanic, D. *Medical sociology,* 2nd Ed. New York: The Free Press, 1978.

Mechanic, D. Nursing and mental health care: Expanding future possibilities for nursing services. In L. Aiken (Ed.), *Nursing in the 1980's: Crises, opportunity, challenges.* Philadelphia: J. B. Lippincott Company, 1982.

Milne, M. A. Training for team care. *Journal of Advanced Nursing,* 1980, *5*(6), 579–589.

Minuchin, S. *Families and family therapy.* Cambridge, Mass.: Harvard University Press, 1974.

Molter, N. Needs of relatives of critically ill patients: A descriptive study. *Heart and Lung,* 1979, *8*(2), 332–339.

Neuhring, E., & Barr, W. Mastectomy: Impact on patients and families. *Health and Social Work,* 1980, *5*(1), 51–58.

Northouse, L. Mastectomy patients and the fear of cancer recurrence. *Cancer Nursing,* 1981, *4*(3), 213–220.

Northouse, L. The impact of cancer on the family. An overview. *International Journal of Psychiatry in Medicine,* 1984, *14*(3), in press.

Northouse, L. & Wortman, C. Models of helping and coping in cancer care. Paper presented at Oncology Nursing Society Annual Congress, San Diego, Calif.: May, 1983.

Novack, D., Plummer, R., Smith, R., Ochitill, H., Morrow, G. & Bennett, J. Changes in physicians attitudes toward telling the cancer patient. *Journal of the American Medical Association,* 1979, *241*(9), 897–899.

Okun, D. What to tell cancer patients: A study of medical attitudes. *Journal of the American Medical Association*, 1961, *175*, 1120–1128.

Orem, D. *Nursing: Concepts of practice*. New York: McGraw-Hill Book Company, 1980.

Parad, H. & Caplan, G. A framework for studying families in crisis. In H. Parad and G. Caplan (Eds.), *Crisis intervention: Selected readings*. New York: Family Service Association of America, 1965.

Pratt, L. *Family structure and effective health behavior*. Boston: Houghton Mifflin Company, 1976.

Rodin, J. & Janis, I. The social power of health-care practitioners as agents of change. *Journal of Social Issues*, 1979, *35*(1), 60–81.

Ruderman, A. Match? In *More cartoon classics*. N.J.: Medical Economics, 1966.

Satir, V. *Peoplemaking*. Palo Alto, Calif.: Science and Behavior Books, Inc., 1972.

Schindler, F., Berren, M., & Beigel, A. A study of the causes of conflict between psychiatrists and psychologists. *Hospital and Community Psychiatry*, 1981, *32*(4), 263–266.

Schulman, B. & Swain, M. A. Active patient orientation. *Patient Counseling and Health Education*, 1980, *2*(1), 32–36.

Silva, D., Clark, S., & Raymond, G. California physicians' professional image of physical therapists. *Physical Therapy*, 1981, *61*(8), 1152–1157.

Staver, S. M.D. learns firsthand about nurses' duties. *American Medical News*, 1982, *25*(1), 13.

Stern, M. & Pascale, L. Psychosocial adaptation post-myocardial infarction: The spouse's dilemma. *Journal of Psychosomatic Research*, 1979, *23*(1), 83–87.

Stone, G. Patient compliance and the role of the expert. *Journal of Social Issues*, 1979, *35*(1), 34–59.

Szasz, T. *The manufacture of madness*. New York: Harper & Row, Publishers, Inc., 1970.

Tagliacozzo, D. & Mauksch, H. The patient's view of the patient's role. In G. Jaco (Ed.), *Patients, physicians, and illness*. New York: The Free Press, 1979.

Taylor, S. Hospital patient behavior: Reactance, helplessness or control? *Journal of Social Issues*, 1979, *35*(1), 156–184.

Templin, E. The system and the patient. *American Journal of Nursing*, 1982, *82*(1), 108–111.

Vachon, M., Freedman, K., Formo, A., Rogers, J., Lyall, W., & Freeman, S. The final illness in cancer: The widow's perspective. *Canadian Medical Association Journal*, 1977, *117*(10), 1151–1153.

Weiss, S. Role differentiation between nurse and physician: Implications for nursing. *Nursing Research*, 1983, *32*(3), 133–139.

Wessen, A. Hospital ideology and communication between ward personnel. In G. Jaco (Ed.), *Patients, physicians, and illness*. New York: The Free Press, 1958.

Weinberger, M., Green, J., & Mamlin, J. Changing house staff attitudes toward nurse practitioners during their residency training. *American Journal of Public Health*, 1980, *70*(11), 1204–1206.

Welch, D. Planning nursing interventions for families of adult cancer patients. *Cancer Nursing*, 1981, *4*(5), 365–370.

Williams, R., & Williams, C. Hospital social workers and nurses: Interprofessional perceptions and experiences. *Journal of Nursing Education*, 1982, *21*(5), 16–21.

Wishnie, H., Hackett, T., & Cassem, N. Psychological hazards of convalescence following myocardial infarction. *Journal of the American Medical Association*, 1971, *215*(8), 1292–1296.

4 Nonverbal Communication in Health Care Settings

To focus exclusively upon the words *humans interchange is to eliminate much of the communicational process from view. . . .* —Birdwhistell, 1970

In recent years, the area of nonverbal communication has received a great deal of attention. Bestsellers such as *Body Language* by Julius Fast (1970) and *Dress for Success* by John Molloy (1975) have helped to popularize the importance of nonverbal communication. People today are interested in being able to understand and to explain their own as well as other people's nonverbal behavior. Health care professionals are also taking an equally strong interest in nonverbal communication (Blondis & Jackson, 1982; Friedman, 1979; McCorkle, 1974; and Weiss, 1979).

So much attention is being given to nonverbal behavior because individuals recognize that it plays a key role in the overall communication process. Birdwhistell (1970), for example, who studied the area of body movement, suggests that 65 to 70 percent of the social meaning of an interaction is transmitted by nonverbal behavior. Mehrabian (1971), another well-known authority on nonverbal communication, estimates that 93 percent of the meaning in a message can be accounted for by nonverbal communication (p. 43). Although these percentages are only estimates, they do indicate that nonverbal behavior is a central aspect of human communication.

To understand the complexities of health transactions among professionals, clients, and family members, one needs to be aware of the contribution made by the nonverbal dimension of the communication process.

Health transactions, as depicted in the health communication model (see Chapter 1), are comprised of both verbal and nonverbal components. The emphasis in this chapter is on the nonverbal component. In this chapter, we define nonverbal communication, describe how it functions in the human communication process, and dispel several myths about nonverbal behavior. In addition, we describe specific dimensions and examples of nonverbal communication.

THE IMPORTANCE OF NONVERBAL COMMUNICATION IN HEALTH CARE

Nonverbal communication has special relevance in health care primarily because patients pay close attention to the nonverbal communication of professionals, and professionals, on the other hand, rely heavily on the nonverbal communication of patients.

Patients' Attentiveness to Nonverbal Communication

Patients and family members are very sensitive to professionals' nonverbal communication for a variety of reasons (Friedman, 1979). First, health care settings evoke considerable fear and uncertainty in patients and family members. To lessen their uncertainty, patients and family members become especially alert to information in their environment and to the nonverbal cues emitted by practitioners. For example, when patients cannot understand the complex medical jargon being used, they focus instead on the professionals' nonverbal behavior as a way of understanding the situation.

Second, patients sometimes believe that health professionals are not completely honest with them. Patients may think that health professionals are trying to protect them from bad news or are hiding their real feelings from them. Nonverbal communication becomes increasingly important during times of illness because many people believe that the truth is often "leaked" through nonverbal channels (Friedman, 1979). For example, even though a clinician may tell the parents of a young child with a birth defect that the defect is minor, the parents will usually scrutinize the clinician's facial expression carefully for some clue as to how serious the clinician *really* thinks that the birth defect is for the child.

Third, patients and family members will sometimes rely on nonverbal observations as a rapid means of gaining information even before any verbal interaction takes place. For example, parents who are anxiously awaiting the results of their child's bone marrow test may quickly scan the clinician's face as he or she enters the room to get a clue to whether they will be receiving good or bad news. This rapid preinteraction observation may help the parents to "get ready" for the verbal interaction that will follow.

Finally, patients often rely heavily on nonverbal communication if they perceive that the practitioner is too busy or is unapproachable. In these situations the patient will use nonverbal cues to supplement the information that is either missing or not understandable from the verbal interaction. These are a few of the main reasons why patients and family members are so attentive to health professionals' nonverbal communication.

Professionals' Attentiveness to Nonverbal Communication

It is not surprising that professionals are usually attentive to patients' nonverbal communication. During their educational experiences, most students are taught about the importance of assessing such things as facial expression, body posture, and gestures. Nursing students, for example, are often required to write extensive process recordings that provide information about *patients'* nonverbal communication as well as their *own* nonverbal communication.

In clinical practice, the practitioner becomes very aware of the need to assess nonverbal communication. In fact, in some cases, nonverbal assessment is the only means of gaining information about the patient's experience. In mental health settings, for example, the psychotically depressed client may be unable to find the words to express the loss, pain, or aloneness that he or she is experiencing. In medical settings, the patient on a respirator will not be able to express concerns to staff members in words. In neonatology units, infants cannot verbally communicate their needs to the nurses. In these situations the health professional needs to rely primarily on the expressions, gestures, and other modes of nonverbal communication to understand and assess the client's needs.

Being attentive to nonverbal communication is also essential for professionals in their communication with each other. Health professionals with busy schedules often do not have the time for in-depth conversations with one another. Typically their conversations are limited and rather brief. In these situations nonverbal communication supplements the verbal interactions and helps professionals to enhance their understanding of each other. Also, health professionals are often in situations in which they are not able to talk. For example, in a crisis situation such as a cardiac arrest, two professionals may share their fears and concerns with one another nonverbally through a quick glance or facial expression and engage in very little, if any, verbal communication.

In light of its importance, understanding the nature, function, and dimensions of nonverbal communication is essential for effective health communication.

THE NATURE OF NONVERBAL COMMUNICATION

Nonverbal Communication Defined

What is nonverbal communication? Is it simply communication without words? Is it communication without sound? Does it include behaviors that have unintended meanings for others? Answers to questions such as these have been the subject of much controversy among researchers of nonverbal communication, because nonverbal communication covers a wide range of overlapping human behaviors.

Although nonverbal communication is a very broad field, it is only a subset of the entire communication process. In Chapter 1, we defined communication as the process of sharing information through a set of common rules. While this same definition can be applied to nonverbal communication, it is important to note that nonverbal communication represents a smaller portion of the communication process—that portion which is free of words. Knapp (1978a) points out that "the term *nonverbal* is commonly used to describe all human communication events which transcend spoken or written words" (p. 38). Other writers have similarly characterized nonverbal behaviors as those behaviors that have the common quality of not being organized by a language system (Eisenberg and Smith, 1971, p. 20). According to Mortensen (1972)

> nonverbal includes nonlinguistic or extralinguistic aspects of behavior that contribute to the meaning of messages: body movement, gesture, proxemics, facial expression, eye contact, posture, and certain paralinguistic cues associated with vocal quality and intonation (p. 20).

In essence, nonverbal communication is *communication without words* and it includes messages created through body motion, the use of space, the use of sounds, and touch.

Although nonverbal communication does not encompass language, nonverbal communication can be either vocal or nonvocal. This may sound surprising, because nonverbal communication is usually thought of as silent. However, vocal sounds that are not language or words fall within the category of nonverbal communication. For example, a groan or a scream of pain by a patient under stress would be *vocal nonverbal* communication, while a smile or frown on a health professional's face would be *nonvocal nonverbal* communication.

In addition, nonverbal communication can be either intentional or unintentional. If a person is communicating an important message to others, she or he will most probably use a facial expression that notes the seriousness of the situation. A community health nurse who maintains a serious facial expression while telling a client about the potential side effects of a new hypertensive drug is using *intentional* nonverbal communication.

Unintentional nonverbal communication would be characterized by a client at a reproductive health center who appears to be carrying on a pleasant, relaxed conversation with the intake clerk but whose facial expressions show fear and uncertainty at the same time. In this situation the client is not aware of her facial expression; it is unintentional nonverbal behavior.

Purposes of Nonverbal Communication

The overriding purpose of nonverbal communication is the effective sharing of information between participants in an interaction. Nonverbal communication performs several identifiable functions in the process of communication, including (1) the expression of feelings and emotions, (2) the regulation of interaction, (3) the validation of verbal messages, (4) the maintenance of self-image, and (5) the maintenance of relationships. At any time in an interaction, one or several of these functions may be operating.

Expression of feelings and emotions
Through nonverbal behavior, individuals express their joy, anger, despair, and fear. Clients and professionals, alike, reveal aspects of their inner states to others by using nonverbal communication. Nonverbal communication allows clients to tell health professionals they feel helpless, they are uncertain, they feel powerless, or they feel anxious. The elderly female who stands in front of a health professional, nervously rubbing her hands together, is communicating some of her inner feelings of anxiety and agitation. Similarly, professionals can tell clients nonverbally that they feel troubled, they feel rushed, they feel positive, or they feel important. Nonverbal communication is a channel for venting and releasing pent-up feelings as well as an avenue for expressing day-to-day feelings.

Regulation of interaction
A second function of nonverbal communication is that of regulating the flow of messages between people. Nonverbal cues, such as a tilted head, intense eye contact, raised eyebrows, a lowered voice, a shift in body posture, or a movement toward or away from someone, all regulate the flow of messages. For example, the clinician who nods his or her head as a client discusses concerns is indicating nonverbally to the client to continue or to carry on. Nonverbal cues regulate an interaction by indicating to others whether individuals want to talk, when they want to talk, whether they want to listen, how long they want to listen, and when a conversation is over. For example, in a home visit, nonverbal communication is used by both the health professional and the client to establish when a formal interview is to begin, how long the interview is to last, whose turn it is to ask or answer questions, and when the interview is completed. The clinician who glances

frequently at a wristwatch near the end of a conversation may be indicating (intentionally or not) that the interaction is concluding. On the other hand, the client who stands up and starts to take coffee cups to the kitchen may be suggesting to the home care nurse that it is time for the conversation to stop.

Nonverbal communication can also be used in professional-professional interactions to regulate communication. In the hospital emergency room a health professional who frequently glances around the room and refuses to maintain eye contact with a community crisis worker who wants to obtain information about a client is controlling the flow of communication. The physician who points to a vacant set of chairs in a conference room as if to invite a social worker to sit down is conveying encouragement or willingness to converse on an issue. In each of these instances nonverbal messages are used to regulate the flow of the interaction.

Validation of verbal messages

It could be argued that of all the functions of nonverbal communication, the main function is validating the verbal dimensions of an interaction. When the words match the individual's expressed feelings and emotions, communication is most effective. If a client says, "I feel great," but looks troubled and angry, the nonverbal dimension of the client's message is incongruent with the verbal dimension. This makes it difficult for others to know how to respond to the client. Or consider the health care administrator who says, "I'm very pleased with how things are going," but has an extremely disgruntled and rather angry facial expression. It is difficult to interpret the administrator's meaning because the nonverbal expressions do not match or correspond with the words. Communication is most effective when the nonverbal dimensions of messages validate the verbal dimensions.

Maintenance of self-image

A fourth function of nonverbal communication is maintaining the self-image of the communicator. While this function of nonverbal communication may not seem as obvious as the other functions just described, it does play an important role in self-preservation, or in assisting us to convey an image of ourselves to others. Goffman (1959, 1963, 1967) has theorized that interaction is much like a stage performance in which individuals assume various roles and act them out. Nonverbal communication assists individuals in performing their roles appropriately in front of others and helps individuals to present the image they want to project to others. Studies on impression formation, for example, highlight the importance of nonverbal communication in shaping our initial impressions of others (Asch, 1946).

In any interaction, individuals have images of themselves they want to maintain. For example, in an extended care facility, an 80-year-old resident who was a banker for 40 years before his retirement may want to be dressed daily in a coat and tie because that is the way bankers dress. His clothes communicate to others that he wants to be seen as a respectable banker. Or consider the newly graduated nurse who wears a stethoscope around her neck during breaks in the coffee shop because she wants to be seen by others as a qualified professional. In both of these examples, the individuals are using nonverbal cues to maintain a role that communicates to others a part of their self-image. Although the nonverbal cues in these examples are obvious to illustrate the point, in many interactions there are subtle and not so subtle nonverbal cues present that individuals give to establish a self-image.

Maintenance of relationships

Finally, nonverbal communication serves the function of defining relationships; nonverbal cues help individuals describe to each other how they feel about their relationship. In Chapter 1, we discussed how communication has both a content and a relationship dimension, and that the meaning in a message emerges as a result of *what* is said (the content) in conjunction with *how* it is said (the relationship). The "how it is said" aspect of a message depends primarily on the nonverbal cues that accompany a message. Nonverbal cues give individuals information about their interpersonal relationship and therefore on how they should interpret the content of a particular message.

Through nonverbal communication individuals convey relational messages to others about such things as inclusion, status, control, or affection. For example, a health professional can often determine his or her level of inclusion in a meeting by looking at the way chairs are set up at the meeting. A nurse educator told us about a treatment planning session at a psychiatric facility where she worked with her students. Staff members sat directly at the oval table in the room and students were asked to sit in chairs behind the staff, away from the table. Although it was never verbally indicated, the larger padded chair at the end of the table was always left vacant for the psychiatrist who ran the treatment planning meetings.

In professional-professional relationships, relational messages concerning status differences can sometimes be observed in how people dress. In some health care settings a long white laboratory coat may indicate high status while a short laboratory coat indicates low status. In other settings professionals who wear street clothes may be viewed as having higher status than personnel required to wear uniforms.

Relational messages about control can also be indicated by nonverbal cues. When a professional sits next to a client, a feeling of shared control is expressed; but if the professional hovers over the client, it implies dominance. Warmth or hostility are also relational messages communicated through nonverbal communication channels. A kind look or caring expression communicates to others a good relationship while an angry look or harsh tone of voice can express to others a cold and more distant relationship. Although one particular nonverbal behavior does not always indicate a particular relationship message, a combination of nonverbal behaviors can often be taken together to provide information about characteristics of the relationship.

Myths About Nonverbal Communication

Several myths have been identified concerning the scope and importance of nonverbal elements in the human communication process (Knapp, 1980). These myths have developed as a result of the recent widespread popular interest in nonverbal communication. It is important to dispel some of these myths so that they do not provide an inaccurate picture of the role that nonverbal communication plays in human communication. The four myths Knapp identifies are (1) the isolation myth, (2) the key to success myth, (3) the transparency myth, and (4) the single meaning myth (p. iv).

The isolation myth

The isolation myth suggests that nonverbal communication is separate and discrete from other aspects of the communication process. It implies that we can treat nonverbal messages in isolation. The problem with this notion is that it fails to see the interrelatedness between nonverbal and verbal communication. Meaning emerges from the interaction between nonverbal and verbal elements in the communication process. To isolate one part of the process from the rest may be appropriate for purposes of teaching or research, but in reality nonverbal communication is closely bound to verbal communication.

The key to success myth

The key to success myth suggests that nonverbal communication is the key to successful interpersonal communication. Implied within this myth is the notion that individuals will indeed be effective communicators if only they stand in certain ways, sit appropriately, and wear the right clothes. The idea overemphasizes nonverbal communication, and regards it as a cure-all for effective communication. Although the potency of nonverbal communication should not be underestimated, neither should nonverbal communication be viewed as the only element contributing to success in human interaction. Nonverbal communication is just one of a multitude of elements comprising the human communication process. To focus on one element as the "key" can distort and misrepresent the overall process of human interaction.

The transparency myth

In many ways the popular newstand-type nonverbal books are directly responsible for the transparency myth—the conception that our nonverbal behavior makes us fully transparent to others. These books purport to provide "quick and guaranteed" ways of accurately assessing people's personalities by focusing on specific nonverbal cues. The faulty assumption made in these books is that an individual's clothes, posture, or stance can totally reveal his or her inner thoughts, feelings, and personality. In reality, each of us gives off a multitude of nonverbal cues in addition to our verbal cues. We can control many of these cues, which means that we can influence how we want to be seen by others. Thus, it is not true that nonverbal cues allow others to "read us like a book." Nonverbal communication is such a complex and often intentional process that no single nonverbal cue or group of cues makes individuals transparent to others.

The single meaning myth

It is also myth to assume that every nonverbal cue has a single, specific meaning. Nonverbal cues are like verbal cues; they have multiple meanings. A scowl can mean an individual is questioning someone else or it can mean an individual is angry. Similarly, a questioning tone of voice can mean an individual is confused or it can mean that an individual disagrees with another person. People who cross their arms in front of their chests may not be trying to shut themselves off from others—they may only be trying to retain a little body heat in a cold room. The point is that the nonverbal communication process is intricate, and each nonverbal behavior can have several meanings depending on the participants and the context in which they are communicating.

DIMENSIONS OF NONVERBAL COMMUNICATION

Nonverbal communication is a complex and multifaceted phenomenon. Researchers have commonly divided the nonverbal communication area into five distinct categories: (1) kinesics, (2) proxemics, (3) paralinguistics, (4) touch, and (5) physical and environmental factors (see Fig. 4.1). Taken together, these categories of nonverbal communication provide a framework for understanding the intricacies of the nonverbal process, and they provide the basis for discussing the clinical implications of sending and receiving nonverbal messages.

Kinesic Dimensions of Nonverbal Communication

Kinesics is the study of body motion as a form of communication. It is the most familiar type of nonverbal communication and it includes such areas as gestures, posture, body movement, facial expressions, and eye

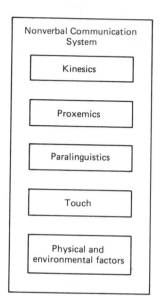

FIGURE 4.1 Dimensions of the nonverbal communication system.

movement. A categorization system for kinesic behavior was developed by Ekman and Friesen (1969), who divide nonverbal behavior into five types: (1) emblems, (2) illustrators, (3) affect displays, (4) regulators, and (5) adaptors (see Fig. 4.2).

Emblems

According to Ekman and Friesen (1969) *emblems* are nonverbal acts that can be directly translated into specific verbal messages having quite specific, agreed-upon meanings (pp. 63–64). Emblems can take the place of words and they are usually easily understood by others. Putting your first finger perpendicular across your lips to say "shhhh" is an example of an emblem. Similarly, gesturing with your head to say "no" or moving your hand to say "come here" are emblems. Another example is the two-finger peace gesture. Essentially, emblems function as substitutes for words. Emblems are used frequently in situations where channels for sending or receiving verbal communication are blocked, such as with deaf individuals or patients who cannot speak.

Illustrators

Illustrators are body movements that have a one-to-one relationship to verbally communicated messages; they are movements that are directly tied to speech and that show with motion what is being said with words (Ekman & Friesen, 1969, p. 68). They usually accompany speech and they help to pictorialize what is being communicated. The gestures one uses while giving directions to another person are called illustrators. A nurse who is teaching a patient how to do a dressing change would most likely show the patient the procedure using a whole series of illustrators. Illustrators are used intentionally to complement and reinforce what an individual is saying.

Affect displays

Earlier in the chapter we said that the first function of nonverbal communication was the expression of feelings and emotions. This function is fulfilled through *affect displays,* which are body movements primarily of the face that indicate the emotional state of an individual. It is affect display that shows whether an individual is feeling mad or glad, weak or strong, and "hyper" or depressed. If a person feels frightened, there is likely to be the expression of fear on that person's face.

Affect displays can be expressed either intentionally or unintentionally, and they may support or contradict verbal messages. Because affect displays are not always intentional nor directly linked to verbal communication, it is important for health professionals to respond to the affect of others with a degree of caution. It is not possible to "read others like a book." Affect displays are subtle and complex, demanding careful response.

Regulators

In a conversation between two individuals, *regulators* are used to adjust and maintain the flow of communication. Regulators are nonverbal movements that establish the pacing for a conversation by regulating the back-and-

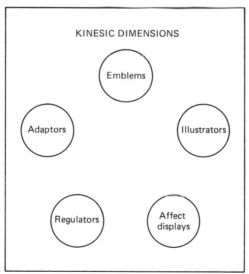

FIGURE 4.2   Ekman and Friesen's classification system for nonverbal behavior acts.

forth speaking and listening between two individuals (Ekman and Friesen, 1969, p. 82). Like affect displays, regulators usually involve movements of the eyes, face, or head; however, hand and arm movements and shifts in body posture can also act as regulators. Sometimes through a head nod we tell another person, "Go ahead and finish what you have to say," or, by raising an eyebrow, we can let them know that, "When you're finished, I'd like to respond to your comments." Eye movements are frequently used as regulators. For example, squinting may signal to another to continue talking, while looking away from another person may signal the end of a conversation. In general, regulators are body movements that assist speakers in controlling the flow of their interaction.

Adaptors

Unlike regulators, which are used by an individual when he or she is involved in a conversation with another person, adaptors are often used when an individual is alone. Adaptors are body movements, such as scratching your head, biting or licking your lips, playing with a pencil, tapping your fingers, or shaking your foot, that are used to satisfy basic physical needs and to manage emotions (Ekman and Friesen, 1969). This kind of nonverbal act usually occurs unintentionally and is not easily defined. Basically, adaptors are learned nonverbal responses that originate from childhood experiences and that allow individuals to adapt to anxiety and stress.

In addition to the types of nonverbal behaviors delineated by Ekman and Friesen in their five-category system, two other common types of nonverbal communication fall within the kinesic domain. These two areas are facial expressions and gaze.

Facial expressions

The human face provides a complex but rich source of information for health professionals and clients alike. Ekman, Friesen, and Ellsworth (1972) point out that

> The human face—in response and in movement, at the moment of death as in life, in silence and in speech, when alone and with others, when seen or sensed from within, in actuality or as represented in art or recorded by the camera—is a commanding, complicated, and at times confusing source of information (p. 1).

For the most part, facial expressions are used to display emotions, either intentionally or unintentionally. However, they are also used by individuals to punctuate conversations or regulate the flow of interaction between two communicators.

It is essential for health professionals to understand clients' emotions and facial expressions because some clients are reluctant at times to express their feelings verbally. Health professionals need to learn to interpret nonverbal facial expressions accurately, but this is no simple task, especially when one considers that facial expression is often controlled by clients and that the human face is extremely complex. Researchers have found, in the laboratory setting, that the muscles of the face are so complex that in only a few hours time the actions of the face muscles can express as many as 1,000 different facial expressions (Ekman, Friesen, and Ellsworth, 1972).

Generally, researchers agree that the expression of some emotions by facial appearances is a universal phenomenon. The position, first proposed by Darwin (1872) in *The Expression of the Emotions in Man and Animals,* has been supported by recent research; facial expressions of some emotions (e.g., happiness, sadness, and fear) are biologically determined, universal, and learned similarly across cultures (Ekman and Friesen, 1975). Although these emotions are universally expressed, there are cultural differences in when a particular facial expression is shown; that is, the rules for displaying a particular emotion are not the same in all cultures (Ekman & Friesen, 1975).

Researchers also agree on a system to categorize the major emotional expressions of the face. Nearly all of the studies in the last 40 years that have focused on emotions expressed by the face have identified the following six emotions: happiness, sadness, surprise, fear, anger, and disgust (Ekman & Friesen, 1975). Figure 4.3 illustrates a simplified and somewhat exaggerated depiction of the six emotions that was created by Harrison (1974).

The task of reading others' nonverbal facial cues becomes difficult and confusing because individuals may simultaneously express different emotions with different parts of their face (e.g., eyes, brows, forehead, mouth, and so on). Facial expressions that combine two or more emotions are called *affect blends* (Knapp, 1978a). A person who simultaneously expresses feelings of either anger and fear, or disgust and surprise, fear and sadness, or happiness and contempt is portraying a blend of affects.

In the book titled *Unmasking the Face,* Ekman and Friesen (1975) provide an elaborate guide based on research findings for recognizing emotions and affect blends from facial clues. They describe distinct *styles* that characterize individuals' facial expressions (pp. 155–157). Perhaps you can recognize your own style or someone else's in one or more of the following categories.

Withholders: These are individuals whose faces rarely signal how they feel. The muscles of their face do not move a great deal; and their faces are unexpressive.

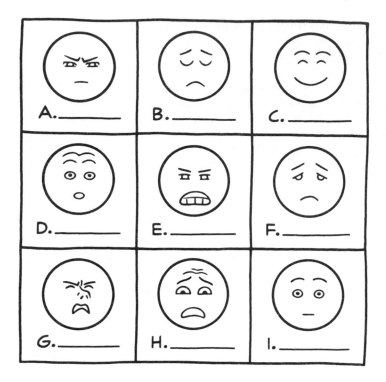

Can you match the above sketches with the correct affects? (1) happy, (2) sad, (3) surprise, (4) fear, (5) anger, (6) disgust.

Answers: A–5, B–2, C–1, D–3, E–5, F–2, G–6, H–4, I–3.

FIGURE 4.3 Cues of the primary affects. (Randall P. Harrison, *Beyond Words: An Introduction to Nonverbal Communication,* © 1974, p. 120. Reprinted by permission of Prentice-Hall, Inc., Englewood Cliffs, New Jersey.)

Revealers: These individuals express their feelings readily, and their emotions are shown all over their face. It is difficult for revealers to control their expressions.

Unwitting expressers: These people show their feelings (usually one or two particular feelings) to others, but they are unaware that they have done so. For example, it is individuals who show anger or contempt on their faces without knowing it.

Blanked expressers: These are individuals who think their faces are expressing a particular feeling or emotion when, in fact, they are blank and neutral. For example, some people say they are happy while their faces show no emotion.

Substitute expressers: These are individuals who display one emotion while they are feeling another. They look mad although they say that they are feeling sad; or they look happy when, in fact, they say they are feeling afraid. These people are usually unaware of the fact that their faces give cues which are incongruent with their real feelings.

Frozen affect expressers: These are persons whose faces consistently express a trace of a particular emotion. They are individuals whose faces always look a bit sad, mad, or glad.

The fact that Ekman and Friesen have been able to delineate so many styles of facial expressions with subtle differences between the styles helps to point out the difficulty in assessing the nonverbal messages in facial appearances. Regardless of the complexity of the face, however, there is strong evidence that facial expression is a useful source of fairly accurate information and that a person can improve his or her skill in assessing nonverbal facial cues (Rosenthal et al., 1979).

Gaze

Gaze is the last type of kinesic nonverbal communication we will consider. Gaze, which is closely linked with facial expressions, refers to how individuals use their eyes in the commmunication process to give information to others, receive information from others, and establish relationships. Gaze plays a central role in nonverbal communication and is an important form of social behavior (Argyle & Cook, 1976).

How does gaze function in social interaction? What is a normal pattern for individuals who attempt to establish eye contact? How should individuals use their eyes when talking with each other? These are the types of questions that have been addressed in research on the functions of gaze and on the normal patterns of gaze.

Functions of gaze. Individuals use their eyes to perform primarily three functions: (1) monitoring, (2) regulating, and (3) expressing (Kendon, 1967, p. 52). *Monitoring* involves assessing or checking out how others appear and how others are responding to us. Both clients and professionals often use their eyes in this way. In a psychiatric setting, a suspicious patient may isolate himself or herself in the corner of a day room and carefully use his or her eyes to monitor the people and events in the room. As we discussed in the beginning of the chapter, clients at times feel vulnerable and have an intense need to observe others' responses to them; they may actively search for visual signs that will give them additional information about their situation. Health professionals, on the other hand, often use monitoring as a primary source of information concerning the client's condition and response to treatment. In intensive care settings, for example, a nurse may gaze closely at a patient to monitor respiratory rates or signs of increasing restlessness that give clues to a change in the patient's condition.

Regulating refers to how individuals use gaze to synchronize their conversation. They use gaze to signal information about whose turn it is to talk and whose turn it is to listen. The regulatory function of gaze allows the speaker and listener to give feedback to each other about how they are proceeding. Hardin and Halaris (1983) reported on the differences in gaze between patients and nurses in videotaped interaction. Although their sample was small, they found that nurses maintain longer and more direct gaze toward patients, while patients tend to look at and away from the nurse more often during the interaction. The way in which gaze helps to regulate interaction between people is described straightforwardly by Harrison (1974):

> In conversation, the speaker is likely to catch the listener's attention. But then, before launching into a long utterance, the speaker will drop his eyes. He will make periodic checks, to see if his listener is still there—and still a listener. But he will avoid eye contact at pauses when, for example, he is trying to think of how to complete his thought. When he is finished, however, he will return his gaze to the listener and prepare to give up the floor (p. 126).

A third function performed by our eyes is *expressing* to others feelings about affiliation, intimacy, and a range of common emotions. Ekman and Friesen (1975) point out that individuals' eyes vary while expressing the basic emotions: surprise, fear, disgust, danger, happiness, and sadness. They contend that these variations in eye expression can be recognized by others.

Normal patterns of gaze.   All of us are familiar with the advice, "When talking to others, it is important for one to establish *good eye contact*." Although this principle is helpful because it stresses the importance of nonverbally acknowledging and confirming others, this advice does not actually describe what is meant by *good* eye contact. Researchers have studied how individuals use eye contact in their ongoing relationships, and several rather interesting findings have been made.

First, researchers have found that, contrary to what one might think, individuals in a typical conversation do not look at one another *all* the time. In fact, the best estimate of the time individuals spend in direct eye contact in a normal conversation is about 50 to 60 percent (Argyle & Ingham, 1972; Cook, 1977; Kendon, 1967). Second, the average length of each gaze is usually less than three seconds, and the average length of mutual gazes has been reported to be less than two seconds (Argyle & Ingham, 1972). Third, speakers spend about 40 percent of their time gazing at the listener and listeners spend about 75 percent of their time looking at the speaker (Argyle & Ingham, 1972). Mutual eye contact occurs during 31 percent of the time in a conversation (Argyle & Ingham, 1972). Fourth, there are differences in how the sexes tend to employ gaze. During interaction, females tend to look more at the other person than males do (Argyle & Cook, 1976).

Given these findings, it becomes easier to interpret the advice to "make good eye contact." Good eye contact means that an individual should look directly at others, but not necessarily 100 percent of the time. Some people seem to operate from the position of "more is better" in regard to eye contact and never shift their gaze from a person during an interaction. Good eye contact does not require long gazes or lengthy mutual gazes. Basically, individuals should try to establish the amount of eye contact with which both participants in an interaction are comfortable. Eye contact, like other kinds of human communication, is a transactional process. Each person affects the other and is affected by the other. Too much eye contact can be uncomfortable and interfere with the normal ebb and flow of an interaction. Too little eye contact may make the individuals feel impersonal, or it may lead to one or both participants feeling disconfirmed or unimportant. "Good" eye contact requires moderate amounts of gazing which are appropriate to the situation.

Before concluding this discussion of kinesics, we would like to consider two additional questions: (1) How can we measure our own, or others' skills in the area of nonverbal communication? and (2) Are some people better at sending and receiving nonverbal messages than others?

A considerable amount of work in finding answers to these questions has been done by Rosenthal and his associates at Harvard University. The majority of their work has centered on developing and testing a tool called the Profile of Nonverbal Sensitivity, or the PONS[1] (Rosenthal et al., 1979). This instrument measures a person's ability to decode nonverbal behaviors. The PONS consists of a 45-minute black-and-white film with 220 numbered segments of nonverbal behavior. A person views the film and then tries to identify the best description of a particular segment of the film from two choices. The segments use a variety of nonverbal channels (e.g., facial cues versus body cues) and affective contents (e.g., positive-dominant behavior versus negative-submissive behavior). After completing the PONS test, a person receives a specific score on reading nonverbal cues from various channels (e.g., face, body, etc.) as well as an overall score for nonverbal accuracy.

[1]The PONS Instrument can be obtained through Irvington Publishers, Inc., 551 Fifth Avenue, New York, N.Y. 10176.

Using the PONS test in many different studies, Rosenthal and his associates identified a number of factors that were related to accuracy in interpreting nonverbal cues. They found that (1) in general, females were more accurate decoders of nonverbal cues than males; (2) accuracy appeared to increase with age and started to level off when people reached 20–30 years of age; (3) intelligence played only a small role in a person's nonverbal accuracy; and (4) the personality profiles of accurate decoders described them as better adjusted, more interpersonally democratic, more extroverted, and more interpersonally sensitive people (Rosenthal et al., 1979). These findings provide an interesting starting point for understanding factors that influence nonverbal accuracy.

Proxemic Dimensions of Nonverbal Communication

Proxemics is a second major component in the nonverbal communication system (see Fig. 4.1). *Proxemics* is a term coined by anthropologist Edward T. Hall to refer to how individuals use and interpret space in the communication process. The seminal work on proxemics is Hall's book *The Silent Language* (1959), a study of the differences in cross-cultural nonverbal communication patterns. This work by Hall and a second, titled *The Hidden Dimension* (1966), are the primary sources for research on proxemics.

Unlike kinesics, which focuses on the individual and the individual's body motion, proxemics is concerned with the space and environment surrounding the individual and with how they affect and are affected by that individual. Proxemics is an area of nonverbal communication that deals with questions such as, How much personal space do clients usually want when talking with a health professional? How close should one be to others in a personal conversation? How does furniture arrangement affect the meaning of messages? Some areas of proxemics that address questions of territoriality, personal space, and distance are particularly relevant to health communication.

Territoriality and personal space

In studying animal life, scientists first observed what has now come to be called *territoriality*—the behavioral process of laying claim to an area of space and then protecting it from intrusion by outside forces. For animals, territoriality provides protection and a place for a species to learn, to play, to hide, and to engage in group activities (Hall, 1966). "One of the most important functions of territoriality is proper spacing, which protects (animals) against over-exploitation" (Hall, 1966, p. 6). Through territoriality, animals establish the boundaries of the space they wish to inhabit.

These studies of animal behavior provide the background for understanding how the concept of territoriality functions in human communication. It is generally believed that humans also show territoriality, although there is debate over whether humans learn territorial behaviors or possess them instinctively (Ardry, 1966; Hall, 1966; King, 1981; Stillman, 1978). Regardless of the origin, "everyone has a need for his personal and private space for thinking, feeling, and communicating with others" (Pluckhan, 1978). Personal space, or one's own territory, is important because it provides people with a sense of identity, security, and control. Individuals feel threatened when others invade their territory because it disrupts their psychological homeostasis, creates anxiety, and produces feelings of loss of control (Allekian, 1973; Stillman, 1978).

In acute care settings, patients frequently experience intrusions into their personal space and territory. As Stillman (1978) so vividly points out:

> Into [the patient's] territory will come a parade of intruders who seem to exhibit more of a right to be there than he does. These trespassers enter often without knocking, carry out activities often without introduction or explanation, and depart, seldom leaving the patient's territory as it was before they arrived. The sick person is often too weak due to his physical and psychological condition to repel the intruders; lack of territory may render him less assertive and unsure of his rights. The patient, in a strict sense, becomes the trespasser on the territory of those health professionals legitimized by society to be within the hospital's walls (p. 1671).

Stillman's comments portray the difficulty patients have in establishing territorial boundaries or in maintaining them if they have been assertive enough to establish them in a health care setting.

How do these intrusions into patients' personal space affect patients? Allekian (1973) reported that moving chairs out of patients' rooms, rearranging bedside tables, or looking through their personal belongings without asking permission were all intrusions of patients' territory and events to which patients responded with annoyance. Allekian also noted that the patients reacted with more annoyance when objects specifically identified with patients (e.g., their belongings in the drawer) were involved versus objects less personalized (e.g., a chair in the room).

Minckley (1968) also observed the reactions of postoperative patients to territoriality issues. She noted that patients often indicated a desire to leave the recovery room and to return to "their own" rooms. In addition, many patients reported less tension when they eventually returned to "their own" beds. Reporting on the problems of obtaining personal space in nursing homes, Tate (1980) reported that residents often share bedrooms, dining areas, lounge areas, and even bathrooms, and for the most part have little space to call their own. As a result, she contends, many residents may engage in aggressive behavior or social withdrawal as a means of coping with an environment that offers them no space to call their own.

When people enter health care settings they are required to give up the personal space and privacy provided by their own homes. They must reside in an entirely new setting and often establish living arrangements with strangers whom they have never seen before. In addition, patients often have to undergo many diagnostic procedures that further compromise their sense of privacy and personal space. Although health professionals may not be able to eliminate these problems of territoriality, there are some fairly straightforward ways to assist patients in lessening the anxiety created by intrusions and loss of space. Stillman (1978) has suggested the following approaches which may be helpful to health professionals.

Give the patient respect. Recognize his or her hospital territory, belongings, and rights to privacy.

Give the patient control. Allow the patient to make decisions about his or her territory. Let the patient have control over whether the door should be open or closed, whether the shades should be up or down, and where the bedside table should be placed.

Give the patient information. Recognize the patient's individuality and provide explanations for activities and procedures which directly or indirectly affect the patient.

Give attention to patients' privacy needs. If possible, protect against leaving the patient's body exposed and minimize the discomfort involved in procedures that require the invasion of privacy (p. 1672).

Distance

A second subarea of proxemics is concerned with how *distance* affects interpersonal communication. As Hall (1959) points out, "Spatial changes give a tone to a communication, accent it, and at times even override the spoken word. The flow and shift of distance between people as they interact with each other is part and parcel of the communication process" (p. 160). In other words, space or distance plays a significant role in how individuals interact. Distance is another nonverbal factor that can influence the comfort and extent of disclosure in an interaction.

In a classic study of distance zones, Hall (1966) attempted to answer the question of whether human beings have a uniform way of handling distance and whether distance could be delineated into specific zones. His study involved interviews and observations of a sample of middle-class adults from the northeastern seaboard of the United States. Although his research cannot be generalized to other classes, racial groups, or cultures, his results provided the basis for a typology of distance zones in human interaction that has become the accepted framework for analysis of this area.

According to Hall, individuals in social situations use essentially four distance zones: (1) intimate, (2) personal, (3) social, and (4) public. For each zone, Hall has provided a description of what commonly occurs.

Intimate distance. For individuals, this distance includes the area in which people are able to touch one another to the area in which they are approximately 1½ feet apart. It is the distance at which individuals engage in such things as protection, comforting, and lovemaking. Talking in this area is usually soft or at a whisper, and topics are usually very personal. Individuals are selective about allowing others within this distance; it is usually reserved for very close friends. Being forced into intimate distance in public places such as in a bus or in an elevator can produce anxiety. Individuals usually react with a tightening-up or rigidly immobile response.

Due to the types of interventions and activities carried out in health care settings, clinicians often need to enter the patient's intimate distance zone. Providing mouth care or perineal care to a patient who is unable to carry out these hygiene measures requires close distance and contact between the clinician and patient. Some patients will accept and appreciate clinicians' willingness to provide needed care within these close distances. However, those situations in which the clinician enters the intimate distance zone by accident or with less attentiveness to the patient may produce more discomfort.

Personal distance. Personal distance ranges between 1½ to 2½ feet between individuals—about arm's length. This is the distance at which individuals can carry on personal conversations with intimates or close friends using soft to moderate voice levels. Significant variations often exist between cultures in the use of personal distance. For example, individuals from one culture may require less space in informal dialogue at this distance than individuals from another culture.

The personal distance zone is commonly used in health care settings in which the practitioner is explaining a procedure to a patient, reading over preoperative instructions, or discussing a matter of personal concern to the patient that he or she does not want others to hear.

Social distance. When individuals are 4 to 12 feet apart, they are establishing social distance. Communication in business and work settings or at casual social events, like parties, is typically carried out at this distance. Offices are commonly arranged to place individuals at social distance. Voice level at this distance is usually moderately loud or normal.

Social distance in health care settings would be characterized by the nurse or physician who stands in the doorway of the patient's room to carry on a conversation. This distance is also common in work areas where professionals are writing progress notes or health assessments.

Public distance.   When people are from 12 to 25 feet or more apart, they are at public distance. At this distance voices are usually amplified, and nonverbal behaviors such as stance and gestures are often exaggerated. Lectures, public speeches, and presentations at large events such as political rallies are examples of places where individuals use public distance. In health care the community health nurse who is presenting a public seminar on hypertension to a group of senior citizens would most likely be using public distance. Similarly, the instructor of an expectant parents class may maintain public distance with the participants while teaching the class, while the couples attending the class are at a social distance from other couples.

Questions that frequently arise regarding distance zones are, how do people choose spatial distance or what accounts for the distance selections people make? According to Hall (1966), individuals choose distance zones according to their feelings, what they are doing, the nature of their relationships, and the communicative transaction itself (p. 120). Burgoon and Jones (1976), who have proposed a theoretical framework for understanding personal space expectations and violations, regard personal distance as a function both of social norms and the idiosyncratic behavior of the communicators. That is, personal distance will vary depending on such things as race, culture, sex, status, age, personality, and the psychological predispositions of the individuals.

We probably become most aware of distance zones in our interactions when the distance used does not seem appropriate for the particular situation. For example some of us might feel uneasy if a stranger walked up to us, stood 6 inches away and started a conversation. Awareness of distance zones is also illustrated by the following example.

> A friend of ours who had recently been diagnosed as having cancer was attending a public lecture being given by a former professor of his. At the end of the lecture as people were leaving the audience the professor happened to glance up into the audience where he saw his former student. The professor yelled out into the audience, "Hi—it's nice to see you. . . . Say, I hear you have cancer. . . .Are you OK?" The former student smiled and yelled back that he was fine. While retelling this story, however, our friend said that he was quite surprised that the professor yelled such a personal question in a public setting with an audience. He also said that he was tempted to yell back to the professor, "By the way, how did your hemorroidectomy turn out?" as a way of humorously sensitizing the professor to the situation.

This rather extreme example of imbalance between distance and content of the interaction helps to point out the need for health professionals and others to keep in mind the distances we use with others and how distance plays a role in the comfort and effectiveness of our communication with others.

There are no strong rules that can be set for health professionals to follow in every health care situation. Nevertheless, it is possible for health professionals to be sensitive to the distance norms for different situations, and to try to allow patients to participate in establishing distance zones when possible. Sensitivity and awareness will enhance the possibility of creating a situation in which effective interaction can take place.

Paralinguistic Dimensions of Nonverbal Communication

A third dimension of the nonverbal communication process is paralinguistics (see Fig. 4.1). *Paralinguistics* refers to the vocal sounds such as "ah" and "um" that accompany spoken verbal communication. These voice sounds run alongside our use of language. Paralinguistics focuses on how the voice plays a role in the interpretation of messages. To understand this area, it is beneficial to consider the elements of paralinguistics and how paralinguistics is related to emotions.

Elements of paralinguistics

Most of the literature on nonverbal communication uses the system suggested by Trager (1958), who divides this area into four major elements: (1) voice qualities, (2) vocal characterizers, (3) vocal qualifiers, and (4) vocal segregates.

Voice qualities. The first aspect of paralinguistics deals with the characteristics of voice including range and control of pitch, lip control, thickness, articulation, rhythm, resonance, and tempo. Each individual's voice is unique and varies in regard to each of these characteristics. For example, some individuals have voices that are deep, thick, and resonant while others' voices are high, thin, and nasal. Our voice quality is a physical characteristic that often makes us recognizable to others.

Vocal characterizers. The second element, vocal characterizers, focuses more specifically on how individuals use their voices when laughing, crying, groaning, moaning, yelling, whispering, coughing, and sighing. Each of us has a rather distinct way of doing each of these and how we laugh or cry is a part and expression of who we are.

Vocal qualifiers. In paralinguistics, three vocal qualifiers have been identified: intensity, pitch height, and extent. *Intensity* refers to the degree of energy or power behind a person's voice—like the volume of a radio. A highly intense voice is overloud; its opposite is oversoft. *Pitch height* has reference to how high or low an individual's voice is perceived to be. *Extent* is the length of time a voice carries and includes voices with long drawling or a short clipping quality.

Vocal segregates.   Vocal segregates are intrusions, interjections, or interruptions in an individual's speech pattern. Examples include expressions such as "uh," "un-huh," "um," "ah," and also voice pauses.

Paralinguistics and emotions

Earlier in this chapter we discussed how facial cues affect the expression of emotions. Now we would like to turn to a discussion of how vocal cues affect emotional expressions. In studying the relative impact of vocal cues, facial expressions, and words on perceived feelings, Mehrabian (1972) and his colleagues have found that vocal cues accounted for 38 percent of the effect, while words contributed 7 percent and facial expressions accounted for the remaining 55 percent. Although Mehrabian's research findings cannot be generalized to all messages in all situations, they do point to the importance of the paralinguistic (or vocal) component in human communication.

Because vocal cues influence emotional expressions, paralinguistics is an area of nonverbal communication to which health professionals need be closely attuned. However, paralinguistic expressions are not always easily and accurately interpreted by listeners. Davitz and Davitz (1959) and Knapp (1978a) suggest that accurate judgments of individuals' emotions by vocal cues is a complex process that is influenced by many factors. The sender, receiver, emotion expressed, and context all influence the assessment made of emotions from vocal sounds.

Although direct and accurate interpretation of vocal cues is difficult, Davitz (1964) has observed that certain emotional cues are often related to certain paralinguistic cues. His observations appear in Table 4.1. By reading the table, one can get a general approximation of the types of vocal expressions (e.g., loudness, pitch, timbre, etc.) that frequently parallel the expression of basic emotions (e.g., affection, anger, boredom, etc.).

Touch: A Special Type of Nonverbal Communication

Touch is a particular type of nonverbal communication. Touch can take a variety of forms and it can convey a variety of meanings. A firm handshake, a gentle squeeze, a sharp pinch, or an enveloping hug are all forms of touch. The meaning of the message conveyed by each of these forms of touch can vary considerably. For example, the stroking touch of a male to a female is often interpreted as a sexual message, while the same touch directed toward a child is often received as a soothing message. Similarly, when one person touches us we may experience comfort and warmth, but when another person does the same thing, we may experience discom-

TABLE 4.1 Characteristics of Vocal Expressions Contained in the Test of Emotional Sensitivity

FEELING	LOUDNESS	PITCH	TIMBRE	RATE	INFLECTION	RHYTHM	ENUNCIATION
Affection	Soft	Low	Resonant	Slow	Steady and slight upward	Regular	Slurred
Anger	Loud	High	Blaring	Fast	Irregular up and down	Irregular	Clipped
Boredom	Moderate to low	Moderate to low	Moderately resonant	Moderately slow	Monotone or gradually falling	—	Somewhat slurred
Cheerfulness	Moderately high	Moderately high	Moderately blaring	Moderately fast	Up and down: overall upward	Regular	—
Impatience	Normal	Normal to moderate	Moderately blaring	Moderately fast	Slight upward	—	Somewhat clipped
Joy	Loud	High	Moderately blaring	Fast	Upward	Regular	—
Sadness	Soft	Low	Resonant	Slow	Downward	Irregular pauses	Slurred
Satisfaction	Normal	Normal	Somewhat resonant	Normal	Slight upward	Regular	Somewhat slurred

Reprinted with permission from J. R. Davitz, *The Communication of Emotional Meaning.* New York: McGraw-Hill Book Company, 1964, p. 63. Copyright © 1964 by McGraw-Hill, Inc.

fort or uneasiness. In this section we will discuss the importance of touch in health care, the factors that influence an individual's degree of comfort or discomfort with touch, and clinical considerations regarding touch.

Importance of touch in health care

Touch has particular relevance to health communication. Touch can be used by a health professional as a bridge to enter a lonely psychiatric patient's world and to decrease a patient's sense of isolation (DeThomas, 1971). In extended care facilities, touch can be used to make contact with a geriatric patient and to assist the patient in maintaining reality orientation (Burnside, 1973). In ambulatory care settings touch is an important tool for assessing and diagnosing health problems (Friedman, 1979). In acute care settings, where sensory deprivation is a major problem for patients who are isolated from close family members, touch plays a special role in providing human contact for patients (Barnett, 1972) and in letting them know that the clinician cares about them (McCorkle, 1974).

Touch and human development.   Touch plays an important role in growth and development. Harlow, in his well-known experiments with infant monkeys, demonstrated the importance of soft contact to the infants during the developmental process (Harlow & Zimmermann, 1959). Harlow constructed two types of surrogate mothers for infant monkeys. One type, made of molded wire, provided nourishment to the infant. A second type was made of the same wire, covered with a soft terrycloth fabric, but it did not provide nourishment. The infant monkeys showed a strong preference for the cloth-covered mother over the wire-covered mother, even though they were not able to receive food from this surrogate mother. Harlow also found that the infant monkeys with cloth mothers formed stronger attachments and had fewer behavioral problems than the infants with the wire mothers. These experiments contradicted earlier beliefs that the infant-mother bond is based primarily on receiving food and highlighted the importance of contact comfort to the mother-infant relationship and to the infant monkey's normal development.

The early work of Spitz (1946) also underscores the importance of contact to normal growth and development. Spitz studied human infants who were institutionalized and whose lives were devoid of human contact. He observed that these infants had a number of behavioral problems which he attributed to their lack of consistent contact with significant others. More recent authors have also reported that touch is essential to human development (Barnett, 1972; Montagu, 1978). There is strong evidence that touch is the earliest and most basic form of human communication for infants and the primary means of communication between the infant and the environment. Early and ongoing tactile experiences appear to be strongly related to an adult's emotional and intellectual development.

Touch and human relationships.   Touch is also valuable in enhancing relationships with others. Aguilera (1967), a psychiatric nurse, studied the usefulness of touch with psychiatric patients. Patients in one group received both touch and verbal communication, while patients in a second group only received verbal communication. Aguilera reported that patients who were touched had more verbal interaction and more rapport with the nurse than those patients who were not touched. In counseling relationships, the therapist's touch contact with the client has been related to increased amounts of self-exploration by the client (Pattison, 1973) and to more positive client evaluations of the counseling session (Alagna et al., 1979). Touch, together with verbal communication, was found to quiet distressed children more than verbal comfort alone (Triplett & Arneson, 1979). These studies are only a few of many that indicate that touch has a positive effect on human relationships. Touch is an important intervention that can be used to supplement verbal communication and to show care and concern toward others.

Touch and healing.   In the last ten years there has been an increase in research on the relationship of touch and healing. For example, a touching technique similar to the ancient healing practice in which practitioners would use a laying on of hands has been developed by Krieger (1975). Krieger's touch intervention involves the healer's becoming aware of his or her own energies, and directing the energy from this "centered" state toward helping the ill person. The clinician places his or her hands on or close to the ill person's body for approximately 10 to 15 minutes (Krieger, 1975). During this time the clinician's energy is directed or "transferred" to the ill person, who is believed to be in a less than optimal state of energy (Krieger, Peper, Ancoli, 1979). In various experiments, Krieger and her associates have reported that this touch intervention has altered patients' hemoglobin rates (Krieger, 1975) and decreased preoperative patients' anxiety levels (Heidt, 1981). Although more in-depth study is needed on the mechanism underlying the effectiveness of touch intervention, Krieger's technique highlights the interest in touch as a special clinical intervention.

Before leaving our discussion of the importance of touch, it is interesting to note that touch interventions have not always been positively received by patients. On the contrary, there are situations in which touch is perceived negatively or at least as *not* helpful. For example, when touch was used with nursing home residents, some of the residents reported feelings of discomfort at being touched by the nurse (DeWever, 1977). Similarly, when the effect of touch on preoperative male patients was studied, patients who were touched responded more negatively on the outcome measures than the men who did not receive the touch intervention (Whitcher & Fisher, 1979). In another study, a majority of postpartum women reported

positive feelings about being touched, but 37 percent of the women reported either neutral reactions or negative reactions to the touch that they
received (Penny, 1979). In light of these reports, it seems clear that touch
will not always be perceived in the same way by each person. Some patients
will regard touch as positive and helpful, while others will view it as negative and not helpful. At times the meaning of touch to the person touching
(such as the nurse) will not be the meaning given to the touch by the
receiving person (such as the client). These mixed responses to and varied
interpretations of touch indicate that health professionals ought to be sensitive and cautious about when and when not to use touch. In the next section, we will discuss four factors that can influence how touch will be interpreted by others.

Factors influencing touch

There are a number of factors that influence not only our comfort with
being touched but also our comfort in touching others. Factors such as our
gender, sociocultural background, the type of touch used, and the nature
of our relationship with the other person can all contribute to our comfort
with touching others or with their touching us.

Gender.   Gender is an important component of our receptivity to
touch. Some men, for example, are comfortable touching women but less
comfortable touching men. Some women, on the other hand, will feel at
ease and natural in touching women, but become uneasy or much less
spontaneous in touching men. In both of these situations, gender becomes
a crucial element in determining whether or not touch is used in the
relationship.

In health care settings, the gender of the patient and the gender of
the health professional can affect receptivity to touch. For example, female
nursing home residents in one study reported more discomfort than the
male nursing home residents to being touched by male nurses (DeWever,
1977). In a preoperative teaching situation, female patients reacted favorably to a touch intervention by a female nurse, while males reacted negatively to the intervention (Whitcher & Fisher, 1979). Although these studies
in no way indicate whether to touch women and not to touch men or vice
versa, they do suggest that the gender of the toucher and the person being
touched are important factors influencing not only receptivity to touch but
also the meaning given to it.

Sociocultural factors.   A second factor that influences our reaction to
touch is our sociocultural background. Some people are born into families
where there is a great deal of touching among family members. Other people have been raised in families where touch is more inhibited among fam-

ily members or limited to task situations. Our family environment and early experiences influence our preferences and comfort with touch as adults.

In addition to family environment, the cultural environment also influences a person's receptivity to touch. Some cultural groups have been referred to as "contact" cultures while others have been referred to as "noncontact" cultures, depending on how much touch they encourage among people (Knapp, 1978a). Montagu (1978) has suggested that there is a continuum of varying preferences for touch among different cultural groups. Montagu places upper-class Englishmen at one end of the continuum (preferring *less* touch) while placing people who speak Latin-derived languages at the opposite end of the continuum (preferring *more* touch). Montagu places Anglo-Saxon Americans between the English, on one side, and Scandanavians, who are in the middle of the continuum. Montagu is quick to note, however, that this continuum is not based on empirical research, but is rather only a way of looking at how culture influences our preference for touch. He believes that differences can be observed between cultures and that these differences influence individuals' comfort with touching and being touched by others. It is important to note, however, that individual differences still exist *within* each culture, even though similarities among people within the cultures have been identified. Taken together, our early family experiences and our sociocultural characteristics are both factors influencing our receptivity to touch.

Type and location.   Although a touch gesture seems relatively uncomplicated and straightforward, each gesture can be characterized by finer discriminations, such as the type of touch, the duration of the touch, and the location of the touch. These specific characteristics influence how a person interprets a particular gesture and whether or not the person will be comfortable with the touch.

The *different forms* of touch—a patting touch, a gripping touch, or a stroking touch—are often associated with different messages. The pat is usually perceived as a friendly or playful form of touch, whereas the stroke is considered a more loving and sexual form of touch (Nguyen, Heslin, & Nguyen, 1975). The *duration* of the touch, that is, whether the touch occurs for a brief or an extended period of time, can also be accompanied by various interpretations (Weiss, 1979). For example, if someone taps your knee briefly, you may interpret the gesture as playful; however, if the person rests a hand on your knee for an extended period of time, the touch may take on meanings of closeness or intimacy.

The *location*, or part of the body being touched, also influences receptivity to touch. Interestingly, researchers have noted that women are especially attuned to the location of touch, whereas men are more attuned to the type of touch that is used (Nguyen, Heslin, & Nguyen, 1975). In addition, while a person may be fairly comfortable with touch to one area of the body, a touch at a different location may produce anxiety or distress. Nursing home residents, for example, said they were most comfortable with a nurse's hand on their arms and least comfortable when a nurse put an arm around their shoulders (DeWever, 1977).

The type of touch can be distinguished not only by its form, duration, and location, but also by the *message* that is conveyed (Heslin & Alper, 1983). Heslin (1974) identified five types of messages that were transmitted through touch (see Table 4.2). The functional-professional type of touch is probably the most common type of touch used in health care, followed by either the friendship-warmth type of touch or the social-polite type of touch. The love-intimacy and the sexual arousal types of touch are probably the least *intentionally* used types of touch, although there are instances in which the touch used by a clinician to a patient or by a patient to a clinician has been interpreted in this manner.

Receptivity to touch depends on both the specific characteristics of the touch gesture (e.g., form, duration, location) as well as on the message conveyed by the particular type of touch. This is illustrated in the following anecdote told by a nurse who was hospitalized for infectious hepatitis. While she was in room isolation, a nurse's aide entered and offered to return later in the evening to give the nurse a back rub. The aide appeared later wearing a pair of rubber gloves to carry out the procedure. The nurse-patient said that although the massage was technically done well, it offered her little soothing comfort because the message she kept being reminded of as the aide's rubber gloves touched her skin was, "You are in-

---

TABLE 4.2   Messages Conveyed by Types of Touch

1. *Functional-professional.* This type of touch usually involves task completion such as touching a patient's arm to take a blood pressure or holding a patient's hand to assist him/her with ambulation. The professional using this type of touch sends the message, "I will assist you."

2. *Social-polite.*   This type of touch is exemplified by a handshake used to greet a new patient who has just been introduced to you. This type of touch characterizes a fairly superficial involvement between two people.

3. *Friendship-warmth.*   This type of touch conveys a liking for the other person. If a patient tells a social worker a humorous story and the social worker laughs and squeezes the patient's arm, the social worker is using a type of touch that conveys the message, "I like you."

4. *Love-intimacy.*   This type of touch signifies a close attachment between two people. It could be characterized by an enveloping hug between two people which transmits the message, "I care deeply for you."

5. *Sexual arousal.*   This form of touch conveys a physical attraction between two people and may be evident in a close physical embrace or a stroking touch. This type of touch sends the message, "I am very attracted to you."

Adapted from R. Heslin, "Steps Toward a Taxonomy of Touching." Paper presented to the Midwestern Psychological Association, Chicago, May 1974, p. 1.

fected and I am afraid of getting your germs." In other words the negative message conveyed by the gloves contradicted the positive intention of the touch.

Nature of the participants' relationship.   The last factor influencing receptivity to touch is the nature of the relationship between the participants. Touch is often a subtle factor that can be used to characterize the nature and boundaries of a relationship. For example, when a clinician touches a patient, it often signifies the helping nature of their relationship; and when a parent touches a child, it may signify the caretaking nature of their relationship. A teacher's touching a student may indicate the supportive nature of their relationship. Touch seems effective in each of these instances because the gesture falls within the guidelines perceived to be appropriate to the relationship. However, when the form of touch used is seen as incongruent with the nature of the relationship or if the norms of the relationship are violated, then discomfort can occur.

The following example illustrates the discomfort that occurs when a touch gesture seems to violate relationship norms.

> A young female nursing student was talking to a young male psychiatric patient who was diagnosed as having an acute schizophrenic reaction. A nursing instructor, who observed the interaction from a distance, noticed that the student touched the patient a couple of times during the interaction. This was not surprising since the student was a warm, caring person who frequently touched people when she conversed with them. However, later in the interaction when the young male patient touched the student's knee, the student appeared uncomfortable and terminated the interaction.
>
> Later the student approached the instructor for feedback on how to handle her uneasiness at her patient's touch and his apparent "attraction" to her. As they talked about this situation, the student said that she had touched the patient to convey emotional support, but that she thought that the patient's touch to her conveyed physical attraction.

This incident illustrates the interrelationship between type of touch, message conveyed, and nature of the relationship. The nursing student believed that she was using a functional-professional form of touch with the client which was compatible with her perception of the relationship. However, she perceived the patient's touch as associated with an intimate or sexual message that was not within the guidelines of the relationship. Although the gesture was the same, the message was interpreted differently according to who touched whom and the context of the relationship.

Touch can also signify lines of power and authority within a relationship. Henley (1973) observed that it is more common for the higher-status person in a relationship to touch a lower-status person, and for men to touch women. The following example may illustrate the relationship between touch and status.

> A young female staff nurse was carrying on a discussion with a middle-aged male hospital administrator about the value of nurses having advanced educational preparation. The administrator, who believed that advanced preparation was unnecessary and too costly, frequently touched the nurse during the discussion. He would touch the nurse's shoulder, make a point, and then withdraw his hand. In addition, he would often touch her shoulder to interrupt her when she made a point to counter his arguments. The conversation continued for some time and became quite heated.
>
> Later when retelling the story, the nurse said, "I felt as if he was treating me like a little girl—touching and interrupting me. When he started touching me less, he seemed to be hearing me out more as an equal." Then with a glint in her eye she said, "When he stopped touching me altogether, I knew that either I had won the argument, totally infuriated him, or changed how he perceived me and our relationship."

In this case, touch was seen as a way to define the power and authority within the relationship. The male administrator, who perceived himself as having more status and authority than the staff nurse, frequently touched the nurse and also used touch to control the flow of the interaction. He thought his position gave him the power to touch the nurse. The nurse, however, defined their relationship differently. She did not want to be touched and did not feel the administrator's position gave him the power to touch her. In effect, the nurse and administrator saw status—exhibited through touch—differently. Overall, receptivity to touch is influenced by many factors. We have identified gender, sociocultural background, type and location of touch, and the nature of the participants' relationship as factors influencing the degree of individuals' comfort and discomfort with touch.

Clinical considerations regarding touch

Unfortunately there is no precise formula for determining when to touch or not to touch patients, and there is no universally accepted meaning that can be given to a single touch. Interpretation and receptivity to touch will depend on many factors.

Although some uncertainty surrounds our understanding of when touch will be most effective with clients, the following statements are general guidelines that can be used to increase the likelihood that touch will be perceived positively in therapeutic relationships.

Use a form of touch that is appropriate to the particular situation.   There are many forms of touch that can be used in a variety of ways. Using a touch gesture that seems compatible with the context will most likely have positive outcomes. For example, a person who has just been told distressing information (e.g., that a son has been injured in automobile accident) may respond positively to the clinician who places his or her hand on the distressed person's arm. On the other hand, this touch may not be well received by a young male patient who is venting anger about having diabetes. The angry patient needs to vent his feelings in this situation. Letting him get the anger out is better than consoling gestures.

Do not use a touch gesture that imposes more intimacy on a patient than he or she desires.   To some people certain gestures may imply a level of intimacy or a degree of closeness. When the gesture suggests a degree of closeness that is not equally shared or implicitly agreed upon by both parties, discomfort may result (Fisher, Rytting, & Heslin, 1976). For example, a suspicious patient who has difficulty forming close personal relationships may be uncomfortable with some forms of touch and the intimacy that the gesture implies. However, when touch is used between a nurse and a geriatric resident who have an established relationship, the touch may be well received because it is in keeping with the nature of their relationship and the level of intimacy that they both desire.

Observe the recipient's response to the touch.   Touch will be most effective when the toucher assesses the impact of the touch on the other person. Assessment is especially important when touch is used in initial meetings with patients and the clinician has no prior knowledge of how the person will respond. Moy (1981) identified behaviors such as the person's pulling away, appearing frightened, or displaying tense facial muscles or other anxious body gestures as negative responses to touch. On the other hand, if the person appears to relax or to seem more comfortable after a touch gesture, then it is likely that the touch is being received positively.

If misinterpretation is likely, supplement the touch gesture with verbal communication.   Sometimes a touch by itself is enough to convey the intended message from one person to another. In other situations, due to the wide range of individual interpretations that can be given to touch, the message may be more clearly understood when words are used along with touch.

In summary, touch is an effective mode of human communication. However, too often touch is used in relationships without attention being paid to what the touch conveys. Health professionals need to be aware of potential negative responses to touch, of situations in which the meaning of touch can be misunderstood, and of situations in which the message conveyed by a type of touch is not compatible with the nature of the relationship. In health care situations in which both the clinician and the client are comfortable with touch, and the use of touch is assessed for its therapeutic effects, touch can be a very valuable means of communication.

Environmental and Physical Factors

Nonverbal communication also includes environmental factors that impact on interpersonal relationships. Environment includes such things as lighting, noise, color, room temperature, furniture arrangement, and building structure. These factors also influence the types of messages that we send to others and the degree of comfort or discomfort that we experience in personal interactions.

Perception of the environment

Each of us can probably recall walking into a person's house or apartment and noticing the warmth that seemed to exude from the setting. Perhaps the type of furniture, the plants, or the newspapers strewn around the room contributed to the impression of warmth. On the other hand, we can recall settings that seemed uninviting, cold or unlived-in, depending on the contents, color, and atmosphere of the various rooms. We also make immediate judgments about hotel rooms, classrooms, hospital rooms, and clinic rooms. Knapp (1978b) has identified six dimensions that people use to assess the environment: formality, warmth, privacy, constraint, distance, and familiarity. While Knapp does not attempt to apply these dimensions to health care settings, these characteristics are useful in describing health care settings as well.[2]

Formality.   According to Knapp, people react to their surroundings based on how formal or informal the setting appears. A large bank in a downtown area, for example, would be placed on the formal end of a continuum, while a small credit union in the suburbs might be placed on the informal end. To some people, large health care institutions in university settings seem more formal, while smaller satellite clinics in rural settings seem informal. In the same way, a meeting in a hospital administrator's office may be perceived as more formal than a meeting in the hospital coffee shop. Knapp notes that the more formal the setting, the more likely that communication will be more superficial, "less relaxed, more hesitant, and generally more difficult" (1978b, p. 73).

Warmth.   Environments can also be perceived in terms of their warmth or coolness. The color of the room and the texture of the upholstery contribute to these perceptions. In health care settings, stark white

[2]The following section is adapted with permission from M. L. Knapp, *Social Intercourse: From Greeting to Goodbye.* Boston: Allyn and Bacon, Inc., 1978.

examination rooms and bright fluorescent lights give an impression of coldness. Knapp believes that psychologically warm environments "encourage us to linger, to feel relaxed, and to feel comfortable" (1978a, p. 88).

Privacy. Partitioned or enclosed environments, where interactions cannot be easily overheard by others, are associated with privacy. In health care settings, six-bed wards offer little personal privacy whereas single-bed rooms do. Curtains pulled around patients' beds offer visual privacy but the next door patient can hear everything. Situations that provide more privacy probably foster more personal communication (Knapp, 1978b).

Constraint. The freedom to enter and leave an environment influences our perceptions of constraint. A locked ward on a psychiatric unit evokes higher feelings of constraint than an unlocked ward. A patient who can move freely about his or her room would probably perceive the environment as less constricting than the patient who is anchored to a bed because of monitors and equipment. Constraint is an important element in patients' perceptions of their environment. Patients in one study ranked being, "tied to the bed with tubes" as the most stressful factor in their intensive care unit environment (Ballard, 1981). Knapp suggests that in environments where physical and psychological constraint is perceived as high, people will be slower to share and to initiate personal disclosures (1978b, p. 75).

Distance. Environmental distance can involve physical distance as well as psychological distance. Hospital rooms at the end of a long hallway may seem both physically and psychologically distant from other patient rooms and the nursing station. Before the recent efforts to sensitize health care personnel to the needs of patients facing death, dying patients were often placed at the end of hallways where they had little attention or communication from others.

Familiarity. A visit from a clinician in the home would be perceived as a familiar environment by patients and family members, while visiting a clinician in a psychiatric setting would be regarded as an unfamiliar environment—especially for patients and family members who have never been in a psychiatric setting. Cautious and hesitant behaviors often occur in new or unfamiliar settings (Knapp, 1978b, p. 74).

Although these six dimensions represent only some of many possible dimensions, they offer a way to look at environments and see how they effect our communication with others. While Knapp (1978a) notes that many of these dimensions overlap and interrelate with one another, in general, more personal communication is often associated with "informal, unconstrained, private, familiar, close and warm environments" (p. 89). Future research is needed to determine more specifically how environmental perceptions affect communication.

Hospital and clinic staff in some specialized areas have worked toward developing comfortable and relaxing environments for patients. In pediatric settings, for example, there have been successful attempts to create an atmosphere of familiarity and warmth; bleak walls have been covered with brightly colored murals of children's favorite cartoon figures, and staff members have replaced sterile white uniforms with more casual and colorful shirts and smocks. The nursing station in one pediatric setting was constructed with lower walls so that small children or children in wheelchairs could talk more easily with staff members (Johnson, 1979). In addition, the nursing station was renamed the "communication station" to eliminate boundaries created by the name "nursing" station.

Family birthing centers are now being constructed in some hospitals, with comfortable furniture, lighting, and homelike atmospheres, as an alternative to the formal and impersonal labor and delivery areas. In oncology clinics, comfortable recliner chairs are replacing desklike chairs and hospital beds as a way of fostering a warmer and more casual environment for receiving chemotherapy. In each of these settings health professionals are demonstrating an awareness of the environment's impact on patient care and interpersonal relationships.

Sound

The clatter of trolleys, the beep of monitors, the click of respiratory equipment, and the rattle of dietary carts all contribute to the sounds of health care facilities. To health care personnel accustomed to this environment, these sounds often go unnoticed. But these sounds often cause patients and family members distress, and they can interfere with rest and recovery (Ogilvie, 1980).

Not all sounds are distressing. Music, for example, has been used in dentists' offices and waiting rooms to relax people and to distract them from potentially stressful events. In intensive care settings, the steady beeps of a cardiac monitor may be reassuring to both the patient and the staff members who are concerned about the patient's status. Sound, in and of itself, is not detrimental to health environments; however, the type and the intensity of sound can have negative effects.

Several research studies have focused on the possible negative effects of sound in health care. Minckley (1968), for example, studied the relationship between noise and the amount of discomfort experienced by patients in a recovery room. She found more pain medication was given to patients during times in which noise levels were very high in the recovery room than during periods of low noise levels. Minckley points out that noise acts as another irritant to the person who is already in pain. Ogilvie (1980), who studied noise levels in a ward in a British hospital, found noise levels during the night shift to be as high as the noise in a person's living room during the day. Similarly, Woods and Falk (1974) studied various types of noise in acute care units and recovery rooms. They reported that the level of noise at times approached the level "in a noisy office or when playing a radio at full volume" and was often at levels that could interfere with patients' rest and sleep (p. 149).

Table 4.3 shows the noise levels generated by various mechanical devices in the acute care unit. For comparative purposes, Table 4.4 shows noise levels of common everyday activities. As shown in the figures, many of the activities on the acute care unit were equal to, or above, the sound levels produced by common "out of the hospital" sources. In addition, Woods and Falk note that medical and nursing personnel in this study often produced noise levels that were greater than those produced by me-

TABLE 4.3   Noise Generated by Mechanical Equipment in the Acute Care Unit and Recovery Room Classified by Source and Noise Level

| | NOISE LEVEL | |
SOURCE OF NOISE	dB(A)	dB LINEAR
Acute Care Unit		
Cardiac monitor (Heartscope HS103)	60–61	82–83
Corbin Farnsworth Scopette	56–58	82–84
2 cardiac monitors, simultaneously	68–70	—'
Bennett respirator MA-1	61–52	81–82
Bennett respirator alarm	66	—
Oxygen outlet	48–50	—
Bedscale operation	66–72	84–85
Computer terminal (4 feet from patient)	58–60	80–82
Recovery Room		
Suction machine, wall outlet		
Not in use, but on	66–68	75–76
In use	68	75
IPPB machine		
At outflow valve	68–70	—
At opposite side	58–60	75–80
Sealy chest suction (water sealed)	56	78
Bedpan washer	69–80	84
Ice machine, dispensing ice	52–64	82
Toilet flushing	74	88
Water running in hopper	74	80
Closing door to operating room corridor (mechanically)	70	76
Telephone	58–60	—

Reprinted from N. F. Woods and S. A. Falk, "Noise Stimuli in the Acute Care Area." Copyright © 1974, American Journal of Nursing Company. Reproduced with permission from *Nursing Research*, March/April, vol. 23, no. 2, p. 147.

TABLE 4.4   Sound Levels in Decibels
            Produced by Common
            Sources

SOURCE	dB(A)
Subway	100
Rush-hour traffic	90
Noisy factory	80
Noisy office	70
Radio at full volume	60
Normal conversation	50
Typical household noise	40
Whisper	30

Reprinted from N. F. Woods and S. A. Falk, "Noise Stimuli in the Acute Care Area." Copyright © 1974, American Journal of Nursing Company. Reproduced with permission from *Nursing Reasearch*, March/April, vol. 23, no. 2, p. 144.

chanical devices. Furthermore, they found that auxiliary personnel produced noise levels at and above the 70 dB level (70 dB is capable of awakening patients from sleep or inducing sensory distortion) while carrying out activities such as emptying the garbage and delivering supplies. Noble (1979) also studied noise levels in the acute care setting. Her findings indicated that noise generated by hospital personnel was greater than the noise generated by machines and equipment.

Noise is an environmental factor that can cause sensory overload and can interfere with effective professional-professional communication as well as with professional-patient interactions. Many suggestions have been made on how to reduce noise in health care environments including encouraging staff to use normal voice tones when conversing, limiting unnecessary interactions during night hours or at times when patients are sleeping, involving health professionals in designing better noise-limiting structures, providing staff with conference areas, and placing equipment (when possible) away from patients' bedsides (Gowan, 1979; Noble, 1979; Woods & Falk, 1974).

Furniture arrangement and structural design

A vivid image comes to mind when considering the importance of furniture arrangement and human communication. If you had visited a large, old psychiatric hospital 20 years or more ago, the most noticeable feature would not have been the high-gloss waxed floors or the cagelike screened porches or the long corridors stretching from one side of the building to the other—but the long rows of rocking chairs placed one behind the other outside the patients' rooms so that a patient sitting in one chair looked at the back of the head of another patient, who looked at the back of someone else, and so on. With this arrangement of chairs, it was not difficult to understand why so little social interaction took place on these wards.

The importance of arranging furniture and designing structures to encourage interaction has received some attention by health professionals. Sommer and Ross (1958) studied the effect of room arrangement on a group of geriatric residents. The researchers found that staff members were reluctant to alter previously established seating patterns because of potential housekeeping problems and because they did not believe it would change ward communication. Patients were also reluctant to have their environment changed and at times would return moved furniture to previous arrangements. In spite of initial resistance, Sommer and Ross found that interactions nearly doubled among the residents when furniture was rearranged to facilitate communication. The authors suggest that staff members who do not arrange furniture to encourage interaction are, in effect, allowing *furniture* to arrange the *patients* and possibly to discourage interactions (p. 133).

Seating arrangements have also been analyzed in other settings. In some types of family therapy settings, family therapists often alter who sits next to whom during a session (Minuchin, 1974). For example, two parents with poor communication are often directed to move their chairs closer to one another so that they can converse more directly. The assumption is that altering seating arrangements will also change interaction patterns in a positive way (Minuchin, 1974). In other settings, such as treatment planning sessions, circular arrangements of chairs are used to facilitate the team members' ability to observe and to interact with one another. Using long tables in these settings has sometimes limited the dialogue among members at different ends of the table and prevented them from reading one another's nonverbal expressions.

The structural design of health care settings also influences communication patterns. In some of the newer hospitals, nursing stations with rooms forming a circle around them have replaced older designs in which the nursing station was the midpoint between two long wings. Other structural changes have included more lounge areas for patients and family members, and various kinds of open and closed areas in the units in which staff can interact with patients as well as other staff members.

Environmental factors do have an impact on our communication with others. The preceding discussion briefly touches on some factors— environmental perception, sound, furniture arrangement, and structural design—that affect human relations and communication in health care settings. Environment does not have a neutral role in health communication. It can facilitate or inhibit communication within a particular setting, and environmental components require close attention by health professionals.

SUMMARY

This chapter has focused on the role of nonverbal communication in the total health communication process. Nonverbal communication is communication without words, a process that can be vocal or nonvocal as well as intentional or unintentional. Nonverbal communication fulfills several purposes in the communication process: to express feelings, to regulate interactions, to validate verbal messages, to maintain self-image, and to maintain relationships. Despite certain myths that frequently surround people's perceptions of nonverbal behavior, nonverbal communication is closely bound to verbal communication; it is one of a multitude of elements comprising the human communication process; it does not make individuals transparent; and nonverbal behavior has multiple rather than single meanings.

Five major dimensions of nonverbal communication are kinesics, proxemics, paralinguistics, touch, and environmental and physical factors. Kinesics is the study of body motion and includes subcategories such as emblems, illustrators, affect displays, regulators, and adaptors. In addition, facial expression and gaze are two other nonverbal areas often considered to be part of kinesics.

The second major dimension of nonverbal communication is proxemics, the study of how people use and interpret space in their interactions. Proxemics focuses on how people deal with territorial issues and invasions of personal space, and how various types of distance (e.g., intimate, personal, social, and public) affect communication.

Vocal sounds and cues that accompany spoken verbal communication are part of paralinguistics, the third dimension of nonverbal communication. Paralinguistics assists individuals in understanding and interpreting messages. This dimension includes elements such as voice qualities, vocal characteristics, vocal qualifiers, and vocal segregates. Vocal sounds are used by individuals to supplement the words and gestures that are used in health interactions.

The fourth dimension, touch, plays a special role in human growth and development, in the development of interpersonal relationships, and in healing. Among the factors that can influence the meaning of touch and a person's receptivity to touch are gender, sociocultural characteristics, type and location of touch, and the nature of the participants' relationships.

The fifth dimension of nonverbal communication, environmental and physical factors, can be analyzed according to the types of perceptions that people form about their environment (e.g., formal or private) and how these perceptions affect interaction in those settings. The effects of sound, object arrangement, and structural design are important factors in creating or detracting from an environment for effective health communication.

REFERENCES

Aguilera, D. Relationship between physical contact and verbal interaction between nurses and patients. *Journal of Psychiatric Nursing*, 1967, *5*(1), 5–21.

Alagna, F., Whitcher, S., Fisher, J., & Wicas, E. Evaluative reaction to interpersonal touch in a counseling interview. *Journal of Counseling Psychology*, 1979, *26*(6), 465–472.

Allekian, C. I. Intrusions of territory and personal space: An anxiety-inducing factor for hospitalized patients—An exploratory study. *Nursing Research*, 1973, *22*(3), 236–241.

Ardrey, R. *The territorial imperative*. New York: Atheneum Publishers, 1966.

Argyle, M., & Cook, M. *Gaze and mutual gaze*. Cambridge: Cambridge University Press, 1976.

Argyle, M., & Ingham, R. Gaze, mutual gaze, and proximity. *Semiotica*, 1972, *6*, 32–49.

Asch, S. Forming impressions of personality. *Journal of Abnormal and Social Psychology*, 1946, *41*, 258–290.

Ballard, K. Identification of environmental stressors for patients in a surgical intensive care unit. *Issues in Mental Health Nursing*, 1981, *3*(1–2), 89–108.

Barnett, K. A theoretical construct of the concepts of touch as they relate to nursing. *Nursing Research*, 1972, *21*(2), 102–110.

Birdwhistell, R. L. *Kinesics and context*. Philadelphia: University of Pennsylvania Press, 1970.

Blondis, M. N., & Jackson, B. E. *Nonverbal communication with patients: Back to human touch*, 2nd ed. New York: John Wiley & Sons, Inc., 1982.

Burgoon, J. K., & Jones, S. B. Toward a theory of personal space expectations and their violations. *Human Communication Research*, 1976, *2*, 131–146.

Burnside, I. Touching is talking. *American Journal of Nursing*, 1973, *73*(12), 2060–2063.

Cook, M. Gaze and mutual gaze in social encounters. *American Scientist*, 1977, *65*, 328–333.

Darwin, C. *The expression of the emotions in men and animals*. London: John Murray, 1872 (Reprinted 1965, University of Chicago Press).

Davitz, J. R. *The communication of emotional meaning*. New York: McGraw-Hill Book Company., 1964.

Davitz, J. R., & Davitz, L. The communication of feelings by content-free speech. *Journal of Communication*, 1959, *9*, 6–13.

DeThomas, M. T. Touch power and the screen of loneliness. *Perspectives of Psychiatric Care*, 1971, *9*(3), 112–118.

DeWever, M. Nursing home patients' perception of nurses' affective touching. *The Journal of Psychology*, 1977, *96*, 163–171.

Eisenberg, A. M., & Smith, Jr., R. R. *Nonverbal communication*. Indianapolis: Bobbs-Merrill Co., Inc., 1971.

Ekman, P., & Friesen, W. V. The repertoire of nonverbal behavior: Categories, origins, usage, and coding. *Semiotica*, 1969, *1*, 49–98.

Ekman, P., & Friesen, W. V. *Unmasking the face: A guide to recognizing emotions from facial clues*. Englewood Cliffs, N.J.: Prentice-Hall, Inc., 1975.

Ekman, P., Friesen, W. V., & Ellsworth, P. *Emotion in the human face: Guidelines for research and an integration of findings*. New York: Pergamon Press, Inc., 1972.

Fast, J. *Body Language*. New York: Murray Evans, 1970.

Fisher, J., Rytting, M., & Heslin, R. Hands touching hands: Affective and evaluative effects of an interpersonal touch. *Sociometry*, 1976, *39*(4), 416–421.

Friedman, H. S. Nonverbal communication between patients and medical practitioners. *Journal of Social Issues*, 1979, *35*(1), 82–100.

Goffman, E. *The presentation of self in everyday life*. Garden City, N.Y.: Doubleday & Co., Inc., 1959.

Goffman, E. *Behavior in public places*. New York: The Free Press, 1963.

Goffman, E. *Interaction ritual: Essays on face-to-face behavior*. New York: Anchor Books, 1967.

Gowan, N. The perceptual world of the intensive care unit: An overview of some environmental considerations in the helping relationship. *Heart and Lung*, 1979, *8*(2), 340–344.

Hall, E. T. *The silent language*. Garden City, N.Y.: Doubleday & Co., Inc., 1959.

Hall, E. T. *The hidden dimension*. Garden City, N.Y.: Doubleday & Co., Inc., 1966.

Hardin, S., & Halaris, A. Nonverbal communication of patients and high and low empathy nurses. *Journal of Psychosocial Nursing and Mental Health Services*, 1983, *21*(1), 14–19.

Harlow, H., & Zimmermann, R. Affectional responses in the infant monkey. *Science*, 1959, *130*, 421–432.

Harrison, R. P. *Beyond words: An introduction to nonverbal communication*. Englewood Cliffs, N.J.: Prentice-Hall, Inc., 1974.

Heidt, P. Effect of therapeutic touch on anxiety level of hospitalized patients. *Nursing Research*, 1981, *30*(1), 32–37.

Henley, N. The politics of touch. In P. Brown (Ed), *Radical psychology*. New York: Harper & Row, Publishers, Inc., 1973.

Heslin, R. Steps toward a taxonomy of touching. Paper presented to the Midwestern Psychological Association, Chicago, May 1974.

Heslin, R., & Alper, T. Touch: A bonding gesture. In J. M. Wiemann & R. P. Harrison (Eds.), *Nonverbal communication*. Beverly Hills, Calif.: Sage Publications, Inc., 1983.

Johnson, M. Toward a culture of caring: Children, their environment, and change. *Maternal Child Nursing*, 1979, *4*(4), 210–214.

Kendon, A. Some functions of gaze-direction in social interaction. *Acta Psychologica*, 1967, *26*, 22–63.

King, I. M. *A theory for nursing: Systems, concepts, process*. New York: John Wiley & Sons, Inc., 1981.

Knapp, M. L. *Nonverbal communication in human interaction*, 2nd ed. New York: Holt, Rinehart & Winston, 1978(a).

Knapp, M. L. *Social intercourse: From greeting to goodbye*. Boston: Allyn & Bacon, Inc., 1978(b).

Knapp, M. L. *Essentials of nonverbal communication*. New York: Holt, Rinehart & Winston, 1980.

Krieger, D. Therapeutic touch: The imprimatur of nursing. *American Journal of Nursing*, 1975, *75*(5), 784–787.

Krieger, D., Peper, E., & Ancoli, S. Therapeutic touch: Searching for evidence of physiological change. *American Journal of Nursing*, 1979, *79*(4), 660–662.

McCorkle, R. Effects of touch on seriously ill patients. *Nursing Research*, 1974, *23*(2), 125–132.

Mehrabian, A. *Silent messages*. Belmont, Calif.: Wadsworth Publishing Co., Inc., 1971.

Mehrabian, A. *Nonverbal communication*. Chicago: Aldine-Atherton, Inc., 1972.

Minckley, B. Study of noise and its relationship to patient discomfort in the recovery room. *Nursing Research*, 1968, *17*(3), 247–250.

Minuchin, S. *Families and family therapy*. Cambridge, Mass.: Harvard University Press, 1974.

Molloy, J. *Dress for success*. New York: P. H. Wyden, 1975.

Montagu, A. *Touching*. New York: Harper & Row, Publishers, Inc., 1978.

Mortensen, C. D. *Communication: The study of human interaction*. New York: McGraw-Hill Book Company, 1972.

Moy, C. Touch in the counseling relationship: An exploratory study. *Patient Counselling and Health Education*, 1981, *3*(3), 89–94.

Nguyen, T., Heslin, R., & Nguyen, M. The meanings of touch: Sex differences. *Journal of Communication*, 1975, *25*(3), 92–102.

Noble, M. S. Communication in the ICU: Therapeutic or disturbing? *Nursing Outlook*, 1979, *27*(3), 195–198.

Ogilvie, A. Sources and levels of noise on the ward at night. *Nursing Times*, 1980, *76*(31), 1363–1366.

Pattison, J. Effects of touch on self-exploration and the therapeutic relationship. *Journal of Consulting and Clinical Psychology*, 1973, *40*(2), 170–175.

Penny, K. Postpartum perceptions of touch received during labor. *Research in Nursing and Health*, 1979, *2*(1), 9–16.

Pluckhan, M. L. *Human communication: The matrix of nursing*. New York: McGraw-Hill Book Company, 1978.

Rosenthal, R., Hall, J. A., DiMatteo, M. R., Rogers, P. L., & Archer, D. *Sensitivity to nonverbal communication: The PONS test*. Baltimore: The Johns Hopkins University Press, 1979.

Sommer, R., & Ross, H. Social interaction on a geriatrics ward. *International Journal of Social Psychiatry*, 1958, *4*(2), 128–133.

Spitz, R. Hospitalism. In A. Freud (Ed.). *The psychoanalytic study of the child* (Vol. 2). New York: International University Press, 1946.

Stillman, J. J. Territoriality and personal space. *American Journal of Nursing*, 1978, *78*(10), 1670–1672.

Tate, J. W. The need for personal space in institutions for the elderly. *Journal of Gerontology Nursing*, 1980, *6*(8), 439–449.

Trager, G. L. Paralanguage: A first approximation. *Studies in Linguistics*, 1958, *13*, 1–12.

Triplett, J., & Arneson, S. The use of verbal and tactile comfort to alleviate distress in young hospitalized children. *Research in Nursing and Health*, 1979, *2*(1), 17–23.

Weiss, S. The language of touch. *Nursing Research*, 1979, *28*(2), 76–79.

Whitcher, S. J., & Fisher, J. D. Multidimensional reaction to therapeutic touch. *Journal of Personality and Social Psychology*, 1979, *37*, 87–96.

Woods, N., & Falk, S. Noise stimuli in the acute care area. *Nursing Research*, 1974, *23*(2), 144–150.

5 Interviewing in the Health Care Context

Interviewing is the key to successful clinician-patient relationships. Skillful interviewing makes possible the communication between patient and clinician that fosters a mutually satisfying relationship and leads to the best possible outcome. . . . It is a skill that should be mastered by all health professionals. —Enelow and Swisher, 1979

Nearly every health professional, at one time or another, has conducted an interview either with a client or with another health professional. For some professionals, interviewing clients is an activity that consumes the majority of their time on any given working day. Acquiring information, discussing results with patients, and monitoring treatment all depend on interviewing (Enelow & Swisher, 1979, p. 4). From intake interviews and initial nursing assessments to discharge planning interviews and home visits, much of the interpersonal communication that takes place in health care settings is carried out through the interview process. In general, interviews play a primary role in the communication of health professionals in all contexts.

Given the prevalence of interviewing in health care, the question this chapter will address is, What is the nature of interviewing and how can it be used most effectively by professionals in health care settings? In essence, we will take the position that interviewing is simply a special type of interpersonal communication. Concepts and theories that apply to interpersonal communication can also be applied to explanations of interviewing. The thrust of our discussion in this chapter will focus on the communication dynamics of the interview process.

Based on the communication assumptions, models, and variables discussed in Chapters 1 and 2, this chapter focuses on the communication dimensions of interviews as they occur in health care relationships. At the outset of the chapter we define interviewing and we describe several common types of interviews that occur in health care settings. Next we discuss what actually goes on during the preparation, initiation, exploration, and termination phases of an interview. In the final section of the chapter we discuss a series of communication techniques that can be used by professionals to make health care interviews more effective.

INTERVIEWING DEFINED

Interviewing is a process that has the same transactional and multidimensional characteristics we discussed earlier in regard to interpersonal communication (see Fig. 5.1). An interview usually takes place between two people in face-to-face interaction and as a rule it involves both verbal and nonverbal messages. Like the communication process, the interview process involves sharing information through a common set of rules. Although all interviews involve interpersonal communication, not all interpersonal communication in health care involves interviewing.

How does an interview differ from other forms of interpersonal communication? What are the specific characteristics of an interview? Interviewing has been defined by Benjamin (1981) as "a conversation between two people, a conversation that is serious and purposeful" (p. xxii). As this definition suggests, one major characteristic of interviewing that differentiates it from other types of interpersonal communication is that it has a specific purpose. Because interviews are intentional, they usually require the participants to keep their conversation focused on particular topics. Figure 5.2 illustrates that the number of different topics brought up for discussion in a general conversation is far greater than the number of topics that are typically discussed in a health interview. In a health interview, the range of topics is restricted primarily to health-related issues. The intentionality or purposefulness that characterizes an interview is summed up in the following statement: "A conversation can go anywhere; an interview, however, must be focused on content that is relevant to your purpose" (Downs, Smeyak, & Martin, 1980, p. 6).

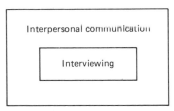

Interpersonal communication

Interviewing

FIGURE 5.1   Interviewing as a subset of interpersonal communication.

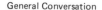

General Conversation

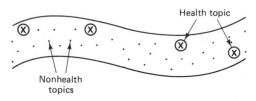

Health Interview

Time ————————➤

FIGURE 5.2 Difference between general conversation and health interviews in regard to the focus of interaction. (Adapted from R. L. Kahn and C. F. Cannell, *The Dynamics of Interviewing: Theory, Technique, and Cases.* New York: John Wiley & Sons, Inc., 1957, p. 15.)

A second distinguishing characteristic of interviews is that they usually involve the use of questions and answers (Stewart & Cash, 1978). Asking and answering questions play a pivotal role in the interview process. Most of the information written about interviewing centers on how to use communication techniques to ask appropriate questions. Later in the chapter we will discuss how different kinds of questions result in different kinds of answers and how questions, if used properly, can make interviews more effective.

Based on the preceding discussion, we will approach interviewing in this chapter using the following definition: Interviewing is a special type of interpersonal communication, usually involving questions and answers, with the purpose of sharing information or facilitating therapeutic outcomes.

TYPES OF INTERVIEWS IN HEALTH CARE SETTINGS

Traditionally, interviews have been divided into *information-sharing interviews* and *therapeutic interviews*. In health care organizations there is an overlap between these two major types of interviews because one of the overriding goals of communication in health care *is* to be therapeutic. Because of this, it is difficult to say that one type of interview is therapeutic and one type is not. For example, a "good" admissions interview focuses on information sharing, but it can also have therapeutic benefits for the client. Although there is some overlap between the major types of interviews, the two categories—information sharing and therapeutic—are used in this chapter to distinguish between interviews that are content focused and of brief duration (information sharing) and interviews that are relationship focused and of longer duration (therapeutic). We now turn to a closer examination of the specific characteristics and dynamics that are distinctive to each type of interview.

Information-Sharing Interviews

Much of what health professionals do involves sharing information through interviews. Information-sharing interviews are designed for the purpose of requesting and providing information, and they emphasize the content rather than the relationship (feeling) dimensions in an interaction. Establishing a good relationship is important in this type of an interview, but it is not the distinguishing characteristic. In health care settings, some of the many examples of this type of interview include admission interviews, history-taking interviews, selection interviews, performance appraisals, journalistic interviews, and research interviews.

Admissions interviews or intake interviews are used in health care agencies to acquire general demographic, biographical, and financial information about the client who has just entered the health care system. In some agencies this information will be collected by clerical staff in an admissions office, while in other agencies this information may be gathered by the health professional. This type of interview is often used to obtain information (e.g., age, address, insurance) about a client.

History-taking interviews are used by some health professionals to gather information about the client's health history. They include obtaining information about the client's hereditary and family background (e.g., allergies, cancer, heart disease, epilepsy), past health problems (e.g., operations, trauma, psychological disorders), and present health status (e.g., respiratory system, neuromuscular system, medications). This information provides the basis upon which subsequent diagnoses and treatment plans are formulated.

Selection interviews are used in a health care organization to obtain information about individuals who are applying for a job, for a transfer, or for a promotion within the organization. In this type of interview, information about the individual is used to determine whether he or she is "the right person" for a new position. Information that is shared in this type of interview usually benefits both the interviewer and the interviewee.

Performance appraisals are interviews used by supervisory staff to provide a formal review and evaluation of an employee's past contributions to an organization and to provide a description of the expectations regarding the employee's future job performance. Information shared in this type of interview is usually evaluative in nature, and often serves as a basis for salary increases, promotions, and planning for the employee's future development (Stano & Reinsch, 1982).

Journalistic interviews are used to gather facts, ideas, and stories to present to others. An example of a journalistic interview in health care would be an interview between a newspaper reporter and a health care administrator about an innovative preventive health program. Another example would be an interview within an organization for an in-house publication between a reporter and a retiring employee about the employee's 45 years of service to the organization. In general, journalistic interviews are relatively rare in health care settings.

Survey interviews are used by researchers to gather information systematically from a group (or sample) of individuals. Survey interviews are usually designed so that data, such as the beliefs, attitudes, or values of a group of people, can be analyzed using standard statistical procedures. The results of survey interviews in health care settings are often used to (1) assess a community's awareness of services offered by a health care organization, (2) evaluate the effectiveness of a recently created health care program, (3) assess the communication climate within an organization, or (4) determine areas of need for new health care services.

These are only a few of many types of information-sharing interviews used in health care. The common goal of each type of interview is to obtain information or share content within a specific area.

Therapeutic Interviews

Whereas the primary emphasis in information-sharing interviews is placed on the acquisition of facts, ideas, and content, the primary emphasis in therapeutic interviews is placed on the development of a supportive relationship—the process dimension (see Fig. 5.3). Therapeutic interviews are designed specifically to help clients identify and work through personal issues, concerns, and problems. Within the context of a therapeutic rela-

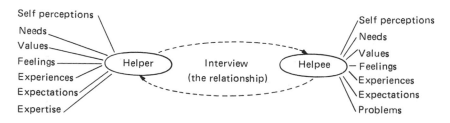

FIGURE 5.3   The helping relationship in the interview. (Reprinted from L. M. Brammer, *The Helping Relationship: Process and Skill,* 2nd ed. Englewood Cliffs, N.J.: Prentice-Hall, Inc., 1979, p. 45.)

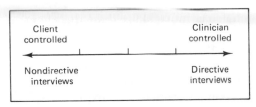

FIGURE 5.4 Continuum of approaches to therapeutic interviews. (From Lewis E. Patterson and Sheldon Eisenberg, *The Counseling Process*, 3rd ed. Boston: Houghton Mifflin Company, 1983, p. 192. Adapted by permission.)

tionship clients can feel free to express their personal thoughts and feelings; they gain new insights about past experiences, develop new problem-solving strategies, and find improved ways of coping with experiences.

Therapeutic interviews are conducted by health professionals in many different types of health care contexts. Social workers, nurses, doctors, chaplains, psychologists, and many others are required to do therapeutic interviews. The therapeutic interviews that we are referring to in this section are most commonly used by health professionals (e.g., clinical psychologists, social workers, or mental health nurse specialists) in settings where patients have personal problems that are primarily emotional or psychological.

There are two basic approaches to conducting therapeutic interviews: *directive* and *nondirective*. In the directive interview, the interviewer (therapist) guides, leads or prescribes solutions for the interviewee (client). In the nondirective approach, the interviewer allows the interviewee to have control and to choose directions in solving his or her own problems. Both approaches can be placed on a single continuum (shown in Fig. 5.4) varying in degree of directiveness or nondirectiveness. Few therapeutic interviews fall at the extreme ends of the continuum because interviews are seldom entirely directive or entirely nondirective (Downs, Smeyak, and Martin, 1980, p. 193).

Directive interviewing

In the directive approach, the health professional often defines the nature of the client's problem and prescribes appropriate solutions for the problem. In this type of interview, the client looks to the professional for direction and guidance because the client perceives the professional as having special knowledge, experience, and expertise that can help the client cope with her or his circumstances. For example, in a directive interview with an overweight client seeking help with weight control, the nutrition specialist would determine what type of a diet plan the client needs to obtain a desired weight. The nutritionist would then provide the client with specific details about the diet. The directive approach is based on the assumption that the professional has more skills than the client in assessing health problems and choosing strategies to work through these problems (Downs, Smeyak, and Martin, 1980, p. 194).

The directive approach has several advantages. First, this approach makes full use of the health professional's expertise. Clients receive help based on the professional's training and experience. Second, the directive approach provides the client with specific, concrete information about the nature of a problem and possible solutions; this can give the client a clear perspective and a sense of direction. Third, the directive approach is much more efficient than the nondirective approach. Directive therapeutic interviews usually focus on the problem, and less time is spent exploring general areas of the client's concerns. In addition, the professional is given the responsibility to assess problems and prescribe solutions; thus the interview seems to proceed more quickly because less negotiation and collaboration occur between client and professional.

Although there are advantages to the directive approach, there are also several disadvantages. First, the directive approach does not fully recognize the ability of the client to provide some useful assessment of his or her problem(s). This assumption that the professional is more competent than the client can belittle or downplay the importance of client observations and experiences. Second, the directive approach can be counterproductive to a client's well being if the recommended advice from the health professional is the "wrong" advice or if it is not compatible with the way the client views the situation. In addition, a directive approach that moves too quickly to formulate solutions without fully exploring the client's situation may lead to ineffective or misdirected solutions. Third, the directive approach has the tendency to force the client into a submissive role while the professional plays the dominant role. When clients do not feel fully involved on an equal basis in an interview, they may not follow through on the solutions suggested.

Nondirective interviewing

In the nondirective approach to therapeutic interviews the client guides the interaction. The nondirective approach originated in Roger's (1951, 1959) client-centered approach to psychotherapy. The health professional, in this type of interview, serves as a facilitator who reacts supportively to the client's own explorations of a particular problem. Through empathic listening the professional establishes a relationship in which the client is able to use his or her own resources to define, confront, and resolve problems. For example, if a client sought the help of a health professional for generalized feelings of anxiety, the therapist using a nondirective approach would provide a supportive atmosphere in which the client could verbalize feelings and develop his or her own understanding of the origins of the anxiety. The nondirective approach is based on the assumption that the client is the person most able to identify and resolve his or her problems.

The nondirective approach to therapeutic interviews has many positive features. It recognizes the innate potential of clients to identify and resolve their own problems. The nondirective approach encourages client involvement in the treatment process and recognizes that clients can affect and change their lives. In addition, this approach increases the chances that the client and the health professional will be addressing the "real" problem being experienced by the client: If the client identifies the problem, there is less chance that the problem will be defined incorrectly and less chance that the "wrong" problem will become the focus of the interview. Furthermore, the nondirective approach gives greater control to the client, who is treated as an equal partner in the interaction. Finally, when clients are active participants in the interview process, the probability increases that they will feel involved in the decision-making process and will follow through on necessary changes.

The nondirective approach to therapeutic interviews also has some unattractive features. A major criticism frequently leveled at the nondirective approach is that it usually requires large amounts of time, a scarce commodity in health care. Some health professionals believe that it is inefficient, costly, and unnecessary to allocate so much time to nondirective interviews. Also, some professionals may feel the nondirective approach does not make full use of their expertise. They may also feel that there are certain situations where it is important and necessary to direct clients toward specific solutions that have been proven to be effective.

Given the advantages and disadvantages of both directive and nondirective approaches to therapeutic interviews, it seems apparent that in some situations a more directive interview will be beneficial, while in other situations a more nondirective interview will be best. Some situations (e.g., an inpatient psychiatric unit) may provide sufficient time for health professionals to use a more nondirective approach, while other situations (e.g., a busy ambulatory clinic) do not. Certain circumstances in clients' lives dictate that professionals be prescriptive (e.g., child abuse situations) while other circumstances suggest less directiveness (e.g., clients with sexual concerns). The situation and the client's needs within that situation will indicate the degree to which the professional's therapeutic approach should be directive or nondirective. Probably the majority of interviews in health care are slightly more directive in focus (see continuum in Fig. 5.4) but also include nondirective aspects.

PHASES IN THE INTERVIEW PROCESS

The interview process can be divided into four phases: (1) preparation, (2) initiation, (3) exploration, and (4) termination. For the purposes of our discussion, each phase will be analyzed separately; however, in actual interviews the phases blend into one another (Benjamin, 1981).

The length of time it takes to move through all four phases of the interview process depends on factors such as the goal of the interview, the severity of the client's problem, the skills of the clinician, and the number of problem areas that emerge (Wilson & Kneisl, 1983). In general, movement through all four phases will occur more rapidly (1) when the goal is information sharing rather than therapeutic change, (2) when the client's personality is well integrated as opposed to severely disorganized, and (3) when there is only a single problem rather than several problems.

The length of time each separate phase will take also varies according to the type of interview. In admission and history-taking interviews, which are usually completed in a single session, only a short time is alloted for each phase. In therapeutic interviews, on the other hand, each phase takes more time and requires more attention. For example, in a therapeutic interview between a psychiatric nurse and a client, it may take two or three sessions to work through the initiation phase of the interview and another three sessions to work through exploration.

In the following discussion of the phases of interviews we will be using the term *interview* to refer to both single-session interviews, such as an admissions interview, as well as multiple-session interviews, such as those utilized in therapeutic relationships. Strictly speaking, an interview occurs at one time and in one place; however, the concepts and theories that apply to specific interview relationships can also be applied to longer term therapeutic clinician-client relationships, which involve a series of interview sessions.

In this section we will describe the characteristics and nature of each of the four interview phases. We will address the tasks that the health professional confronts in each phase, and we will also discuss some of the common problems that occur during each of the phases.

Preparation Phase

The preparation phase involves anticipating and planning for the actual interview. Sometimes the importance of this phase is minimized or even ignored. We have included it as one of the major phases because the planning or lack of planning has a significant impact on subsequent interview phases.

During the preparation phase, participants often develop preconceived ideas about each other and about how the interview will go. Clinicians seldom approach an interview without some notion about the clients with whom they will be meeting. At a walk-in clinic, for example, a clinician can learn the client's name, age, and ethnic background from the intake sheet. In emergency health care settings, information about a patient is often sent ahead of the patient's arrival. In a community health setting, a nurse who receives a referral from another agency may have considerable information about the client before their first interaction. In each of these examples, the health professional has acquired information that will affect his or her feelings about the interview process.

Clients, like clinicians, also actively anticipate their first meeting with the health professional. Some clients learn the professional's name, find out about his or her specialty, and obtain information on the professional's competence prior to their first meeting. Other clients may go through an extensive process of consulting friends, relatives, or other professionals in order to locate a professional with a certain expertise. Still others may spend time gathering information about a clinician's interpersonal style, therapeutic approach, or success in helping others. Based on the preinteraction information they obtain, clients form images and expectations about the clinician and about the first meeting.

A major task for the health professional in the preparation phase is to *plan for the first meeting with the client* (Stuart & Sundeen, 1983). Interviews are more likely to be effective if the clinician is prepared and if the physical setting is also ready. Preparation can include studying about recent advances in treatments, getting assessment forms ready, having educational materials available, or locating an appropriate place to meet. In Chapter 4, we stressed the importance of the environment on the participants' communication. During the preparation phase the clinician can arrange for a comfortable setting that will make it easier to communicate effectively—for example, reserving a conference room, obtaining enough chairs to accommodate an entire family, or making sure that the interview will not be interrupted.

The second task of the preparation phase is to *assess one's own strengths and limitations* and to work through any personal anxieties (Stuart & Sundeen, 1983). Clients have many types of problems, and not all of them are easy for health professionals to handle. For example, some clinicians may have difficulty dealing with a client who is returning for a second abortion. Other clinicians may find it hard to handle a client who has made repeated suicide attempts. Still other clinicians have problems helping a client whose alcohol intake has caused traumatic injuries to others. Health professionals need to be aware of which client problems are difficult for them to face or to deal with. Self-assessment in the preparation phase means that the clinician sorts through personal feelings and biases and, if necessary, gets help in resolving personal anxieties related to problem areas.

If there is not enough preparation, difficulties are bound to occur in later phases. For example, if there is lack of adequate planning for room arrangements, the participants' interaction may be interrupted. Similarly, if a professional is unable to work through personal anxiety about a client's problem, considerable tension may pervade the initial meeting with the client. Thus, planning and self-assessment before the interview prepare the professional and the client for the first face-to-face encounter.

Initiation Phase

The initiation phase begins when the professional and client make their first contact with each other (e.g., a telephone conversation) or have their first meeting. Sundeen and her associates (1981) point out that the initiation phase is especially important because it sets the tone and creates the climate for the professional-client relationship. Although the initiation phase is considered extremely important, surprisingly little research has been conducted in this area (Saltzman et al., 1976; Wilson & Kneisl, 1983).

During the initiation phase, the preconceived notions and expectations that clients and clinicians have developed in the preparation phase are either confirmed or revised. The following example illustrates how a client sometimes needs to change and revise preinteraction expectations about having an interview with a professional.

> Joyce was a little apprehensive about her first meeting with a psychologist. A friend had given Joyce the psychologist's name and recommended him highly to her. Her friend had described the psychologist as a perceptive, understanding person in his early fifties, with many years of clinical experience. Joyce formed a visual image of the psychologist as a rather gray-haired fatherly man, and she looked forward to her first meeting with him.
>
> When Joyce arrived for her first session she was immediately taken aback by his appearance. He was dressed casually in a crewneck sweater and corduroy pants, and he appeared much younger and more attractive than Joyce had anticipated. Joyce felt disappointed and anxious during the first part of the session. She thought that her friend had misguided her and that she would not be able to relate to this young, attractive man, who was very different from the person she was expecting. As the interview continued, however, she found that in spite of his young appearance, the psychologist was understanding and empathic.

Although in this example it is the client who adjusted her expectations, it is equally important that professionals are able to adjust their own preconceptions of clients in the initiation phase.

After reconciling initial expectations, one of the first tasks for professionals in the initiation phase is *to establish a therapeutic climate that will foster trust and understanding*. A supportive atmosphere is particularly helpful at the beginning of the interview because it reduces the client's anxieties about new situations and relationships. A nonthreatening interview atmosphere makes it easier for clients to share their worries and concerns.

Communication plays an important role in creating a supportive interview climate. One type of communication that is often used to put participants at ease in the initial stage of an interview is phatic communication. Phatic communication refers to "small talk," such as the weather (e.g., "Did you have any trouble driving here through the snow?"), the parking (e.g., "Were you able to find a parking spot?"), or the setting (e.g., "Is that chair comfortable for you?"). A brief period of commonplace talk gives participants time to adjust to the setting and to each other before getting into a discussion of more personal information (Barnlund & Haiman, 1960). Phatic communication is used more frequently in professional-professional interviews (e.g., in selection interviews) and it is used less often in therapeutic professional-client interviews. Too much of it can sidetrack an interview, or make an interview seem phony, or produce an awkward atmosphere as the participants become unsure of how to move from superficial topics to more important issues.

Certain types of specific communication techniques such as open questions, reflection, restatement, and clarification also add to the development of a supportive atmosphere during the initial phase of an interview. These techniques are described and discussed at greater length in the last section of this chapter.

The second task of the initiation phase is *to clarify the purpose of the interview*. Benjamin (1981) encourages the interviewer to state clearly the purpose of the interview. He points out that ambiguous statements such as, "I think that we both already know why we are meeting today," can lead to second guessing or poor communication between participants. In addition, if the purpose of the interview is not stated, the participants may be unsure about their relationship (e.g., whether it is social or therapeutic) and it can hinder the focus of their interaction. In an information-sharing interview, a statement such as, "I am a discharge planning nurse, and I would like to talk with you about what kind of care you are going to need at home," immediately lets the client know the clinician's expectations for the session. In a therapeutic interview, a statement such as, "Perhaps you could share some of the concerns that brought you here today and then we can decide which area would be most helpful for us to pursue," helps to identify the purpose of the interview. In both types of interviews, clarifying the purpose gives a structure to the relationship and gives a sense of direction for the interaction that is to follow.

The third task for professionals in the initiation phase is *to formulate a contract with the client*. A contract is a mutually agreed upon statement that provides specific guidelines about the nature of the interview. Essentially, a contract lets both participants know what to expect from one another during the relationship (Langford, 1978). The contract often includes specific information such as the time and place of meetings, the length of each session, the number of sessions, the confidentiality of issues discussed, and plans for termination (Sundeen et al., 1981). The details included in a contract vary with the type of interview being conducted. In a single-session information-sharing interview, such as a diet-planning meeting, the contract is less formal and mainly includes what is going to be covered in the present meeting and how long it will last. However, when there will be a series of interviews, the contract is often more formal and confidentiality and termination issues need to be discussed specifically.

Contracts can be either verbal or written. Most contracts are established through verbal interaction, although the participants may never use the word *contract* in their conversations (Sundeen et al., 1981). A clinician or client may find the word *contract* too formal and may prefer to describe the contract as "a mutual expectation" or "mutual agreement." However, some clinicians prefer written contracts to verbal contracts. Steckel (1982), for example, believes that written contracts provide an observable, tangible mechanism to establish accountability between the clinician and client. Whether contracts are verbal or written, they clarify the details and structure of the interview process.

The fourth task of the initiation phase is to *establish mutual goals*. In brief interviews, goal setting is often not emphasized, or it is assumed that goal setting is a part of the general purpose of the interview. In therapeutic interviews that often involve several sessions, goal setting is essential. Mutual goal setting fosters collaboration between the client and the professional, and prevents either individual from imposing goals on the other (Boettcher, 1978). The goals that are established during the orientation phase provide a sense of direction and readiness for the exploration phase that follows.

During the initiation phase, several communication problems may arise which will hinder the development of the interview process. Sayre (1978, pp. 176–177) has identified several common errors that nursing students often make during the initiation phase of a nurse-patient interaction. The following examples illustrate these errors:

Clinican uses vague introductions to explain the purpose of the interview.

Clinician moves too quickly to get the patient to disclose uncomfortable information.

Clinician has difficulty dealing with the client's request for personal information about the professional.

Clinician is unsure of how to proceed with an interview after the initial introductions and moves instead into social conversation.

Potential problems in the initiation phase are more likely to occur when the clinician does not create a supportive climate or clarify the purpose of the relationship. In addition, the lack of a contract and setting mutual goals can often leave participants floundering early in their relationship. Although participants may feel a little awkward as they try to get to know each other, the four tasks of the initiation phase are crucial because they provide a structure and direction for moving into the exploration phase.

Exploration Phase

After the structure and direction of the interview are established, the participants are ready to enter the exploration phase. Because of their increased familiarity with one another, the participants are often more comfortable about their relationship during this phase (Sundeen et al., 1981). As their feelings of trust and rapport increase, clients feel more secure to disclose personal thoughts and feelings. The exploration phase is often called the *working phase* because it is the phase of the interview in which the client and the clinician try to confront, analyze, and work on the client's problems. During this working phase the health professional tries to assist clients to master their anxieties, increase their sense of independence and responsibility, and acquire new coping abilities (Stuart & Sundeen, 1983).

A major task for professionals in this phase is *to help clients explore their personal problems*. During this phase, the clinician and the client can begin discussing more emotionally charged topics. Benjamin (1981) contends that in the exploration phase a client's initial concern is often replaced by a different, more central concern. For example, a client may send out a trial balloon (a minor concern) in the initiation phase to see how the clinician responds to it. If the clinician seems to handle the first concern with sensitivity, the client then proceeds to share a more pressing concern. In addition, the goals formulated during the earlier phase are often modified as new information surfaces in the exploration phase. The following example illustrates this process.

A nursing student sought counseling to work through the tensions that she was experiencing at school. During the first session the student said that she was having problems with low motivation, an inability to concentrate, and difficulty meeting classroom deadlines.

At a later session, however, when the student was feeling more comfortable with the counselor, the student said that her real worry was her father's alcoholism and abuse of the younger children in her family. She said that these home problems were interfering with her ability to study. Based on this new information, she and the counselor agreed on different goals and discussed new ways of coping with the family stresses.

The task of exploration does not necessarily proceed at a smooth, consistent pace (Benjamin, 1981); the process has many stops and starts, ups and downs, advances and detours. As a rule, though, general themes and patterns emerge in the exploration phase that provide the basis for growth and positive change for the client.

Health professionals often utilize communication techniques more directively in the exploration phase. For example, it is common for health professionals to ask for clarification, to question inconsistencies, and to offer their own interpretations of client problems during this phase of the interview process.

A second task of the exploration phase is *to help clients manage feelings* generated by the discussion of stressful issues. The disclosure of personal and private information by clients during an interview session can generate anxiety. Clients may wonder if they have said too much, if the clinician will accept them, or if their feelings are typical of others who have experienced the same problems. In addition, for clients, the discussion of personal information may also bring out a wide range of feelings such as fear, anger, sadness, or hopelessness. In an atmosphere of acceptance and support, the clinician can help clients to manage and express these feelings.

The third task for health professionals in the exploration phase is to help clients *develop new coping skills*. Through the process of exploration, clients may question their previous behaviors, their usual ways of responding, and their rigid patterns of thinking. Even in short interviews (such as an intake interview) clients can become aware of their strong values or beliefs. The underlying goal of exploration is to help clients build their skills in coping with problems and stress.

The exploration phase is not easy for clients or professionals. Clients may be hesitant to discuss personal feelings, and clinicians may be uncertain about how to explore clients' feelings. Several common communication errors that can occur during this phase have been identified by Sayre (1978, pp. 178–180). They are listed below.

> Clinicians are unable to maintain a sustained focus on an important issue. They prematurely change topics or give clients insufficient feedback to continue on a topic.
>
> Clinicians frequently offer inappropriate advice, approval, or reassurances.
>
> Clinicians respond in stereotyped ways to clients. They overuse the same communication techniques (e.g., reflective statements).

The errors cited by Sayre are just a few of many of the communication errors that can be made in the exploration phase.

There are no perfect ABC guidelines for the exploration phase. The direction and flow of the conversation will vary considerably depending on the participants and the topics being discussed. Through the ongoing interaction the exploration process unfolds, goals are accomplished, and the termination phase begins.

Termination Phase

It is the termination phase that has been written about the most often, especially as it applied to therapeutic interviews (Lego, 1980). Perhaps so much has been written about this phase because termination evokes so many mixed feelings in people. Sundeen and her associates (1981) point out that at the close of a successful relationship, the satisfaction experienced by both participants at having met their mutually agreed upon goals must be balanced against the realization that they have to end a meaningful relationship. Termination is seldom easy for participants because it can evoke feelings of sadness, fear, or uncertainty at saying "goodbye."

Although it is sometimes difficult, termination is an essential phase of effective interviews. In this phase, the professional assists the client in finding closure to problems and concerns that have been discussed in the interview. Termination signals to the client that the purpose of the interview has been accomplished, the goals have been reached, and the end of the interview relationship is near.

The major task of this phase is to *plan for closure of the interview.* Ideally, the planning for termination begins in the initiation phase when the clinician and the client establish a contract (Nehren & Gilliam, 1965). The fact that the interview is moving toward a conclusion is reinforced at various times throughout the other phases. At the very least, in interviews that continue for several sessions, termination issues should be considered in one or two sessions before the final meeting. In single-session interviews, termination issues should be discussed prior to the last few minutes of the interview. In either situation, the reminder that the interview is coming to an end enables the participants to reorient themselves and to tie up unfinished areas in the time that remains. In a single-session interview, participants may want to finish covering a particular topic or complete a particular area of assessment. In an extended series of interviews, the participants may plan how they intend to use the remaining sessions. Some clinicians suggest elaborate planning for the final session as a way of ensuring a good "goodbye" (Koehne-Kaplan & Levy, 1978).

Planning for termination also involves making arrangements for needed follow-up resources. In a single-session interview, the participants may not have enough time to address some of the specific concerns that have been raised, and the clinician may need to refer the person elsewhere. For example, a school nurse who has the opportunity to meet only once with a troubled parent of a student who uses drugs may find it essential to refer the parent to another community resource for further help. In therapeutic interviews that have a number of sessions, the clinician may identify a follow-up resource person and link the client with the new resource person before the final meeting. For example, a student who is working with a client in a community mental health agency may plan one or two joint meetings between the client and the new resource person before the actual termination of the student-client relationship.

A few other factors should be included in plans for termination. At times it is helpful to decrease the frequency of the sessions or the length of each session as termination approaches. For instance, participants may decide to meet every other week rather than every week, or for one-half hour rather than an hour. Also, as termination approaches it is helpful for clinicians to direct clients toward discussion of topics that are less emotionally charged (Benjamin, 1981). Emotionally laden topics create anxieties in participants that can impede the closure process. Bringing up new topics that create new emotional struggles works directly against the purpose of closure.

The second task of the termination phase is *to summarize issues and accomplishments*. The summary can be made by either the clinician or the client, but it is best when both people share in the process. It is helpful to clients to summarize areas that have been fully or partially resolved, as well as to summarize and repeat any "homework" assignments. Summaries are more beneficial if they are brief and specific, and if they underscore the movement in a relationship and in an interview.

The final task of the termination phase is *to assist clients to express their feelings about termination*. We mentioned earlier that termination often causes mixed feelings. Even if the termination is desired and the goals have been reached, it is fairly common to find feelings such as sadness, anger, abandonment, guilt, and helplessness during the termination process (Nehren & Gilliam, 1965; Sundeen et al., 1981). These feelings may be heightened in either the client or the clinician if the person has gone through previous unresolved separations. Perhaps it is not surprising that at times participants choose to extend the time set for termination, or skip the termination session altogether. However, by creating a climate and opportunity to work through these feelings, the clinician can bring the interview to a satisfying closure.

Several communication errors that can lead to ineffective movement through termination have been identified by Sayre (1978, pp. 182–183). She points out that students frequently make the following errors:

Clinician prematurely terminates the interaction because the client is not responding in the expected way.

Clinician does not allow enough time for termination and therefore deals with termination issues only superficially.

Clinician brings up emotionally charged issues that should have been dealt with in an earlier phase.

Clinician avoids dealing with termination issues because the clinician thinks he or she has not been helpful to the client.

These brief examples highlight some of the difficulties that can occur during termination. Many of these errors can be eliminated by attending to the tasks of termination.

In general, it is best when termination can be planned and carried out after all the other phases have been completed. In reality, however, termination is not always neatly planned or perfectly timed. Terminations often occur unexpectedly when clinicians change jobs, students leave their clinical rotations, emergencies arise on a unit, or clients are transferred to another health care setting. In each of these cases, a departure terminates the participants' interaction.

Obviously, unexpected terminations or terminations with nebulous timelines are difficult to plan. For example, sometimes the actual termination date may be in limbo for several days, as in the case of a patient in an acute care hospital who has to wait for an available room in a rehabilitation center. In situations such as this, it is not unusual for the patient to be transferred suddenly, with little or no time to terminate relationships with the hospital staff. Furthermore, if the patient's primary nurse or social worker is off work on the departure day, termination with these health professionals may be missed altogether. In situations such as these, where sudden and unplanned departures are a real possibility, it is important for health professionals to discuss aspects (e.g., resource planning or expression of feelings) of the termination process early.

All four phases of the interviewing process and the specific tasks associated with each phase are listed in Table 5.1. Like other developmental processes, the development of the interview relationship takes time. Each interview situation is different and each interview develops over time in unique ways. However, nearly all interviews proceed either directly or indirectly through the four phases. By attending to the tasks of each phase, health professionals can reduce the possibility of problems occurring during the interview and also improve the quality of the health care interview.

COMMUNICATION TECHNIQUES IN INTERVIEWS

Earlier in the chapter we pointed out that interviewing is a special type of interpersonal communication that utilizes questions and answers and that is intended to acquire information or facilitate therapeutic outcomes. In this section of the chapter we will describe specific communication techniques that are used by health professionals to conduct interviews. The

TABLE 5.1   Phases and Tasks of the Interview Process

PHASES	TASKS
Preparation	Plan for first meeting Assess strengths and limitations
Initiation	Establish therapeutic climate Clarify purpose Formulate contract Establish mutual goals
Exploration	Explore problems Manage feelings Develop coping skills
Termination	Plan for closure Summarize issues Express feelings

Adapted from G. W. Stuart and S. J. Sundeen, *Principles and Practice of Psychiatric Nursing*, 2nd ed. St. Louis: The C. V. Mosby Company, 1983, p. 75.

techniques we will discuss are open and closed questions, silence, restatement, reflection, clarification, and interpretation. These are *only* techniques and their use does not guarantee that the interview will always fulfill its purpose. However, if these techniques are used together with the communication variables discussed in Chapter 2—trust, empathy, and confirmation—it is more likely that the interview will be effective.

Questions

The interviewer's ability to ask appropriate questions is the technique that is most important in effective interviews. Asking questions is the principal mode of carrying out interviews or, as Benjamin (1981) suggests, it is "the basic tool of the interviewer . . . " (p. 71). In general, there are two types of questions that can be used: closed questions and open questions. Each type is used for different purposes in interviewing. A closer examination of each type of question will clarify how each can contribute to or detract from effective interviews.

Closed questions

Questions that limit and restrict clients' responses to specific information are called *closed questions*. Closed questions have been likened to true-or-false and multiple-choice examination questions since the respondent can only give specific or limited responses. Probably the most common type of closed question is one to which the client is asked to answer yes or no. In health care, closed questions are often used to gather demographic data, medical histories, or diagnostic information. Closed questions are used more frequently in information-sharing interviews than in therapeutic interviews.

The following examples are illustrations of closed questions:

Do you think your breathing is better, worse, or about the same as yesterday?

How many weeks ago did you first notice these symptoms?

Are you feeling anxious about what the laboratory reports might reveal about your condition?

Do you have a history of heart problems in your family?

Do you think you could get out of bed and do some more walking today?

Does being sick make you angry?

Are you afraid that if you express your true feelings you might be rejected by others?

Do you think you have the time to do these exercises we have prescribed for you?

It has not been easy for you in the past. Would you like to learn how to change your behaviors?

Clients could respond quickly to each of the preceding closed questions with straightforward and specific answers.

The main advantage of closed questions is that they can be used by professionals to get quick answers. They are efficient. In addition, this type of question does not demand deep introspection on the part of the client, while at the same time it provides the health professional with valuable information. However, there are also disadvantages to closed questions. Closed questions do not allow the client to explain feelings or emotions or give additional information. Thus, closed questions inhibit client communication and lessen the client's sense of control.

Open questions
Open questions do not restrict clients' responses; they allow clients to give extended and unlimited answers. As Benjamin (1981) points out, "The open question is broad; . . . allows the interviewee full scope; . . . invites him to widen his perceptual field; . . . [and] solicits his views, opinions, thoughts, and feelings" (p. 73).

Open questions are frequently used in therapeutic interviews as the

TABLE 5.2   Classification of the Advantages and Disadvantages of Closed versus Open Questions

	TIME AND EFFICIENCY	BREADTH AND DEPTH	EMOTIONS AND FEELINGS	CONTROL FOR CLIENT
Closed questions	Yes	No	No	No
Open questions	No	Yes	Yes	Yes

From *Human Behavior* by Bernard Berelson and Gary A. Steiner, © 1964 by Harcourt Brace Jovanovich, Inc. Reprinted by permission of the publisher.

primary means of encouraging clients to explore their personal thoughts and feelings. This type of question draws clients out, allows for catharsis, and assists clients to express pent-up emotions.

Open questions are illustrated in the following examples:

You seem upset. What are you feeling right now?

Describe what you think is going to happen.

You have had trouble following this diet. What do you think about the diet?

How did you feel when you first learned of your diagnosis?

You've had this problem for sometime now. What do *you* think is behind it?

I think you've made considerable progress. What are your thoughts and feelings about how you're doing?

In each of the preceding examples, the questions are phrased so as to encourage the interviewee to talk and to describe his or her own frame of reference on a topic.

Open questions are advantageous and essential in therapeutic interviews. Clients have a sense of control because they have the freedom to answer in whatever way they choose. In other words, clients can select what they want to say, how much they want to say, and how they want to say it. Open questions are also valuable because the interviewer obtains more information and description from the client. With the added information the interviewer can gain a better understanding of how the client thinks and feels. The only disadvantage of open questions is that they often require more interview time.

From the preceding discussion of open and closed questions, it is apparent that there are advantages and disadvantages of both types of questions. Table 5.2, summarized from the work of Berelson and Steiner

(1964), compares the advantages and disadvantages of closed and open questions. In general, open questions give clients more control and they encourage responses that have more breadth and more feelings, while closed questions are more time efficient.

Silence

We have all heard the phrase, "Silence is golden." Silence can play a very valuable role and have very positive effects in the interview process, but it is not *always* positive. Sometimes silence is negative and counterproductive to effective communication. The major questions that confront interviewers are *when* to use silence and *how* to use silence most effectively.

Baker (1955) has proposed a model of silence that illustrates two kinds of silences: positive silence and negative silence (see Fig. 5.5). In Baker's model, silence that is negative (indicated by the notation S−) occurs when the participants in an interaction (person A and person B) feel uncomfortable and when tension is high in their relationship. In addition, silence is also regarded as negative when no reciprocal identification (e.g., no empathy) is experienced by the participants for one another during the silence. As we move from left to right on the model, silence becomes more positive (indicated by S+), when tensions are reduced and the reciprocal identification between the participants increases. Baker suggests that positive silence is silence "in which arguments and contentions, whether expressed or not, have vanished, to be replaced by understanding acceptance on the part of the hearer (or hearers) and satisfied contentment on the part of the speaker" (p. 161).

Generally, silence is used less frequently in the initiation and termination phases of interviews and more often in the exploration phase. During the initiation phase, the clinician and client are trying to establish a rela-

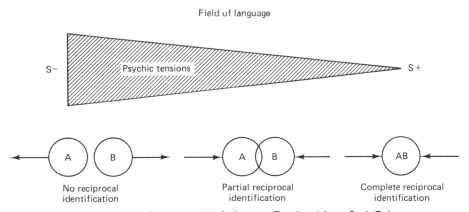

FIGURE 5.5 The Baker model of silence. (Reprinted from S. J. Baker, "The Theory of Silences." *Journal of General Psychology*, 1955, *53*, 159.)

tionship through conversation, and excessive use of silence detracts from this process. At the end of an interview, silence may imply that the work of the interview has halted prematurely, which could work against a sense of planned closure. During the exploration phase, the use of silence by clinicians is more common because it provides a time for both the client and the clinician to think about the issues that they are actively exploring.

In an interview, silence can be used appropriately by a clinician to give a client the message, "Carry on and continue talking." The following example illustrates how silence can be used to stimulate the client to elaborate and expand upon a topic.

> CLIENT: I'm really not sure I've done the right thing by deciding to put Mom in the nursing home. I feel like I should be taking care of her myself—at home. (*Client has wrinkled forehead.*)
> CLINICIAN: Mm'hm. (*Clinician nods.*)
> CLIENT: You know . . . going to a rest home is the last thing she would have chosen. She was normally so interested in everything we were doing. Our family is so close. It seems like we're just dropping her off and getting rid of her. (*Sighs.*)
> CLINICIAN: So you wish you could care for her yourself?
> CLIENT: Yes. But, I just can't do it. I should, but I don't think I can with all the problems she has. She can't walk by herself, she needs to be fed, she can't go to the bathroom alone, and she is confused most of the time. I don't know what to do. If only. . . . (*Pauses.*)
> CLINICIAN: (*Remains silent. Continues to look at client.*)
> CLIENT: . . . If only she hadn't had this stroke. I feel so guilty about not spending more time with her. But I guess I don't have any other good alternative at this point.

In the preceding example the clinician's silence allows the client time to collect her thoughts and to think through the feelings that she has about placing her mother in a nursing home. In effect, the silence of the clinician is saying to the client, "Carry on. I'm with you on this. Do you have more you'd like to say? I'll listen." Silence is a useful technique that allows both the clinician and the client to collect their thoughts and ideas. Although long pauses for this purpose can be uncomfortable, shorter silences are an important element in effective interviews.

Although silence has several positive purposes, silence also has some drawbacks—it is *not* always golden. As is indicated in the Baker model, silence will create tension in situations where the interviewer and the client do not strongly identify with each other. For example, when two people are uncertain about what the other person is thinking during a silence, the silence may increase their discomfort and anxiety. Overuse of silence can also create a sense of directionlessness in interviews. Too many pauses or silent periods can result in participants feeling that the purpose of their conversation is unclear and unfocused. Finally, excessive use of silence may make clients feel that they are getting insufficient feedback on a topic.

Overall, it is important to be aware of both the positive and the negative effects that silence can produce in interviews. Effective interviewing requires clinicians to be sensitive to clients' needs and to use silence in situations where it will lead to positive outcomes.

Restatement

In Chapter 1 we discussed communication as a process in which there is feedback between the source and the receiver. In interviewing contexts, restatement acts as a feedback mechanism between the clinician and the client. Through restatement the clinician can communicate to the client that the clinician is listening and that the clinician understands what the client has said. Benjamin (1981) suggests that restatement is a way of giving the following message to the client:

> "I am listening to you very carefully, so carefully, in fact, that I can restate what you have said. I am doing so now because it may help you to hear yourself through me. I am restating what you have said so that you may absorb it and consider its impact, if any, on you. For the time being, I am keeping myself out of it" (p. 119).

Restatement is a technique that confirms clients because it directly acknowledges their point of view. Restatement gives clients a sense of validation—a feeling that they have been heard by another human being. The underlying assumption of restatement is that as clients feel validated or understood, they will also feel encouraged to continue speaking and examining their concerns (Benjamin, 1981).

As a communication technique, restatement involves paraphrasing or repeating the client's message. Although technically the clinician may restate the exact words of a client, it often seems more empathic and less mechanical to restate the message in slightly different words. In general, the clinician using restatement acts like a sounding board for the client. The following example illustrates how a clinician might use restatement:

CLIENT: It is very hard for me to think about how my epilepsy is going to affect my wife and kids. I really wish they would carry on as if these seizures had never happened, but I'm concerned that my condition will upset them.

CLINICIAN: It is difficult for you to think about the fact that your epilepsy will influence your family situation. You wish they could act as if everything was normal but you are worried that your potential to have more seizures will bother them and make things unnatural.

CLIENT: Yes. I care an awful lot about them and I don't want to worry them.

CLINICIAN: You really love your family and want the best for them.

CLIENT: I sure do. They mean everything to me. That's why I'm feeling so down about this sickness. I just don't want it to affect them in any way.

In the preceding example the clinician is paraphrasing or restating what the client has verbalized without adding any of his or her own personal feelings or thoughts.

In using restatement, health professionals often preface their responses to clients with phrases such as, "I hear you saying . . .," or, "It sounds as if you feel . . .," or, "Let me see if I understand you; you're saying. . . . " Prefaces such as these are useful in restatement because they help the clinician move into an other-directed frame of mind, and they help clients by expressing the intentions of the clinician to restate what the client has verbalized. At times, the prefaces to restatements can be overused or used inappropriately. Consider the following example:

CLIENT: I'm sorry I'm late for this interview.

CLINICIAN: I hear you saying you're sorry for being late for this interview.

Obviously this preface and even the restatement itself, are unnecessary. The clinician's response sounds phony and insincere. However, when restatements are used at the right time, in response to significant client concerns, they are a valuable communication tool that can make interviews more effective.

Reflection

As a communication technique, reflection is very similar to restatement. Both techniques aim to help clients to understand their thoughts and feelings, and both techniques also require the interviewer to act as an echo or sounding board for the client's expressions. In neither technique does the interviewer express her or his own perspectives. However, reflection is different from restatement and it does require a different approach on the part of the interviewer.

In reflection, the interviewer acts as a mirror for the expressed and sometimes unexpressed emotions and attitudes of the client. Unlike restatement, which centers on *what* the client has said (the content), the focus in reflection is on *how* something has been expressed, or the feeling dimension. "Reflection consists of bringing to the surface and expressing in words those feelings and attitudes that lie behind the interviewee's words" (Benjamin, 1981, p. 123). Reflection helps clients get in touch with their feelings and assists them in identifying and describing them.

Reflection is more difficult than restatement because it requires listening empathically for emotions and feelings. Clients are not always able to identify specifically their own emotional states. Reflection is a means of helping them in this process. To accurately understand clients, health professionals need to be attuned to the general emotion the client is expressing and the intensity of that emotion. In addition, health professionals need to be able to accurately communicate back to the client the precise feeling that has been expressed (Hammond, Hepworth & Smith, 1977, pp. 85–86).

The following example of a professional-client interview illustrates how reflection can be used to help the client get in touch with feelings that are present:

CLIENT: This hospital really makes me mad. One person tells me one thing and the next person tells me exactly the opposite. I wonder what's going on around here. (*Shakes head, throws hands in the air.*)

CLINICIAN: You are feeling pretty confused and angry by it all.

CLIENT: Boy, am I! All my reports seem mixed up and everyone tells me something different. I just can't believe it has to be this way. (*Looks down.*)

CLINICIAN: It seems that all the uncertainty over your reports is upsetting to you and that you feel helpless about how to respond.

CLIENT: I guess so. I know they're doing everything they can—I just feel out of control and that worries me.

As the preceding example shows, in essence, reflection is a technique that helps clients to identify feelings that are enmeshed in the descriptions of their experiences. In short, reflection is a technique that helps clients get a handle on their feelings.

To use reflection effectively, health professionals themselves must have a broad vocabulary of feelings. In Table 5.3 we present a vocabulary of feelings developed by Hammond, Hepworth, and Smith (1977) which may be useful as a resource in identifying feelings. The vocabulary provides a list of feeling words that are strong, moderate, and mild variations of ten basic feeling categories (e.g., happy, depressed, lonely). Sometimes it is less threatening for clients to acknowledge mild feelings and more threatening for them to acknowledge strong feelings. For example, a client who is hesitant to discuss feelings may respond more readily to a clinician's reflection that the client is feeling "worried" (a mild feeling) than that he or she is "terrified" (a strong feeling) about a situation. As their relationship develops and the client experiences more trust in the clinician, the client may be comfortable enough to acknowledge stronger feelings. Being aware of the diversity of feeling words and the various levels of intensity of these words can enhance one's ability to accurately reflect the feelings that a client is experiencing.

TABLE 5.3   Vocabulary of Feelings

LEVELS OF INTENSITY	HAPPY	CARING	DEPRESSED	INADEQUATE	FEARFUL
Strong	Thrilled	Affection for	Dejected	Worthless	Terrified
	Ecstatic	Attached to	Hopeless	Powerless	Frightened
	Overjoyed	Devoted to	Bleak	Helpless	Intimidated
	Excited	Adoration	In despair	Impotent	Horrified
	Elated	Loving	Empty	Useless	Desperate
Moderate	Cheerful	Caring	Downcast	Inadequate	Afraid
	Light-hearted	Fond of	Sorrowful	Incompetent	Scared
	Happy	Admiration	Demoralized	Inept	Fearful
	Serene	Concern for	Discouraged	Deficient	Apprehensive
	Aglow	Close	Pessimistic	Insignificant	Threatened
Mild	Glad	Warm toward	Unhappy	Lacking confidence	Nervous
	Contented	Friendly	Down	Unsure of yourself	Anxious
	Satisfied	Like	Low	Uncertain	Unsure
	Pleasant	Positive	Sad	Weak	Hesitant
	Pleased	toward	Glum	Inefficient	Worried

Clarification

Clarification is a technique that can be used by clinicians to assist clients in moving from broad, elusive areas of discussion to narrower, more pinpointed areas of concern. Clarification serves as the vehicle that gets participants on the same wavelength and helps them find a common frame of reference about a particular set of events. In health care interviews, clarification helps the clinician to understand the client more clearly and helps the client to understand his or her own thoughts and feelings better (Benjamin, 1981).

The process of clarifying can take many different forms. It may involve eliciting more specific descriptions from a client who is talking in generalizations. For example, the clinician may ask the client to describe exactly *who* was involved, *what* was involved, *where* it occurred, or *when* it occurred (Peplau, 1960). Clarification can also involve asking the client who is vaguely describing a concern to give an *example* of the situation so that both the clinician and the client can share the same point of reference in their subsequent discussion. Clarification is also useful when the client raises several concerns at one time and the clinician is not certain which issue is most relevant or which problem the client feels is most pressing. In this situation, the clinician can ask the client which topic is of most concern to him or her so they can spend their time discussing it first.

TABLE 5.3 (Cont.)

LEVELS OF INTENSITY	CONFUSED	HURT	ANGRY	LONELY	GUILT-SHAME
Strong	Bewildered Puzzled Perplexed Confounded Befuddled	Crushed Destroyed Devastated Disgraced Humiliated	Furious Enraged Seething Infuriated Violent	Isolated Abandoned All alone Forsaken Cut off	Sick at heart Humiliated Disgraced Degraded Exposed
Moderate	Mixed-up Foggy Adrift Lost Disconcerted	Hurt Belittled Overlooked Abused Depreciated	Resentful Hostile Annoyed Agitated Mad	Lonely Alienated Estranged Remote Alone	Ashamed Guilty Remorseful Demeaned To blame
Mild	Uncertain Unsure Bothered Uncomfortable Undecided	Put down Neglected Overlooked Minimized Unappreciated	Uptight Disgusted Perturbed Chagrined Dismayed	Left out Excluded Lonesome Distant Aloof	Regretful Wrong Embarrassed At fault In error

Adapted from D. C. Hammond, D. H. Hepworth, and V. G. Smith, *Improving Therapeutic Communication.* San Francisco: Jossey-Bass, Inc., Publishers, 1977, pp. 86–87.

Examples of clarification are illustrated in the following interaction:

CLIENT: I can't ever get along with him. (*Shakes head.*)

CLINICIAN: Who do you have trouble getting along with? (*Looking at client.*)

CLIENT: My boss. I've tried all sorts of ways to get along with him and to try to get him to like me, but I still feel like he is putting me down all the time. (*Frowns.*)

CLINICIAN: You sound frustrated about your relationship with your boss. What situation, recently, has been especially difficult for you?

CLIENT: (*Pauses and thinks a moment.*) I guess . . . the time when I returned from my vacation. While I was gone all sorts of work had piled up and. . . .

In the preceding example, the clarifying techniques enable the clinician to get a better understanding of what exactly is bothering the client. Clarification also gives the client a chance to sort through general feelings of frustration and discomfort and attach these feelings to specific events. In general, clarification is a helpful technique for pinpointing an area of concern and for increasing the accuracy of communication between the participants in the interview.

Interpretation

Unlike the preceding communication techniques, all of which keep the focus of the interview on the client, interpretation is a technique in which the focus of the interaction shifts temporarily back to the interviewer. Interpretation is a process in which the clinician offers an explanation about the expressed concerns of the client. The goal or intention of interpretation is to offer the client a new frame of reference or a new way of looking at her or his experience, which will help the client to understand that experience better. Interpretation is not typically used in informal, information-seeking interviews but more commonly used by experienced therapists in psychotherapeutic settings, particularly during the exploration phase of an interview.

When interpretation is used, it is important that the client be given the opportunity to accept or reject the perspective offered by the clinician. Sometimes it is helpful if the interpretation is offered as the clinician's hypothesis or "hunch" about what is happening to the client (Brammer, 1973). This tentativeness gives the client the chance to react to the validity of the interpretation. In the end, the interpretation needs to make sense to the client if it is going to be useful.

Although it is difficult to illustrate interpretation without an elaborate case description of a client's history and circumstances, the following example provides a sense of how a clinician uses interpretation:

CLIENT: You know . . . before I retired . . . I used to be very busy. I'd see people in my office as late as 8:00 P.M. every night. But what was it all for? What difference does it make? Now I sit here, read a little, eat a bit, and that's it.

CLINICIAN: I understand you to say that you devoted your whole life to helping people and now because you've retired it is difficult to find things to do that are meaningful. Is it possible that you are feeling the emptiness and loneliness of not being able to help or affect others' lives anymore?

CLIENT: You could be right. The difference between my life now . . . and then . . . is like night and day. You know, my practice used to be one of the largest in the area. Now, I just sit, think, and reflect on how things used to be. It is nice not having the pressure that comes with knowing you always have to go to the office the next day. But I do miss it. . . .

As the example indicates, interpretation can be a useful tool in helping the client gain a different insight into his or her circumstances.

If interpretation is used appropriately, it can have a strong and positive impact on the client. To use interpretation appropriately, the following guidelines have been suggested by Brammer (1973):

1. Look for the *basic message(s)* of the [interviewee].
2. *Paraphrase* these to him [her].
3. Add *your understanding* of what his [her] message means in terms of your theory or your general explanation of motives, defenses, needs, styles, etc.
4. Keep the *language simple* and the *level close to his [her] message*. Avoid wild speculation and statements in esoteric words.
5. *Introduce* your ideas with some kind of statement indicating that you are offering *your ideas tentatively* on what his [her] words or behavior means. Examples are, "Is this a fair statement . . . ?" "The way I see it is. . . . " "I wonder if. . . . " "Try this one on for size. . . . "
6. Solicit the (interviewee's) *reactions* to your interpretations.
7. Your main goal is to *teach the [interviewee]* to do his [her] own interpreting. Remember, you can't give insight to others (p. 106).

With these guidelines in mind, interpretation can be a useful communication technique that will clarify and amplify clients' understanding of their situations.

In this section, we have discussed the major communication techniques that can assist the clinician in the interview process. Although our intention has been to focus on communication techniques that facilitate effective interviews in Table 5.4, we have listed some common responses such

TABLE 5.4   Communication Techniques That Block Effective Interviewing

RESPONSE	EXAMPLE	OUTCOME
Probing	"Why are you feeling so depressed about your son's situation?"	Puts client on the defensive and asks for information that the client may not have.
Advice-giving	"If I were in your situation, I would call him back and try to convince him that. . . ."	Centers the interaction on the professional's needs and perspective rather than on the client's needs and perspective.
False Reassurance	"Everything will work out eventually—I know it will."	Smooths over client's concerns and does not help the client to solve a particular problem.
Moralizing	"You acted too hastily; you should have thought through the consequences before you got involved."	Does not move interaction forward. Blames client and stagnates interaction.
Belittling	"I think that you're overreacting. Things aren't as bad as you make them seem."	Makes evaluative judgment about the client and restricts further discussion of client's concerns.

as putting clients on the defensive, glossing over their concerns, or making evaluative judgments about them, which can block effective interviewing (Bernstein & Bernstein, 1980; Peplau, 1960). Communication techniques that focus on the client, that demonstrate understanding of the client's perspective, and that facilitate the client's ability to understand and work through areas of concern will enhance the professional-client relationship and promote an effective interview process.

SUMMARY

Overall, conducting interviews plays a prominent role in the communication of health professionals. *Interviewing* is defined as a special type of interpersonal communication, usually involving questions and answers, for the purpose of sharing information or facilitating therapeutic outcomes.

In health care settings there are two general types of interviews: information-sharing interviews and therapeutic interviews. Information-sharing interviews involve requesting or providing information. In this type of interview the focus of the interaction is on purposeful content in a specific area of interest. Included in this category of interviews are admissions interviews, history-taking interviews, selection interviews, performance appraisals, journalistic interviews, and survey interviews. Therapeutic interviews are concerned with helping clients identify and work through personal issues and concerns. More emphasis is placed on building a supportive relationship, in this type of interview. Therapeutic interviews can be conducted by health professionals using directive as well as nondirective approaches.

The four phases of the interview process are preparation, initiation, exploration, and termination. The preparation phase occurs prior to the actual interview dialogue, and it involves anticipating and planning for the interview. During this phase, the major tasks of the health professional are to engage in self-assessment and to plan for the first meeting with the client. In the second phase, initiation, the stage is set for the rest of the interview. During this phase the clinician's responsibilities focus on establishing a therapeutic climate, clarifying the purpose of the interview, formulating a contract with the client, and establishing mutual goals. The third phase, exploration, is often called the "working" phase. During this phase, the clinician and client confront, analyze, and struggle with the client's concerns. The clinician tries to assist the client in analyzing problems, managing feelings, and in improving coping skills. The termination phase signals to the client that the end of the interview relationship is near. During this phase the clinician's responsibilities include planning for closure, summarizing major issues, and assisting the client in expressing feelings about termination.

Special communication techniques that are directly related to interviewing include closed and open questions, silence, restatement, reflection, clarification, and interpretation. Closed questions are questions that elicit yes or no answers. They take less time but only provide a restricted amount of information. Open questions elicit elaborate in-depth answers from clients and require more time. Silence is used to encourage further response from the client. It can be positive or negative depending on how much empathy or tension exists between the participants. Restatement is used to repeat or paraphrase the content of a client's message, while reflection is used to focus on the feelings that the client is expressing beneath the words. Clarification moves the interaction from generalities to specifics, and interpretation offers the client a tentative new way of looking at his or her situation. In general, appropriate use of these techniques can make health care interviews more effective.

REFERENCES

Baker, S. J. The theory of silences. *Journal of General Psychology*, 1955, *53*, 145–167.

Barnlund, D. C., & Haiman, F. S. *The dynamics of discussion*. Boston: Houghton Mifflin Company, 1960.

Benjamin, A. *The helping interview*, 3rd ed. Boston: Houghton Mifflin Company, 1981.

Berelson, B., & Steiner, G. A. *Human behavior: An inventory of scientific findings*. New York: Harcourt, Brace & World, Inc., 1964.

Bernstein, L., & Bernstein, R. *Interviewing: A guide for health professionals*. New York: Appleton-Century-Croft, 1980.

Boettcher, E. G. Nurse-client collaboration: Dynamic equilibrium in the nursing care system. *Journal of Psychiatric and Mental Health Services*, 1978, *16*(12), 7–15.

Brammer, L. M. *The helping relationship: Process and skills*. Englewood Cliffs, N.J.: Prentice-Hall, Inc., 1973.

Downs, C. W., Smeyak, G. P., & Martin, E. *Professional interviewing*. New York: Harper & Row Publishers, Inc., 1980.

Enelow, A. J., & Swisher, S. N. *Interviewing and patient care*, 2nd ed. New York: Oxford University Press, 1979.

Hammond, D. C., Hepworth, D. H., & Smith, V. G. *Improving therapeutic communication*. San Francisco: Jossey-Bass, Inc., Publishers, 1977.

Kahn, R. L., & Cannel, C. F. *The dynamics of interviewing: Theory, technique, and cases*. New York: John Wiley & Sons, Inc., 1957.

Koehne-Kaplan, N. S., & Levy, K. E. An approach for facilitating the passage through termination. *Journal of Psychiatric Nursing and Mental Health Services*, 1978, *16*(6), 11–14.

Langford, T. Establishing a nursing contract. *Nursing Outlook*, 1978, *26*(6), 386–388.

Lego, S. The one-to-one nurse-patient relationship. *Perspectives in Psychiatric Care*, 1980, *18*(2), 67–89.

Nehren, J., & Gilliam, N. R. Separation anxiety. *American Journal of Nursing*, 1965, *65*(1), 109–112.

Patterson, L. E., & Eisenberg, S. *The counseling process,* 3rd ed. Boston: Houghton Mifflin Company, 1983.

Peplau, H. Talking with patients. *American Journal of Nursing,* 1960, *60*(7), 964–966.

Rogers, C. R. *Client-centered therapy.* Boston: Houghton Mifflin Company, 1951.

Rogers, C. R. A theory of therapy, personality, and interpersonal relationships, as developed in the client-centered framework. In S. Koch (Ed.), *Psychology: A study of science, Vol. III. Formulations of the person and the social context.* New York: McGraw-Hill Book Company, 1959, 184–256.

Saltzman, C., Leutgert, M. J., Roth, C. H., Creaser, J., & Howard, L. Formation of a therapeutic relationship: Experiences during the initial phase of psychotherapy as predictors of treatment duration and outcome. *Journal of Consulting and Clinical Psychology,* 1976, *44*(4), 546–555.

Sayre, J. Common errors in communication made by students in psychiatric nursing. *Perspectives in Psychiatric Care,* 1978, *16*(4), 175–183.

Steckel, S. B. *Patient contracting.* Norwalk, Conn.: Appleton-Century-Crofts, 1982.

Stano, M. E., & Reinsch, Jr., N. L. *Communication in interviews.* Englewood Cliffs, N.J.: Prentice-Hall, Inc., 1982.

Stewart, C. J., & Cash, Jr., W. B. *Interviewing: Principles and practices,* 2nd ed. Dubuque, Iowa: William C. Brown Co. Publishers, 1978.

Stuart, G. W., & Sundeen, S. J. *Principles and practice of psychiatric nursing,* 2nd ed. St. Louis: The C. V. Mosby Company, 1983.

Sundeen, S. J., Stuart, G. W., Rankin, E. D., & Cohen, S. A. *Nurse-client interaction: Implementing the nursing process.* St. Louis: The C. V. Mosby Company, 1981.

Wilson, H. S., & Kneisl, C. R. *Psychiatric nursing,* 2nd ed. Menlo Park, Calif.: Addison-Wesley Publishing Co., Inc., 1983.

6 Small Group Communication in Health Care

In a strong group, the members recognize that they form a unit; they want to belong to that unit, and they unstintingly provide whatever services the unit needs from them, working hard in its behalf and conforming to its demands.   —Zander, 1982

During the last decade, the health care field has seen groups take over functions that once were performed on an individual basis, or not at all. The number of self-help groups, for example, has increased dramatically in recent years. Estimates indicate that there are approximately 500,000 different self-help groups in the United States (Naisbitt, 1982). In addition, many other types of groups are now being used to teach clients how to maintain health as well as how to overcome illness. Fitness groups, relaxation groups, nutrition groups, health education groups, and support groups are just a few of the many client-oriented groups that are part of health care today. Groups are also being used more and more among health professionals. Interdisciplinary groups, advisory groups, task forces, management groups, stress reduction groups, and care-for-the-caregiver groups are some of the growing number of these professional-oriented groups. During a typical week it is not uncommon for a health professional to be involved in several planned group meetings plus other informal groups.

With the increased use of groups in health care, it has become increasingly important for health professionals to understand how groups work and how members communicate within groups. In self-help, task, and therapy groups, effective communication is essential. In essence, when the communication in a group works well, the group has a good chance of working well. Communication is the process that connects members to one another and enables them to work interdependently.

The purpose of this chapter is to present, explain, and discuss communication concepts and theories that apply to small groups in health care. We begin by providing a definition of small group communication and then we provide a discussion of three different types of health care groups. Next, we describe the central components that are common to most groups, and the four major phases that occur during the development of groups. The chapter concludes with a description of techniques for decision making in small groups.

DEFINITION OF SMALL GROUP COMMUNICATION

Before defining small group communication, it is useful to consider the question, What is a small group? Answers to this question have been provided by members of several professions including social work, psychology, sociology, administration, nursing, speech communication, and public health, to name a few. Although each profession has focused on groups from its own unique perspective, there are certain basic elements of small groups that are commonly identified by nearly all of these professions.

Generally speaking, a small group refers to a set of three or more individuals whose relationships make them in some way *interdependent* (Cartwright & Zander, 1968; Loomis, 1979; Zander, 1982). A more specific definition of a group is provided by Tubbs (1978) who suggests that "a group is a collection of individuals who influence one another, derive some satisfaction from maintaining membership in the group, interact for some purpose, assume specialized roles, are dependent on one another, and communicate face to face" (p. 7). Cartwright and Zander (1968) indicate that individuals in groups usually exhibit one or more of the following characteristics:

They engage in frequent interaction.

They define themselves as members.

They are defined by others as belonging to the group.

They share norms concerning matters of common interest.

They participate in a system of interlocking roles.

They identify with one another as a result of having set up the same model-object or ideals in their super-ego.

They find the group to be rewarding.

They pursue promotively interdependent goals.

They have a collective perception of their unity.

They tend to act in a unitary manner toward the environment (p. 48).

As Cartwright and Zander point out, there are many qualities that can be used to characterize small groups.

Small group communication refers to the verbal and nonverbal communication that occurs among a collection of individuals whose relationships make them to some degree interdependent. Stated in another way, it refers to how a group of individuals who are dependent on each other share information and meanings through a common set of rules. As Goldberg and Larson (1975) point out, the focus in studying group communication is on "communication phenomena in small groups" (p. 12). This includes developing a better understanding of the communication process in small groups, being able to predict what communication outcomes will occur in small groups, and then learning to improve the communication among group members. Throughout this chapter we will discuss the transactions that occur in small groups and also factors that influence these transactions.

TYPES OF HEALTH CARE GROUPS

The communication focus is different in different types of groups. By distinguishing between various types of groups, the communication implications for different groups in health care can be better understood. In this section we will provide a general overview of types of groups and a specific typology that distinguishes types of groups according to the group objective, size, leader behavior, and member behavior. While there are other ways to delineate various types of groups, the following approaches are especially useful for understanding the communication focus of groups in health care.

A General Perspective

A general way of viewing the numerous groups in health care settings is according to whether they are process oriented or content oriented (Loomis, 1979). Throughout this book the terms *process* and *content* have been used frequently to describe the components of a communication message. In group activity, the time spent discussing tasks and goals is referred to as the *content focus* of the group and the time spent relating and getting along with people is referred to as the *process focus* of the group (Loomis, 1979). Although *all* groups have both content and process ele-

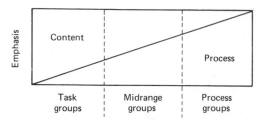

FIGURE 6.1 The empasis on content and process in different types of groups. (Adapted from M. E. Loomis, *Group Process for Nurses*. St. Louis: The C. V. Mosby Company, 1979, p. 102.)

ments, groups vary in the degree to which one or the other of these elements is emphasized.

Figure 6.1 illustrates types of groups along a content-process continuum. *Task groups,* which appear on the left end of the continuum, focus nearly all of their efforts on substantive issues such as the goal of the group, the activities that the group needs to accomplish, or the procedures the group will follow. A committee that is formed to revise staff policies is typical of a task group that is mainly concerned with content issues. *Process groups,* which appear at the right end of the continuum, focus on group members, how they are related, and how they communicate with each other. A therapy group in a hospital psychiatric unit would be a familiar example of a process group. In a therapy group, most of the time is spent discussing how members feel about themselves, about other members of the group, and the group as a whole. Many groups fall midway between the two extremes of the task and process groups. These groups, referred to as *midrange groups,* have a blend of task and process (Loomis, 1979). For example, groups set up for ostomy patients generally emphasize content (e.g., physical care of ostomy) as well as processing feelings among members (e.g., concerns about self-disclosure).

The content-process continuum provides a general way of differentiating groups into those that are more content oriented and those that are more process oriented.

A Specific Typology

A more specific approach to differentiating types of groups is provided in a typology developed by Betz, Wilbur, and Roberts-Wilbur (1981) (see Fig. 6.2). This typology parallels the more general content-process perspective just discussed. The typology developed by Betz, Wilbur, and Roberts-Wilbur divides groups into three basic clusters or group types:

GROUP DYNAMICS

	The Clusters and Their Elements	Objective	Size	Leader Behavior	Member Expectations and Behavior
TYPE I The Task-Process Cluster	Committee Task Force Staff Conference Retreat Action Group Pot Boiler Meeting	EXTRA-PERSONAL To accomplish a task, complete a project or produce a product.	Variable and Related to size of task	Directs group to the charge, examines interferences to movement, moves for consensus and terminates process.	Problem solving activities are the responsibility of all. Responsibility for production between sessions are assumed.
TYPE II The Socio-Process Cluster	Guidance Group Social Group Work Discussion Group Human Potential Group Guided Group Interaction Recovery, Inc. Life Style Group	INTER-PERSONAL To cause examination of attitudes, values and beliefs and to inform and criticize.	UL 20 LL 6	Focuses topic or area of concern, encourages expression from all, promotes understanding and communication and exercises judgment in exhaustion of topic.	Discussion of etiology, consequences, alternatives and personal experiences center about mutual topics of concern to the group. Thrust is social and familial role.
TYPE III The Psycho-Process Cluster	Group Counseling Group Therapy Marathon Conjoint Family Therapy Encounter Group Attack Group Group Psychotherapy	INTRA-PERSONAL To change or modify behavior by focusing that behavior in the group.	UL 10 LL 5	Causes group to focus on itself and its problems, assists in the solution of group and individual problems within system of behavior change.	More freedom to choose personal content of material. Affect laden and personal; at times repressed and unconscious material rises. Learn as a group to change own behavior.

FIGURE 6.2 A typology of group processes. (From R. Betz, M. Wilbur, and J. Roberts-Wilbur, "A Structural Blueprint for Group Facilitators: Three Group Modalities." *The Personnel and Guidance Journal*, 1981, 60 (1), 31–37. Copyright ©1981 by The American Personnel and Guidance Association. Reprinted with permission.)

task-process, socio-process, and psycho-process.[1] Betz and his associates hypothesize that these three categories of groups can be distinguished from each other by four variables: (1) objective, (2) size, (3) leader behavior, and (4) member expectations and behavior. These variables appear across the top of the model in Figure 6.2. Although this typology is developmental in nature, each of the three categories of the typology will be helpful in understanding various types of health care groups. The boundaries between the categories should not be viewed as rigid or discrete. At times the categories may overlap one another, and some health care groups with numerous objectives may fit into more than one category or vary between the categories at one time or another during the life of the group.

Task-process groups

As its name implies, the primary purpose of a task-process group is the accomplishment of a task or completion of a preassigned charge. As illustrated in Figure 6.2, committees, task forces, staff conferences, and planning meetings are examples of task-process groups. The *objective* or focus of task-process groups is *extra*personal, which means the communication in these groups is directed toward accomplishment of a goal or objective rather than toward individuals' feelings or group members' relationships.

The *size* of task-process groups can vary from very small, such as a task force of 3 members, to very large, such as a long-range planning committee of 25 members. For the most part, the size of these groups is related to the nature and complexity of the task being considered.

In a task-process group a *leader's behavior* includes responsibilities such as clarifying goals, structuring of task activity (e.g., time of meeting, place, purpose, agenda, expected outcomes, and record keeping), removing obstacles to goal accomplishment, assisting members in the decision-making process, and finally terminating the group as it completes its task.

Member behavior includes those activities in which individuals try to solve problems and proceed through various steps in their efforts to reach group goals. In this regard, Betz, Wilbur, and Roberts-Wilbur point out that it is important that group members maintain an extrapersonal focus. If members focus on intrapersonal or interpersonal needs (individualism), it can work against or create resistance to the group's extrapersonal function of goal accomplishment. If a group can work through and resolve struggles between member individualism and group task activity, the group's cohesiveness and achievement will increase.

In health care settings professionals are often required to spend time

[1]It should be noted that the word *process*, which appears in each of three major types of groups in the Betz, Wilbur, and Roberts-Wilbur typology, is being used to denote a series of actions or operations that occur in groups. It is *not* being used as it is often used in a clinical way to denote the activity of talking about feelings and relationships—group maintenance behavior.

working in task groups. Unit reports, treatment planning meetings, agency staff meetings, program development meetings, and budget priority meetings are some examples of this category of groups in health care. The typology suggests that the communication focus (objective) of these groups needs to be extrapersonal. For example, when a nurse is giving report to a group of staff members, it is important for the staff members to focus their discussion on patient care concerns and not become sidetracked talking about personal or social topics. According to Betz, Wilbur, and Roberts-Wilbur, the key to making task-process groups work effectively is to encourage group members to realize that their *primary* goal is not to address individual and interpersonal needs but to concentrate communication on the group goal.

Socio-process groups

The socio-process category includes those groups that have an interpersonal focus. In other words, as the name *socio-process* implies, these groups foster communication *between* members so that members can share values and beliefs and learn from one another and the group. The typology indicates that guidance groups, discussion groups, and self-help groups (e.g., Recovery Inc.) fit into this socio-process category. For the most part, a majority of the client-oriented groups that health professionals lead are socio-process groups. Support groups, stress reduction groups, preoperative education groups, health discussion groups, and socialization groups are just some of the many types of health care groups that fall into the socio-process category. The *objective* of these groups is to allow individuals to communicate with each other for the purpose of sharing information and examining beliefs, attitudes, and values. Essentially, the focus of socio-process groups is on helping members cope more effectively with life circumstances; the focus is not on changing their personality. For example, women who have participated in postpartum support groups have reported that they joined these support groups so that they could meet and share ideas with other women having a similar experience (Cronenwett, 1980). The women also reported that the groups helped them learn to cope and problem-solve more effectively. Similarly, members of a staff group to prevent burnout have reported that they learned ways to become more assertive and to cope with problems (Forsyth & Cannady, 1981). When members of these groups are identified as having concurrent and intense personal problems, they are often referred for additional counseling to other professionals rather than encouraged to deal with these problems in the socio-process group.

The *size* of socio-process groups usually ranges from a lower limit (LL) of 6 to an upper limit (UL) of 20 members. In groups with more than 20 members it becomes difficult for all members to have the opportunity to participate in the group within the allotted period of time.

The *leader* in a socio-process group is responsible for promoting discussion, exploration, and interaction among group members. Although a leader may at times provide information to group members (e.g., health education groups), for the most part the leader's role is to assist members to understand how they can integrate this information into their lives. In addition, the leader tries to create an atmosphere in which there is open communication and nonjudgmental listening. The leader's goal is to get members to participate.

Group members are expected to share their ideas in a socio-process group. For example, in cancer education groups such as "I Can Cope," members discuss their mutual experiences related to cancer such as when they first got cancer, what their treatment involved, and how it affected their families. Members of these cancer groups typically offer one another suggestions about ways to cope with various aspects of the disease. In addition, members often find that the group helps them to alter their beliefs and attitudes. The focus in socio-process discussions is on the interpersonal dimension of sharing. Attempts by members to be extrapersonal (e.g., focus on issues outside of the group) or intrapersonal (e.g., focus on in-depth personality problems) work against the effective functioning of socio-process groups.

Psycho-process groups

The third cluster of groups in the typology is psycho-process groups. Group counseling, group therapy, encounter groups, and conjoint family therapy are examples of groups that fall into this category of the typology. In health care the psychotherapy groups in inpatient psychiatric settings or the therapy groups in outpatient mental health agencies would typify this category of groups. The *objective* of psycho-process groups is to assist group members in changing or modifying their own behaviors by focusing on those behaviors in the group. The communication emphasis in this type of group is placed on feelings and intrapersonal issues.

Psycho-process groups usually range in *size* from a lower limit of five to an upper limit of ten members. The upper limit size of a psycho-process group is smaller than either of the other two groups because of the intensity of the group and the personality alterations that are being sought within this particular group.

As in the other two types of groups, the *leaders* in psycho-process groups are responsible for structuring the group session. Leaders of psycho-process groups are expected to intervene in the group process and to encourage members to confront problems. In addition, they are expected to assist individuals to start changing their behavior within the security of the group. As in the other types of groups, leaders are also responsible for helping group members in the termination process.

Members usually enter psycho-process groups with the expectation that they will need to confront their own behavior patterns. They expect to deal with emotions and feelings, and they also expect to be free to choose what aspects of their own behavior they are going to change. Group members who attempt to operate on the extrapersonal level rather than on the intrapersonal level may be perceived as resisting the goal of the group. Effective psycho-process groups nurture individual behavior change by focusing on specific individual feelings and behaviors within the group.

In summary, the typology of groups proposed by Betz, Wilbur, and Roberts-Wilbur provides a system for classifying groups in health care according to four variables: objective, size, leader behavior, and member expectations and behavior. The three major types of groups that emerge from this typology (task-process, socio-process, and psycho-process) are evident in various health care contexts.

A major strength of this typology is that it provides a fairly easy way of thinking about the many kinds of health care groups. It is a useful organizing framework. Another strength of the typology is that it provides the practitioner with direction on how leaders should approach communication in the different types of groups, depending on the purpose for the group and member expectations. In other words, the typology highlights that task-process groups focus communication primarily on *extrapersonal* issues, socio-process groups emphasize communication that has an *interpersonal* focus, and finally, psycho-process groups are concerned with communication that is focused on *intrapersonal* issues. Although groups in health care seldom focus their communication entirely on one set of issues, this typology highlights the primary emphasis in the various kinds of groups.

The major weakness of the typology presented by Betz, Wilbur, and Roberts-Wilbur is that it deemphasizes the important role that group-maintenance behavior plays in task and socio-process groups. Issues regarding personal feelings and group member relationships always arise in groups, whether it is a therapy group or a task force, yet this typology implies that affective issues are of concern primarily in psycho-process groups. Finally, this typology is a blueprint and it is still unknown whether in fact the proposed structure is fully accurate. The conceptual basis for the model still needs to be tested empirically by research.

COMPONENTS OF SMALL GROUPS

In the preceding section we discussed the various types of groups that exist in health care. Now, we will look more closely at the various *components* of a group such as the goals, norms, cohesiveness, leader behavior, member behavior, and curative factors that influence group functioning.

Goals

Every group needs a reason for its existence or else there would be no need for individuals to come together. Goals provide the rationale and motivation for people to form a group. Cartwright and Zander (1968) refer to goals as inducing agents that motivate members to perform certain goal-directed activities.

Two types of goals can operate in groups: individual goals and group goals. *Individual goals* are based on the particular needs and desires of each group member and may or may not be related to the goals of the group. *Group goals,* on the other hand, are shared (to some extent) by group members and involve some element of interdependence among the members. Both individual and group goals often operate simultaneously within a group. For example, a new employee may join a task force to study the parking problem at an agency as a way to get to know some other employees (individual goal) and also because of an interest in improving parking at the agency (group goal). Similarly, a nursing student may offer to co-lead a preoperative class for patients because the student is interested in helping the patients prepare for surgery (group goal) but also because the student wants to develop his or her own leadership skills (individual goal).

Problems can occur, however, when the individual goals held by one member are not *compatible* with the goals held by another member. This situation often leads to competition among group members especially when goal achievement by one member blocks the goal achievement of another member (Shaw, 1976). In addition, members' incompatible goals can disrupt the flow of communication and reduce the degree of collaboration and the amount of friendliness among group members (Deutsch, 1968). In contrast, mutually shared goals lead to greater cooperation among the participants in a group.

Group goals also need to be *realistic.* When goals are set unreasonably high, members often feel overwhelmed by trying to reach the goal or frustrated when their attempts are unsuccessful. Yalom (1983) contends that therapists who set overly ambitious goals in groups can create antitherapeutic effects: Members are set up for a situation in which they are likely to fail. On the other hand, goals that are too simplistic also present problems. Members of a task group, for example, may have difficulty getting interested or motivated in working in a group whose goals offer little interest or challenge (Zander, 1982). Group goals need to be realistically attainable within the time available to the group.

Another important issue to be considered regarding group goals is their degree of *clarity.* Clarity refers to the amount of certainty that members have about the nature of group goals and about how they should go about meeting those goals. In order for people to work together, they need to have a common understanding about the mission of the group (Loomis & Dodenhoff, 1970). Ambiguous or vague goals can lead to uncertainty and annoyance among group members (Marram, 1978; Raven & Rietsema, 1957). For example, Klein (1981) reported that the lack of clear goals can be especially problematic in patient-staff community meetings in a psychiatric unit. He observed that an inability to specify clear goals for the group leaves members wondering how long the meeting should last, what topics are appropriate for discussion, and what type of participation is desired from patients and staff. In addition, he observed that when goals and task boundaries are not clearly established, topics in the meeting shifted rapidly and unpredictably, the level of disclosure varied, the meetings lacked continuity, and group members' anxiety increased.

Goal clarity can be enhanced if the leader helps members to identify group goals and removes the obstacles to meeting these goals (see Chapter 7 on path-goal leadership). For example, in a health education group for diabetics, the leader can outline the general goals of the group before the meeting so that clients can determine if the proposed group will meet their needs. In a psycho-process group, the leader and members can jointly determine how to use the group, and they can review and modify the goals as the group develops. When the goals of a group are clear, realistic, and shared by group members, the group will function more effectively.

Norms

Norms are the rules of behavior that are established and shared by group members to ensure consistency in the behavior of group members. Norms often suggest what type of behavior is appropriate or *should* be exhibited by group members (Shaw, 1976), thus adding to the predictability within a group. Norms do not emerge on their own—they are the outcome of people interacting together (Stech & Ratliffe, 1976). However, a group does not develop norms for every single behavior within a group, only for those behaviors that are important to the group (Shaw, 1976).

Norms can be overt or covert. *Overt norms* are usually verbally agreed-on rules that are generally known to all members. For example, a group of health professionals may agree not to smoke during their weekly treatment planning meetings. In this group, not smoking becomes the norm and new members who enter the meetings are quickly reminded of this rule of behavior. *Covert norms* are not usually verbally acknowledged by group members. For example, a communication norm that often operates in groups is that when one person talks, all others should listen. Group members who violate this norm often receive disapproving glances or other nonverbal messages from group members. Another example of a covert norm could be the seating arrangement in a group. If everyone knows where he or she is "supposed" to sit without its being discussed, a covert norm is operating within the group.

Norms can also be enabling or restrictive (Loomis, 1979). *Enabling norms* assist the group in meeting its goals. For example, in a task group, the norm that "all members do their homework and come to the meeting prepared" enables the group to make decisions more efficiently. In a socio-process group, such as a parent effectiveness group, the norm that "members share experiences and offer constructive feedback to one another" enables members to learn more about parenting from one another. *Restrictive norms* hinder the group's movement toward goals. When norms develop in a group that allow members to attack one another verbally or to be chronically tardy, the group is restricted from accomplishing its goal. The following example illustrates how the restrictive norms in a group can hinder group development.

> Two students were asked to assume a leadership role in an ongoing group in a community mental health center. The group consisted of clients from the state psychiatric hospital who were presently living in the community. The group was called a "relating" group and was designed to improve the members' interpersonal skills. Prior to taking over as leaders of the group the students observed several sessions of the group and became aware of norms operating in the group. They observed that several members frequently arrived 15 to 30 minutes late for the meeting. Other members made frequent trips to the bathroom or to the coffee machine during the meeting.
>
> Due to the constant movement of members in and out of the group, members who left the group were unsure about what topic was being discussed when they returned. Members who remained in the meeting were constantly interrupted by members who were returning. Although "relating" was the title of the group, little interpersonal relating went on in the group.
>
> Over a period of time the new student leaders, with the help of a few influential group members, tried to change the norms in the group. They limited the entry of late members to the group, encouraged members to take bathroom and beverage breaks before the meeting, and also complimented members on their increased attentiveness to one another. Under the new leadership, norms gradually changed in the group.

In the above situation the norms operating in the group were restrictive; they interfered with the group goal that members learn how to relate to one another. New norms gradually developed that enabled the group to meet its goals.

Generally, there is some latitude in the amount of conformity demanded by group members of other group members. Groups seldom demand 100 percent conformity. Although groups may tolerate more deviance from some norms (e.g., punctuality) than from others (e.g., no smoking), individuals who deviate considerably from important or highly valued norms will receive reprimands from other group members.

Norms are an important component of group functioning. Group leaders and members need to attend closely to early norm development and try to shape norms that will maximize group effectiveness.

Cohesiveness

Cohesiveness is often considered an elusive but essential component of groups. Group members frequently have an intuitive sense of when there is a high degree of cohesion in their group, but they have difficulty describing what cohesiveness is or how it developed. Cohesiveness is often described as a sense of "we-ness," the cement that holds groups together, or as the *esprit de corps* that exists within a group. Festinger (1968) refers to cohesiveness as "the resultant of all forces acting on members to remain in the group" (p. 185). Based on this definition, cohesion is viewed not as an isolated factor but as the result of a combination of factors that influence members to stay in a group. It should be pointed out that groups are neither cohesive nor uncohesive in an absolute sense, but rather have varying degrees of cohesion (Jones, Barnlund & Haiman, 1980). Groups without *any* cohesion would most likely cease to exist.

Cohesion has been associated with a number of positive outcomes for group members (Cartwright, 1968; Shaw, 1976). First, high cohesiveness is frequently associated with increased participation and better interaction between members. People tend to talk more readily and to listen more carefully in very cohesive groups (Zander, 1982). Second, in highly cohesive groups, group membership tends to be more consistent. Members are attracted toward one another and will want to attend group meetings. Third, highly cohesive groups are able to exert a strong influence on group members. Members conform more closely to group norms and engage in more goal-directed behavior for the group. Fourth, member satisfaction is high in cohesive groups; members tend to feel more secure and find enjoyment in participating in the group. Last, members of a cohesive group usually are more productive than are members of a less cohesive group. Members of groups with greater cohesion can direct their energies toward group goals without spending extensive time working out interpersonal relationship issues.

Recognizing the importance of cohesiveness, what factors influence the development of cohesiveness in a group? Cartwright (1968) has identified several factors which are summarized in Table 6.1. While some of these factors may be more influential in one type of group than another, attention to these factors and the way in which they are helping or hindering cohesiveness increases group effectiveness.

In addition to factors that foster the development of group cohesiveness, there are also factors that threaten cohesion. Loomis (1979) has identified four *threats to cohesiveness* that she encountered in health care

TABLE 6.1   Factors That Influence Group Cohesiveness

Group goals	Clear goals, based on similar member values and interests, motivate members to seek or maintain group membership.
Similarity among members	Members are frequently attracted to other members who share similar values and beliefs. There are some instances, however, in which people are attracted to people who are dissimilar in values and attitudes.
Type of interdependence among members	Groups that function in a cooperative versus competitive manner tend to have higher cohesion among members.
Leader behavior	For the most part, democratic styles of leadership are associated with higher group cohesiveness than other styles of leadership are (e.g., autocratic).
Communication structures	Decentralized communication structures, characterized by increased member interaction, are associated with increased morale and satisfaction among members.
Group activities	Members who are asked to perform group activities that they believe are above their capabilities will feel less attraction toward the group, while members who believe group activities are within their capabilities will feel more attracted toward the group.
Group atmosphere	Members are frequently attracted to groups that help members to feel valued and accepted.
Group size	Group size should match the number of members needed to complete the task. Larger groups, in which the group size interferes with group goals, can lessen cohesiveness.

Data from "The Nature of Group Cohesiveness" by Dorwin Cartwright in *Group Dynamics: Research and Theory*, 3rd ed., edited by Dorwin Cartwright and Alvin Zander, pp. 91-109. Copyright 1953, © 1960 by Harper & Row, Publishers, Inc., Copyright © 1968 by Dorwin Cartwright and Alvin Zander. By permission of Harper & Row, Publishers, Inc.

groups: (1) unstable membership, (2) group deviants, (3) subgrouping, and (4) leadership problems. According to Loomis, cohesiveness is threatened in groups with *unstable membership* because members are uncertain about the goals and the norms of the group. This threat would seem especially likely to occur in "drop-in" groups or in an inpatient setting such as a crisis unit where the clients stay in the setting for only a short period of time. *Group deviants,* the second threat identified by Loomis, hinder group cohesiveness because they vary so much from the group norms and group goals. Other members often have to expend considerable time and energy to get the deviant to conform to the group. *Subgrouping* also threatens cohesiveness because members can become more committed to the needs of the subgroup rather than those of the whole group. Subgroups or cliques often form within a large group when the needs of many members cannot be adequately addressed and satisfied. The last threat identified by Loomis is *leadership problems.* She contends that if the leader lacks the ability to develop the group's cohesiveness, it is likely to diminish.

Cohesiveness, like norms and goals, is an important component in ef fective group functioning. Cohesion does not develop instantaneously but is created gradually as members communicate with one another (Jones, Barnlund, & Haiman, 1980). Group effectiveness is enhanced when health professionals focus on helping groups to build cohesiveness.

Leader Behavior

Leader behavior is a fourth component that influences group func tioning. The leader plays a pivotal role in guiding the group to meet its goals, in developing group norms, and in facilitating communication among group members. There are many ways to view the broad area of leadership and these are detailed at length in Chapter 7. In this section, we will provide a more limited discussion of specific leader behavior in groups.

Leader behavior in groups was studied extensively by Leiberman, Yalom & Miles in 1973. They studied the behaviors of encounter group leaders and identified four dimensions that they believed explained leader behavior in therapy or personal growth groups. The four behaviors were (1) emotional stimulation, (2) caring, (3) meaning-attribution, and (4) exec utive function.

Emotional stimulation is characteristic of a leader who assumes an active role in encouraging members to express feelings, assists members in con fronting their ideas and values, and models ways to share concerns in the group. *Caring* includes those behaviors in which the leader demonstrates kindness, warmth, openness, and sincerity with group members. *Meaning- attribution* involves cognitive activities in which the leader provides expla nations or helps members to understand why they are acting or feeling a certain way. Meaning-attribution also involves assisting group members to look at either the meaning of the group's behavior as a whole or at the meaning of the behavior of individual members within the group. *Executive functioning* describes the managerial aspects of a group in which the leader sets limits, monitors rules, and attends to various procedures in the group.

Lieberman, Yalom, and Miles found there were certain amounts of these four leader behaviors that were related to effective group outcomes. The most effective leadership style was associated with leaders who exhib ited *moderate* amounts of emotional stimulation, *high* levels of caring, *high* levels of meaning-attribution, and *moderate* levels of executive function. Less effective leadership styles were associated with leaders who used ei ther too much or too little stimulation, did not demonstrate high degrees of caring toward members, offered little interpretation of the experiences of group members, and used either too much or too little executive function. Lieberman and his associates emphasized that two leader behaviors— caring and meaning-attribution—were critical to successful group leader ship. Although this study has relevance to groups in health care, it should be noted that this study was based on outcomes in encounter groups. Further research is necessary to determine whether these findings would be applicable in other kinds of health care groups.

Leader behaviors can also be discussed in terms of how the behavior of the leader should vary in different types of groups. In the typology formulated by Betz, Wilbur, and Roberts-Wilbur, which was discussed earlier in this chapter, leader behaviors were suggested for different types of groups. According to Betz and his co-authors, the leader of a task group helps group members move toward accomplishing their tasks with minimal interference. The leader of a socio-process group focuses primarily on facilitating interaction among group members, and the leader of a psycho-process group assists group members in analyzing thoughts and feelings, and guides members in changing their behavior. In essence, leader behavior is based primarily on the goals or objectives of the group.

This approach helps the leader of groups in health care to realize that different leader behaviors are indicated for different types of groups. For example, the leader of a community task force to improve interagency communication would be concerned with structuring the meeting so that members could hold a discussion on the problems and formulate solutions within a given period of time. If, however, the same leader were leading a socio-process group with dialysis patients, the leader would be more concerned with establishing a group climate that would foster sharing and supportive interactions among group members. In other words, the leader uses different behavior in different types of groups.

A drawback of looking at leader behavior in relation to group goals alone, is that members can vary considerably within various types of groups. For example, members of one task group may be motivated, prepared and eager to work in their group, while members of a different task group may be bored, uninterested, and unmotivated. The leader would need to adjust his or her behavior according to the needs and behaviors of members who comprise the particular group. As discussed in Chapter 7, leader effectiveness depends on the leader using an approach that is compatible with the needs of members and a particular situation (e.g., task, socio-process, or psycho-process group).

Member Behavior

Member behavior is just as important to effective group functioning as is leader behavior. Too often, however, the responses of group members toward one another are often overlooked or considered of only minor importance to group functioning. It is not uncommon, for example, to hear students blame a boring seminar entirely on a student leader. While blaming only the leader, students overlook the way in which their behavior (e.g., failing to participate) contributed to the ineffective and boring group.

Similarly, health professionals sometimes complain about a leader who allows a group to get sidetracked on an irrelevant issue that consumes much of the committee's allotted time. Like the students, these individuals have minimized their role in group functioning and have placed responsibility solely on the leader. Effective group functioning is influenced by *both* leader and member behavior; it is a shared responsibility.

Member behavior in small groups has been assessed in a number of ways. In this section, member behavior will be examined by looking at the roles and interaction patterns among group members.

Member roles

Early work on *member roles* in small groups was conducted by Benne and Sheats (1948), who classified the roles of group members into three broad categories: (1) group task roles, (2) group-building and maintenance roles, and (3) individual roles. Although Benne and Sheats's work was reported a number of years ago, their role categories are still recognized as useful in understanding group functioning, especially in task groups. Benne and Sheats believed that group members often fulfill more than one role in a particular group and that the various roles can be played by either the leader or individual group members.

The first category, *group task roles*, include members' roles that contribute to the group's performing its task. These roles are concerned primarily with members' obtaining and sharing information so that they can solve particular problems. The names of the group task roles and a brief description of each role are listed below:

1. *Initiator contributor:* Suggests new ideas or a new way of viewing the group task.
2. *Information seeker:* Asks for clarification or for additional information about the problem being discussed.
3. *Opinion seeker:* Asks for clarification of values that may be involved in the goal or task that the group is discussing.
4. *Information giver:* Offers facts or personal experiences that are related to problems being discussed in the group.
5. *Opinion giver:* States his or her personal beliefs that are pertinent to the group's discussion.
6. *Elaborator:* Expands on ideas being discussed by offering an example or the rationale for a suggestion.
7. *Coordinator:* Pulls together various ideas and suggestions made by group members or tries to coordinate group activities.
8. *Orientor:* Defines the present position of the group in relation to its goals or raises questions about the direction in which the discussion is moving.

9. *Evaluator-critic:* Considers the practicality or logic of suggestions offered in the group.

10. *Energizer:* Stimulates the group toward an action or decision.

11. *Procedural technician:* Assists group movement by carrying out routine tasks for the group.

12. *Recorder:* Writes down suggestions or activities decided on by the group.

As the names of these various group task roles indicate, these members' roles assist the group in meeting its task or goal obligations.

The second category, *group-building and maintenance roles,* includes roles that promote cohesiveness among group members and enhance members' ability to work together as a group. These roles focus more on developing good working relations among the members rather than on the particular task of the group. The specific roles in this category are as follows:

1. *Encourager:* Provides praise and acceptance of other members' contributions.

2. *Harmonizer:* Mediates the differences among various group members.

3. *Compromiser:* Offers to modify his or her position to maintain group harmony.

4. *Gatekeeper:* Regulates the flow of communication, facilitates quiet members' contributions, and limits the comments from members who are dominating the discussion.

5. *Standard setter:* Reminds group members of the standards they are trying to achieve.

6. *Group observer:* Comments on the various aspects of group process that are operating within the group and, in doing so, enables members to be more aware of how well they are functioning as a group.

7. *Follower:* Goes along with the movement of the group.

The third and last category of group roles described by Benne and Sheats includes *individual roles.* Unlike the previous two categories of roles that facilitate the effective functioning of groups, these roles are nonfunctional and unhelpful to the group. Individual roles are used by group members to satisfy their own particular needs. These roles do not help the group to accomplish its task (group task roles) or to facilitate good member relationships (group-building roles). The roles in this category are listed below:

1. *Aggressor:* Attacks or disapproves of others' suggestions, feelings, or values.

2. *Blocker:* Resists, without good reason, or becomes extremely negative to others' suggestions.

3. *Recognition seeker:* Calls attention repeatedly to own accomplishments and diverts the group's attention.

4. *Self-confessor:* Uses the group's time to express personal, non-group-oriented feelings or comments.

5. *Playboy-playgirl:* Plays around and displays other behavior that indicates he or she is not involved in the group process.

6. *Dominator:* Tries repeatedly to assert own authority and often interrupts other group members.

7. *Help seeker:* Tries to elicit sympathy from other group members.

8. *Special interest pleader:* Speaks for a particular group or person (e.g., "the union," "the unemployed") but is really using the group to meet personal needs and to cloak personal biases and prejudices.

According to Benne and Sheats, it is helpful when group members are able to fulfill a variety of roles so that they can meet the group's needs at various points in time. They also believe that some roles will be more helpful to a particular group at one time and less useful at another. For example, a newly formed task group may have a higher need for an initiator-contributor than for an evaluator-critic. The evaluator-critic role may be more helpful later when members start to weigh pros and cons of various alternatives.

How, then, can these three categories of group member roles be helpful to health professionals interested in group process? First, these categories remind health professionals that as members of various groups, they can influence group functioning by the type of role that they assume. Second, these categories can serve as a useful assessment tool to help professionals identify the roles that they tend to assume in groups or the roles that they *need to* utilize more in groups (see Fig. 6.3). Third, these categories can help leaders and members to diagnose group problems. For example, if a curriculum committee is repeatedly unable to get at its task of resolving curriculum problems, the members (either alone or as a group) can analyze roles that are counterproductive in the group and concentrate on developing new roles that will increase group productivity. These role categories do not prescribe or offer a formula for determining which roles at which time will assure optimal group functioning. They do, however, provide a way of looking at how various roles assumed by group members can influence group process.

Communication networks

Member behavior in small groups can also be understood by analyzing interaction patterns or the *communication networks* that exist among group members. Communication networks indicate whether communication is

ROLE ASSESSMENT CHECKLIST

Roles	Roles I usually play in groups	Roles I need to practice in groups
Group Task Roles		
1. Initiator-contributor		
2. Information seeker		
3. Opinion seeker		
4. Information giver		
5. Opinion giver		
6. Elaborator		
7. Coordinator		
8. Orienter		
9. Evaluator-critic		
10. Energizer		
11. Procedural technician		
12. Recorder		
Group Maintenance Roles		
1. Encourager		
2. Harmonizer		
3. Compromiser		
4. Gatekeeper		
5. Standard setter		
6. Group observer		
7. Follower		
Individual Roles		
1. Aggressor		
2. Blocker		
3. Recognition seeker		
4. Self-confessor		
5. Playboy/playgirl		
6. Dominator		
7. Help seeker		
8. Special interest pleader		

FIGURE 6.3 Checklist of role behaviors adapted from the role categories described by K. D. Benne and P. Sheats, "Functional Roles of Group Members." *Journal of Social Issues,* 1948, *4* (2), 41–49.

centralized (all messages flow to one person) or decentralized, and whether channels are open or closed between participants. Communication networks do not describe who sits next to whom in a group but rather the lines of communication between members.

Several common communication networks are portrayed in Figure 6.4. The symbol "o" represents a person and the line(s) connecting the "o's" represents channels of communication between participants. The *circle* pattern illustrates a decentralized pattern of communication. A group member can send a message either to the person on the left or right, but a one-

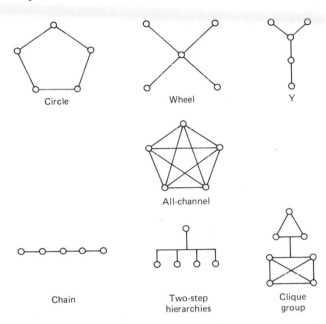

Circle   Wheel   Y

All-channel

Chain   Two-step hierarchies   Clique group

FIGURE 6.4 Types of communication networks. (From *Small Group Communication* by Michael Burgoon et. al. Copyright © 1974 by Holt, Rinehart and Winston, Inc. Reprinted by permission of Holt, Rinehart and Winston, CBS College Publishing.)

to-one communication channel does not exist between members who are on opposite sides of the circle. The *wheel* pattern illustrates that all members send their communication to and through the person who is in the center of the wheel. It is a highly centralized pattern of communication. The Y pattern is similar to the wheel, in which one member occupies a central position in the apex of the Y, but also has one member at the bottom of the Y, who is on the periphery and must send messages through another person in order to reach the most central member. The *all-channel* pattern, often considered the most desirable pattern, has open communication channels among all members. It is a decentralized pattern, and no one person retains the central position. The *chain* pattern illustrates another centralized pattern because the middle members tend to receive more communication than outside members. No direct communication link or feedback mechanism exists between members on the far ends of the chain. The *two-step hierarchies* are a form of centralized communication because individuals in the lower-status group talk primarily to the individual above them. The *clique group* shows that open communication channels generally exist among members of a subgroup but that only one channel is open between the lower subgroup and the upper subgroup.

Considerable research has been done on the impact of these various communication networks on member satisfaction and group effectiveness.

In general, there are advantages and disadvantages to each pattern. Group morale is usually better in decentralized networks such as the circle or all-channel networks than it is in the centralized networks such as the chain or wheel (Shaw, 1976). More centralized communication networks, however, are often more efficient when the group is working on a simple problem, while decentralized networks are more efficient for resolving complex problems (Burgoon, Heston, McCroskey, 1974). In addition, group members who occupy central positions in the communication channel are usually more satisfied with their position than are members who occupy distant positions that have limited communication (Shaw, 1976). While the all-channel network is often the preferred pattern, this pattern is not necessarily the best pattern at all times in all group situations. The communication network within a group needs to be compatible with the goal of the group, the complexity of the task, and the desired outcomes for group members.

Communication networks are useful for understanding how people interact in health care groups. By observing communication patterns, health professionals can become more aware of which channels are open or closed in a group. Individuals may not always be able to change a particular communication network, but by being aware of existing channels they can work toward opening new channels and closing others (Burgoon, Heston, & McCroskey, 1974). In addition, health professionals may find that one type of communication network is more effective with a specific type of group than is another. For example, the all-channel network, with high interaction among members, is often considered more effective in a *therapy* group than is a wheel pattern, in which all communication is directed through the leader (Yalom, 1975). On the other hand, a wheel or Y pattern may be the most useful network for transmitting information in certain health care situations where time is limited and the issue is not complex. Not all groups will fit into the patterns that have been identified. Only some of many patterns that have been described by communication specialists have been presented in this chapter.

Another way of looking at the interaction patterns of group members is to draw a *sociogram*. A sociogram provides a means of charting "who is talking to whom" and "how often" in a small group setting. Figure 6.5 is a sociogram depicting the interaction patterns of a group of health care members during one treatment planning session. Each line indicates that a verbal interaction has taken place between group members. Arrows indicate who sent the message. In this sociogram, the physician and psychologist direct most of their communication toward one another. Only occasionally do they direct communication toward the group as a whole or to other team members. The diagram also illustrates that the student and dietitian are quiet members; the dietitian directed only one comment to the group and the student did not send or receive any comments. In addition,

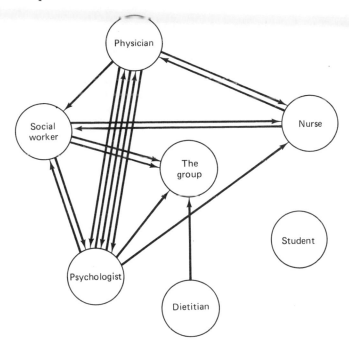

FIGURE 6.5 Sociogram of an interdisciplinary treatment planning conference.

the sociogram shows that most of the communication occurs between physician, nurse, social worker, and psychologist. For the most part, members direct their comments to specific members; little communication is directed to the group as a whole. Assuming that the goal of this particular group is to resolve a unit problem that requires input from all group members, this sociogram suggests that the dietitian and student need to be drawn into the discussion, the physician and psychologist need to direct less communication toward each other, and all members need to direct more communication to the group as a whole.

Figure 6.6 illustrates a sociogram of a group of clients in a newly formed group for adolescent single parents. In this group the leader occupies the central position where he or she receives the majority of member interaction. Very little communication is occurring between group members. If the goal of this group is to have members share experiences and concerns about single parenting, then the leader needs to move out of the central "switchboard position" and encourage more member-member or member-group interaction.

Diagrams illustrating interaction patterns among group members, whether in the form of *common communication network* diagrams or *group-specific sociograms*, help to illustrate the flow of communication in small groups. These diagrams help members to understand another important

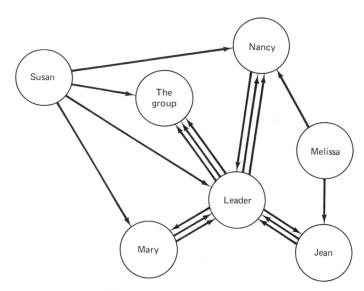

FIGURE 6.6   Sociogram of a client group.

aspect of member behavior which ultimately influences how well the group functions.

Therapeutic Factors

How do groups help people change? What interpersonal processes in groups are beneficial to members? Are there specific factors in groups that can be called "therapeutic"? Questions such as these have motivated researchers to study various groups in an effort to identify those factors that have a positive influence on group members. These studies have identified a series of positive forces, often referred to as curative factors, that operate in groups (Corsini & Rosenberg, 1955; Lieberman, Yalom & Miles 1973; Yalom, 1975). Yalom (1975) has written most extensively about these curative factors and his writing will be used as the primary source for the following discussion.

Based on his research and clinical experience, Yalom identified 11 curative factors that are crucial to the process of change. In his more recent writings Yalom has a new term for curative factors—*therapeutic factors* (1983). Yalom states that some of these factors are actually mechanisms of change while others exist more as conditions for change. The curative factors can be viewed as a cluster of factors that, taken together, in varying combinations, exert a positive "therapeutic" influence on group members. Any one factor by itself is not sufficient to create change. These therapeutic factors are generally thought of as forces operating within therapy groups, but some of these factors can operate in other groups as well.

The first therapeutic factor is called *instillation of hope*. It is essential in groups, especially during the initial phase of the group when members are not sure if the group will be able to help them. Members often become hopeful as they meet others in a group who have been in a similar situation (or worse) and who have been able to overcome their difficulties. For example, new hemodialysis patients often feel more hopeful about their ability to adjust to hemodialysis after talking with "veteran" dialysis patients (Steinglass et al., 1982). From the realization that others have succeeded, or from the encouragement that they get from other group members, the individual gains optimism that he or she will also be able to overcome similar hurdles. Self-help groups such as Recovery Incorporated and Alcoholics Anonymous rely heavily on providing hope. In these groups, seasoned members give testimonies to new members about how they were able to stop drinking or to cope with mental stress in spite of numerous difficulties.

Universality, the second therapeutic factor, occurs as group members realize that they are not alone—that their circumstances are shared by others. Universality is similar to instillation of hope but places more emphasis on the fact that, although each individual is unique, human problems are universal or shared to some extent by other people. This curative factor helps to break down the isolation that people often experience as a result of their problems. A person with cancer, for example, may frequently feel that he or she is the only person struggling with a life-threatening illness. However, when this person enters a Make Today Count group, the person realizes that he or she is not alone; others are also struggling with a serious illness.

Imparting information includes the advice, suggestions, educational information, and other ideas that the leader or members give to one another. In health care groups this therapeutic factor is frequently evident when clients are offered health teaching or practical suggestions from others. For example, a nurse may provide information on infant care to a group of new parents, or a person who has already had cardiac bypass surgery may tell patients being oriented to a cardiac surgery unit what to expect. Information becomes curative when it gives people a greater sense of control and knowledge of what to expect in their experiences or circumstances.

Altruism occurs when one group member assists another and feels good about having helped. According to Yalom, this therapeutic factor is often minimized by group members who frequently wonder how they can possibly help others when they are so absorbed and overwhelmed by their own problems. Altruistic behavior helps the giving individuals to realize that in spite of their own difficulties or concerns they still have the strength and capability to help others. Altruism reinforces the positive resources that people retain even in times of stress.

The *corrective recapitulation of the primary family group* also serves as an important therapeutic factor in groups. During group experiences, some members often respond to other group members or to the group leaders in ways that are similar to how they responded to parents or other family members. For example, in an inpatient therapy group a young male adolescent may play the male co-therapist against the female co-therapist in much the same way that he pitted his father against his mother. The adolescent also uses the same tactics to create tension in the group as he did to create tension in his family. As these parallels surface, group members can gain awareness of how they respond to family members outside the group, and they can use the group to practice new ways of behaving.

The *development of socializing techniques* also can occur within the group setting. In some groups (e.g., "relating" groups or "social awareness" groups), the development of social skills will be the primary focus of the group. In other groups, such as problem-solving groups, the development of socializing skills will not be the main focus, but it will still occur as members continually interact with one another about how to make decisions and learn to solve problems. For instance, the development of socializing techniques was evident in one group in which a young woman was initially very withdrawn and never contributed to the group. During the course of the group, other group members frequently drew the client into the group discussion and complimented her on her insightful observations. Through the assistance of group members, the woman was encouraged to participate more, and in doing so she gained more confidence and skill in socializing with others.

Imitative behavior occurs in groups when group members start to model their behavior, appearance, or language after the leader or other group members. For example, the behaviors of the therapist of a battered women's group were often imitated by members of the group. The therapist, who was also battered at one time in her life, spoke assertively in the group and demonstrated respect for herself as well as for others. Members frequently would adopt this woman's mannerisms and dress. One explanation that Yalom (1975) offers for the curative effect of imitative behavior is that it enables members to break out of old patterns and try on new behaviors so that they can determine if the new behaviors will also work for them.

Interpersonal learning occurs as members provide one another with feedback about their interpersonal behavior. Some members may seldom have received constructive feedback from others. With this new information, members can alter their behavior or learn more effective ways of interacting with others. To illustrate, a student was referred to the counseling center at the university because of the trouble she was having communicating with clients during her clinical rotation. The student set high standards for herself as well as for others, and she frequently treated clients in a condescending manner. During the group experience the student received feedback that she frequently displayed disgust (nonverbally) toward group members when they did not behave or respond in exactly the way that she desired. From this feedback and from the other things she learned in the group the student became more aware of how she often gave negative interpersonal cues to others and how this behavior could interfere with her communication with clients.

Cohesiveness is another therapeutic factor discussed by Yalom and which was discussed earlier in this chapter. Yalom states that group cohesion facilitates the development of many positive outcomes in group members such as acceptance, belonging, and feeling valued as a human being. According to Yalom (1975) group cohesiveness is not merely a curative factor but a "necessary pre-condition for effective therapy" (p. 47).

Catharsis, as a therapeutic factor, means more than just the expression of pent-up feelings. Catharsis becomes an important therapeutic factor when the ventilation of feelings is coupled with interpersonal learning. Yalom believes that "learning how to express feelings" or acquiring the skill of expressing feelings is more important than the mere act of getting them out. For example, Mr. B., a first-time criminal offender, was attending weekly group sessions at a rehabilitation center. At one meeting Mr. B. started to cry and told the group about some of his traumatic childhood experiences that he had never told anyone before. Mr. B. received a great deal of support from other members, and he learned that it was important and acceptable for him—a man—to cry and to express feelings.

Existential factors are the last of the therapeutic factors identified by Yalom. Group members realize that life is sometimes not fair, that pain cannot always be escaped, and people need to take responsibility for the way that they live their lives. Part of this curative factor is the need for people to grapple with issues of responsibility, choice, and meaning in life. Existential factors can play an important role in groups where members have terminal or progressive illness. Existential factors become curative to the extent that members are supported as they struggle with existential concerns and find their own answers to difficult questions and meaning in their circumstances.

For health professionals working in groups, it is important to assess which therapeutic factors are operating and which factors can be fostered to increase the benefit of the group for clients. Yalom (1975) states that some factors will be more important in one phase of the group than others. For example, instillation of hope and universality are especially important during the early phase. In addition, some curative factors will be more useful to some members than others (Yalom, 1983). For example, certain members may benefit a great deal from socializing techniques while other members may benefit more from imparting information. All in all, the therapeutic process of groups is strongly influenced by these 11 factors that often operate in a group setting.

In this section we have discussed the various components that influence how various groups function. In general, groups will function more effectively with clear group goals, facilitative norms, a leader who is attuned to the needs of group members, and members who occupy roles and use interaction patterns that assist the group to complete its goal. In addition, effective groups will try to build group cohesiveness and will use some of the therapeutic factors that can have a positive influence on group members.

PHASES OF SMALL GROUPS

In the previous section, we described the make-up or components of small groups. Now we would like to shift our discussion to an explanation of how groups develop and proceed over time—the phases of small groups.

Several models have been proposed to explain the phases that occur in small groups (Bales & Strodtbeck, 1951; Bennis & Shepard, 1956; Fisher, 1974; Schutz, 1958; Tuckman, 1965; Yalom, 1975). Some of these models have been constructed by assessing the various stages in task groups and others have been constructed through observations of different phases in therapy (process) groups. Considered together, this research provides a basis for suggesting that most groups go through a consistent sequence of identifiable phases. As Shaw (1976) points out, "It is probable that the kind and sequences of phases in group development are similar for all groups, although the content and duration of phases vary with the kind of group and with the group task" (p. 97).

Generally, small groups proceed through five phases: (1) orientation, (2) conflict, (3) cohesion, (4) working, and (5) termination. The time it takes to complete a single phase may vary from group to group. For example, short-term ad hoc groups may proceed through all five phases in a single session, while long-term therapy groups may spend many weeks in a single phase. Movement from one phase to another usually occurs in sequence, even though the group may return to a previous phase at one time or another. Although each phase has identifiable characteristics and qualities that make it distinct from other phases, the phases often overlap and blur into each other (Yalom 1975).

Orientation Phase

The beginning period in the small group process is called the orientation phase. During this phase, individuals spend time assessing their purpose for joining the group and also figuring out where they fit in the group. The focus of communication in the orientation phase is on questions of "in or out" (Schutz 1958). In other words, members are often trying to determine how included or excluded they are in the group. Yalom (1975) points out that during the orientation phase "members wonder what membership entails. What are the admission requirements? How much must one reveal himself or give of himself? What type of commitment must one make?" (p. 304). These concerns are illustrated by the comments made by one woman in a mastectomy support group.

> When I first read about this group in the newspaper, I wasn't sure that the group was for someone like me. I felt that I had adjusted well to my mastectomy and I wondered if the group was more for women who were having a hard time accepting their mastectomies. I also was unsure what happens in a "support" group. I had never been to one before and didn't know what to expect.
>
> At the first session I still felt uncertain about why I was there, how I would fit in with the rest of the group, and what we were going to do.
>
> After the meeting, I felt more comfortable. The leader helped to make me feel at ease. It helped to meet the other women and talk to them. Each of us had a different story to tell. I still felt unsure of myself, but I knew I was going to continue on in the group.

Schutz (1958) suggests that in the orientation phase members want to become included in the group as unique individuals; they want to belong and be related to the group but they do not want to lose a sense of who they are. Members need to feel that they can retain their unique identity even though they are joining in a group experience with others.

Tuckman (1965), whose perspective is derived from a synthesis of 50 articles on the sequential phases of groups, has labeled the orientation stage of groups the *forming phase*. He suggests that during the forming phase, members engage in testing the other members and the leader to determine what is appropriate and acceptable behavior within the group. Tuckman points out that members often express a strong sense of dependence on the leader or some other important group member for guidance regarding appropriate boundaries in a new situation. In a task group, for example, members spend time at this point trying to identify the nature of the task and the ground rules operating within the group. They frequently ask and give information about the group goal and also look to the leader for direction.

Communication during the orientation phase is often stereotypic and restricted (Yalom, 1975). Group members, who are unsure about their position in the group or the norms of the group, do not want to "rock the boat" at the beginning. As a result, members frequently introduce safe topics of conversation. For example, Schutz (1958) says it is common for new groups to engage in conversations about "goblet issues" during this early phase. The term *goblet issue* originates from a description of cocktail party conversations when people (with goblets in hand) talk about seemingly unimportant, ritualistic subjects such as the weather or common acquaintances (e.g., "Do you know so and so?"). Goblet issues serve a valuable function; they allow individuals to size up others and to determine how others will respond to them. Goblet issues give members the chance to communicate in ways that have little risk, while they simultaneously determine where they fit in the group. In general, communication during the orientation phase remains at a superficial level and there is little self-disclosure until members gain more trust in one another and feel more secure in the group setting.

Leadership in the orientation phase is directed toward helping group members satisfy their needs for belonging. It requires helping them to feel a part of the group but also to feel a sense of privacy and independence. In addition, an effective leader provides a degree of structure for the group, establishes group guidelines, shapes group norms, and assists group members in understanding the role they play in the overall purpose of the group. If the leader can help members through some of the discomfort in the orientation phase, the work of group members in subsequent phases becomes easier.

Conflict Phase

The second phase in the developmental sequence of group process is called the *conflict phase*. During this phase, members become less interested in orientation issues, such as how they are fitting into the group, and more interested in control issues, such as how they are influencing the group. Each member wants to be perceived by others as a competent group member with something to offer others. Members are concerned during this time with the relative amount of control and authority they have, compared to other members and the leader, on the decisions that are made by the group. Communication in this phase focuses on issues of "top or bottom," that is, who will have more influence in the group (top position) and who will have less influence in the group (bottom position) (Schutz, 1958). According to Schutz, during this stage there are often leadership struggles and increased competition among members. In addition, frequent discussions typically occur about what task needs to be completed, which rules of procedure will be followed, and how decisions will be made in the group (p. 171).

Conflicts resulting from struggles for control are common as a group develops. As Yalom (1975) states, "The struggle for control is part of the infrastructure of every group: it is always present, sometimes quiescent, sometimes smoldering, sometimes in full conflagration" (p. 306). In psychotherapy groups, conflicts between group members and the therapist are inevitable during this phase (Yalom, 1975). In addition to leader-member conflicts, struggles for control can also cause the development of coalitions or subgroups (Bennis & Shepard, 1956). Coalitions represent members' needs to express their own power within a subframework of the group.

The following example illustrates a task group in the conflict phase of group process.

> A task group was meeting for the second time to discuss the implementation of primary care nursing on a unit that had previously used functional nursing assignments (e.g., medication nurse, treatment nurse). Although in the first meeting there seemed to be agreement and excitement among members about implementing the primary care system, in this second meeting there was considerable conflict among members. Disagreements arose over *how* the new system should be implemented and even *if* the new system should be implemented.
>
> As the meeting progressed, one subgroup formed among staff from the day shift, who argued for implementation of the proposed plans as soon as possible. Another subgroup formed among the evening shift who argued that implementation be delayed. The evening staff contended that the recent reduction in evening personnel would make implementation of primary care impossible on their shift. The full group was unable to reach a consensus during this meeting; they had reached an impasse. Additional meetings were needed to resolve their conflicts and to reach agreement on the primary care plan.

In the Tuckman (1965) schema, the conflict phase is called *storming*, which refers to the stormy intragroup conflicts that typically occur during this phase. Tuckman suggests that members' hostility during this phase is an indication of their resistance to forming a new group structure. Members want to maintain their individuality while they struggle with the unknown of a new set of interpersonal relationships. In regard to task issues, members during this phase exhibit a greater degree of emotional response to what the group task demands of them as individuals. Specifically, members weigh options more carefully and consider how changes will affect them personally. The members of the task group mentioned earlier, for example, started expressing concern about how the new primary care system would affect them on their particular shift.

Leadership in this phase is directed toward helping the group members accept and work through group conflicts. Group members often fear that conflict and criticism will harm cohesiveness (Fisher, 1974). Members also worry that group debates and indecision are symptomatic of poor group functioning. Leaders can help members realize that increased emotional expression or conflict is normal during this phase (see Chapter 8). Leaders can also help members understand that group decisions take time and that a "mulling-over time" helps groups to make high-quality decisions (Fisher, 1974).

Furthermore, leaders can assist group members to satisfy their needs for control or influence within the group during the conflict phase. Some members may want a lot of responsibility and influence, while others may prefer less (Schutz, 1958). Leaders can help both types of group members. For example, a leader could give a special assignment to a member who wants more influence and have that member report back to the group in the following session. Leaders can also allow other members with lower desires for control to maintain lower profiles in the group during this time. As members satisfy their needs for control, conflicts eventually lessen and the group moves to the third phase.

Cohesion Phase

The third phase in the development of groups, the *cohesion phase,* usually follows on the heels of the control struggles and conflicts. This phase can emerge for a variety of reasons. For example, members of a task group may become aware of time pressures and realize that they need to start moving toward consensus in order to meet their objectives. Members of a therapy group may become more understanding of one another's differences and more able to accept these differences in the group. Still others may observe the splits and factions of the previous stage and feel the need to move closer rather than farther away from others. Essentially, members want to develop more unity during this phase.

Communication in this phase often focuses on issues of "near or far" (Schutz, 1958). Group members want to maintain close positive relationships with each other but they also do not want to become too intimate. As group members start feeling more positive about each other and the group, they also feel more secure expressing their opinions; members now think that others will listen and be supportive of them. Yalom (1975) points out that during this phase there is an increase of morale among members; their trust in one another builds and they dare to tell others more about themselves (p. 311). In addition, during this phase it is not unusual for group members to suppress negative comments and feelings for the sake of group unity.

The cohesion phase is similar to the *norming phase* in Tuckman's model. Tuckman (1965) points out that during the norming phase, group members accept the idiosyncrasies of fellow group members and they try to maintain and perpetuate the group and its norms. For example, a group member may shrug off a bizarre comment or an eccentric behavior by another group member and say, "Oh, that's just the way he acts when he's nervous." Members also attempt to protect the uniqueness of the group and to ensure harmony within the group. During this phase there is greater expression of ideas, opinions, and observations on task issues.

Leadership during this phase poses fewer problems than during other phases because of the positive feelings and the unified sense of direction in the group at this time. The leader can put the group on "automatic pilot" during this phase as members work in harmony on group objectives.

The leader provides guidance and direction only as needed during this phase and essentially assumes a nondominant role (Schuurmans, 1964).

Working Phase

The fourth phase in group development is called the *working phase*. This phase is similar to the cohesion phase but it involves more time, greater depth, and increased disclosure among group members (Yalom, 1975). There can be considerable variability in this stage from one type of group to another. In long-term therapy groups, this phase can take a couple of months to develop. In some short-term task groups, a distinct working phase may never be clearly observable; the work of this phase may actually be carried out in the conflict and cohesion phases.

Tuckman (1965) calls this phase the *performing phase,* because members now perform the work they have set out to do. At this point members feel secure to express both positive and negative emotions in task groups, yet communication usually remains positive, even to the point of members joking and praising each other (Fisher, 1974). The group spirit and the feeling of unity among members are often high during the working phase.

Little directive leader behavior is needed in task groups during this phase since members are actively solving problems and working with one another in goal-directed activity. In therapy groups, leader behavior will vary according to the various issues in the group (see Yalom, 1975, for a more extensive discussion of the therapist's responsibilities during the working phase). Some groups will require more intervention by the therapist while others will not.

Termination Phase

The last phase is called the *termination phase.* This phase usually occurs when the goals of a group have been fulfilled or when the allotted time has run out and the members begin to consider the implications of ending the group. Yalom (1975) points out that "the end of the group is a real loss; patients gradually come to realize that it can never be recovered, that even if they continue a relationship with one member or a fragment of the group, nevertheless the entire group will be gone forever" (p. 374). As we discussed in Chapter 5, termination is a time when individuals experience a whole range of emotions, from guilt to fear, depending on their own unique previous experiences with the termination process.

Schutz (1958) contends that groups often go through a cycle during termination that is the reverse of what they experience during the formative phases. He suggests, for example, that during this disintegration phase of groups, members first deal with their *affectional* ties; they express positive and negative feelings about the group. Next they focus on *control* is-

TABLE 6.2   Typical Kinds of Communication in Different Phases of Groups

ORIENTATION	CONFLICT	COHESION	WORKING	TERMINATION
Safe topics	Disagreements and debates	Supportive comments	Positive comments	Summary of discussions
Goblet issues	Discussions about rules and procedures	Greater self-disclosure	Consensus statements	Expression of feelings
Little self-disclosure	"Top or bottom" discussions	Suppression of negative feelings	Problem-solving comments	Closure statements
"In or out" discussions		"Close or far" discussions	In-depth self-disclosure	

sues; they consider their relationships to the leader. Lastly, they discuss issues related to *inclusion* as a group member; they discuss their commitment to group members and contemplate what it will be like to no longer be in the group (Schutz, 1958, p. 174).

During the termination phase, leaders nee ₁ to summarize the work of the group, emphasize goal accomplishmen' , and help group members find a sense of closure as they confront their feelings about the approaching end of the group and the members' relationships. Each group member will confront termination in a unique way and the leader can help the group by being sensitive to these differences. Finally, leaders also need to express their own feelings about the group's coming to an end.

In summary, most groups progress through five phases: orientation, conflict, cohesion, working, and termination. Table 6.2 summarizes the communication that often occurs during each phase, although at times there is overlap between the phases. By being aware of these phases and the issues that frequently surface in each phase, health professionals can increase their capacity to work effectively in groups.

TECHNIQUES FOR DECISION MAKING IN SMALL GROUPS

How does a small group of people arrive at a decision? What procedures increase the chance that a group will choose the best solution to a problem? These questions will be considered in this final section of the chapter. There are a variety of techniques that can be used to make decisions and arrive at solutions in small groups. Probably the most familiar technique is Dewey's creative problem-solving procedure (1910), which is described at length in Chapter 8 as a win-win approach to decision making in conflict situations. In this procedure group members proceed through five steps: (1) define the problem, (2) identify solutions, (3) evaluate solutions, (4) select the best solutions, and (5) implement and evaluate the solution. This technique provides a series of steps for group members to follow in decision-making situations and is a commonly used approach to solving problems in health care.

In addition to Dewey's creative problem-solving technique, there are several other effective decision-making procedures that can be used by groups. Three of these procedures seem particularly useful for understanding decision making in health care task groups: (1) brainstorming, (2) the nominal group technique, and (3) the Delphi method. Each procedure provides a different but practical approach to group decision making.

Brainstorming

Brainstorming is a discussion technique developed by Osborn (1957) to stimulate the production and generation of creative ideas in groups. Brainstorming enhances creative thinking and expands the imaginations of group members by allowing them to express their ideas freely without being inhibited by the fear of criticism. The assumption that underlies brainstorming is that if group members feel uninhibited about expressing their ideas, more ideas and better ideas will emerge from the group.

The brainstorming technique is relatively easy to use in small group discussions. The rules for brainstorming are provided in Table 6.3. Although all the rules are important, rule 3—withholding criticism—deserves special attention. For brainstorming to work effectively, group members must not judge or criticize the ideas expressed by others. This nonjudgmental approach is often difficult to master because most people are conditioned to evaluate the pros and cons of a new idea as soon as it is introduced in a group. Criticism, however, is counterproductive to the overall goal of brainstorming because members who fear criticism will most likely express conventional solutions and withhold "wild" or innovative ideas.

Brainstorming provides a practical tool to assist a group in developing a multitude of ideas, some of which may be very creative, regarding an issue, problem, or solution. For example, brainstorming was used by a group of health professionals at a mental health conference. Participants were

TABLE 6.3   Rules for Brainstorming

1.	Generate numerous ideas about an issue.
2.	Welcome free thinking and facilitate open expression of ideas.
3.	Withhold any evaluation or criticism of the ideas that are expressed.
4.	Build and improve on ideas already expressed.

asked to think of ways to provide services to an increasing number of psychiatric clients who were being discharged from a long-term psychiatric hospital at the same time state revenues for mental health services were being reduced. Members were divided into a number of small groups and instructed on the guidelines for creative brainstorming. From this process a number of innovative ways for combining community services and decreasing agency overlap were generated.

In addition to encouraging group members to think creatively, brainstorming can also create positive feelings and trust among group members. For example, in the situation just described many of the professionals from the different agencies did not know one another before the conference. The brainstorming technique became an enjoyable activity that enabled members to participate in the group and get to know one another without having their competence evaluated with each suggestion they made. As a result members gain a sense of having had an impact on the group process, and they feel more a part of the group.

Nominal Group Technique

The nominal group technique was developed by Delbecq and Van de Ven (1970) based on their studies of decision making in various groups. This technique is designed to promote the expression of many high-quality ideas from members who initially work *independently* and then share their ideas with the group (Van de Ven & Delbecq, 1974). Unlike the freewheeling expression of ideas in brainstorming, this technique uses a more systematic procedure that ensures that each member will have the opportunity to present an idea to the group for consideration. The overall goal of the nominal group technique is to arrive at a group decision that represents a *pooled* judgment that is based on the independent ideas of all group members.

Table 6.4 presents the format for using the nominal group technique. It usually takes approximately 1½ hours for a group to complete all four steps of this process. The format utilizes both the independent thinking of members (e.g., writing down ideas) and group interaction (e.g., discussing the ideas) in order to arrive at a joint decision. The nominal group method is used when individuals can be brought together at one location and when the problem requires a relatively quick solution. Stech and Ratliffe (1976) point out that this procedure can be used by a group to define problems, to delineate criteria for a solution, to actually develop solutions, or to assess the quality of proposed solutions. In health care, this approach can be useful for determining program priorities or for identifying needed program content in areas such as staff development (Cooper, 1982).

As a decision-making procedure, the nominal group technique has several advantages (Van de Ven & Delbecq, 1974). First, when members

TABLE 6.4   Format for the Nominal Group Technique

1.   Group members, without any discussion, *independently* write down their ideas about a problem or task.

2.   Each group member presents an idea to the group without discussion. This process continues around the table until all ideas have been expressed. The ideas are then summarized and listed on either a chart or a chalkboard.

3.   Members discuss each of the recorded ideas for the purpose of clarification and evaluation.

4.   Members independently give their own priority rankings of ideas. These independent rankings are added together and averaged. The final group decision emerges from the pooled outcome of the independent rankings.

Based on A. H. Van de Ven and A. L. Delbecq, "The Effectiveness of Nominal, Delphi, and Interacting Group Decision Making Processes." *Academy of Management Journal, 1974, 17* (4), 605–621.

are given the opportunity to write down their own ideas independently, their ideas tend to be more problem-centered and of higher quality. Second, the technique allows all members an *equal* opportunity to express their views and also an *equal* opportunity to vote on the group decision. This technique prevents a group discussion from being dominated by a few influential members. The structured format of the nominal group technique helps group members gain a sense of accomplishment as well as a sense of closure regarding the group process. On the negative side, this technique can be time consuming and somewhat difficult to implement in all situations.

Delphi Method

The Delphi method of decision making was initially developed by Dalkey and his associates (1963, 1969), who used this method to gather data from groups of experts for the purpose of making forecasts about future events. More recently, in health care, the Delphi method has been employed to determine priorities in such areas as nursing research (Western Interstate Commission, 1974) and cancer nursing (Oberst, 1978). In this method the participants are usually in different geographical locations and they do not meet for face-to-face interaction as they typically do in the brainstorming and nominal group technique procedures. The Delphi method structures the group communication process so that a large group of individuals can work together as a whole and solve a complex problem (Linstone & Turoff, 1975, p. 3).

The Delphi method consists of soliciting information from a group of individuals through a series of sequential questionnaires about a particular topic (see Table 6.5). For example, in the Oberst cancer nursing study (1978), questionnaires were sent to 575 cancer nurses asking them to identify 5 important questions about the nursing care of cancer patients. The

TABLE 6.5   Procedures Followed in the Delphi Method of Group Decision Making

1.	Group members are sent a questionnaire which asks them to identify important questions or issues on a specific topic.
2.	Members' responses are compiled and a second questionnaire is administered which asks members to assess and prioritize the list of responses derived from the first round.
3.	Step 2 is repeated in subsequent rounds. Each time the priorities of members are summarized and narrowed down to those which are the most important. The results are returned to each group member for further ranking and evaluation.
4.	In the last phase, a final summary and ranking is provided to each member of the group. This represents a synthesis of the series of sequential rankings completed in all prior rounds.

Based on A. H. Van de Ven and A. L. Delbecq, "The Effectiveness of Nominal, Delphi, and Interacting Group Decision Making Processes." *Academy of Management Journal,* 1974, *17* (4), 605–621.

first round of questionnaires produced 1,800 questions, which were then grouped into 101 new items by the monitoring team. Next the cancer nurses were sent a second questionnaire which asked them the following three questions concerning the newly grouped 101 items:

1. Should nursing assume research leadership in this area?
2. How much value would researching this problem have for practicing nurses?
3. What impact on patient welfare is the solution to this problem likely to have? (Oberst, 1978, p. 282)

Generally, after three or four rounds of questionnaires a summary evaluation is generated that indicates the degree to which the group has reached consensus in their priority rankings. In the Oberst study, after a third round of questionnaires was returned, the data were analyzed and the ten patient care items receiving the highest ranking by cancer nurses were identified.

The major advantages of the Delphi method are that it produces a large quantity of high-quality responses, it is free of pressures for respondents to conform, and it provides a moderate degree of closure to group members (Van de Ven & Delbecq, 1974). The method also makes it possible to collect the ideas of people in a variety of geographic locations who normally would be unable to commit time and resources to attend a group meeting.

The major disadvantages of the Delphi method are that it does not allow for the development of emotions and feelings in the group, and it does not allow for face-to-face feedback and clarification (Van de Ven & Delbecq, 1974). Overall, however, the Delphi method is a very useful, though time-consuming, decision-making technique.

The group decision-making techniques discussed in this section are only a few of many methods that can be used by health practitioners. The techniques presented here are fairly straightforward and practical means of facilitating creative decision making among various groups of health professionals.

SUMMARY

Small group communication refers to the verbal and nonverbal communication that occurs among a collection of individuals whose relationships make them to some degree interdependent.

Many different types of small groups exist in health care settings. The various types of health care groups can be distinguished in a general way according to the degree to which they are content oriented or process oriented. A more specific typology divides groups into three categories: task-process groups, socio-process groups, and psycho-process groups. The three categories are further distinguished from one another according to the group's objective, size, leader behavior, and member behavior and expectations. In task groups the communication focus is extrapersonal, in socio-process groups the focus is interpersonal, and in psycho-process groups the communication is focused on intrapersonal issues.

There are several components of small groups that can affect the functioning of small groups. Goals provide the reason and motivation for people to form a group. In general, it is important for goals to be clear, realistic, and shared to a considerable extent among group members. Norms are the rules established by group members that indicate what types of behaviors are appropriate within the group. Norms can be overt or covert, and they can facilitate or restrict the group's activity. Cohesiveness is the sense of "we-ness" shared by group members that stimulates members to stay in a group. Leader behavior plays an important role in guiding the group, developing norms, and facilitating communication. Specific leader behaviors such as emotional stimulation, caring, meaning-attribution, and executive functioning are related to effective group functioning. Member behavior, which is often overlooked, is also an important component. Member behavior can be described in terms of the roles occupied by group members (task roles, group-building and maintenance roles, and individual roles) or in terms of the interaction patterns used by group members. Therapeutic factors, often referred to as curative factors, are also an important component in group functioning. Eleven therapeutic factors that can have a positive influence on group members have been identified as operating in groups at one time or another.

Groups commonly progress through five phases: orientation, conflict, cohesion, working, and termination. The orientation phase occurs at the beginning as members try to determine how they are related to each other and to the group goal. Communication usually stays on safe topics with limited amounts of self-disclosure during this phase. The conflict phase centers around issues of authority and control as members try to determine how much influence they have in the group. In this phase, communication is frequently marked by disagreements and dissent among members. The cohesion phase is a time when group members draw closer together and develop a greater sense of unity. Members often suppress negative communication and become more supportive of one another during this time. The working phase is marked by greater disclosure and more profound discussion of group issues. The termination phase occurs at the end of the process as the group completes its tasks or goals. During this time, issues are summarized and members' feelings toward one another and the group are expressed.

Practitioners who work in health care groups can select from among several different decision-making techniques. Three specific techniques are brainstorming, the nominal group technique, and the Delphi method. Brainstorming is a discussion technique that stimulates the generation of creative ideas in groups. It allows group members to express their opinions freely without being inhibited by the critical evaluations of others. The nominal group technique is designed to promote high-quality independent opinions and ideas in groups that meet face to face. It allows a group to arrive at a joint decision that is equally representative of all group members. The Delphi method is often used with groups that cannot meet face to face and when there is considerable time available. In this method a series of sequential questionnaires elicit members' priority rankings about a given topic, and a mutual consensus is the result.

REFERENCES

Bales, R. F., & Strodtbeck, F. L. Phases in group problem-solving. *Journal of Abnormal and Social Psychology,* 1951, *46,* 485–495.

Benne, K. D., & Sheats, P. Functional roles of group members. *Journal of Social Issues,* 1948, *4*(2), 41–49.

Bennis, W. G., & Shepard, H. A. A theory of group development. *Human Relations,* 1956, *9,* 415–437.

Betz, R. L., Wilbur, M. P., & Roberts-Wilbur, J. A structural blueprint for group facilitators: Three group modalities. *The Personnel and Guidance Journal,* 1981, *60*(1), 31–37.

Burgoon, M., Heston, J. K., & McCroskey, J. *Small group communication: A functional approach.* New York: Holt, Rinehart & Winston, 1974.

Cartwright, D. The nature of group cohesiveness. In D. Cartwright & A. Zander (Eds.), *Group dynamics: Research and theory,* 3rd ed. New York: Harper & Row, Publishers, Inc., 1968.

Cartwright, D., & Zander, A. (Eds.) *Group dynamics: Research and theory,* 3rd ed. New York: Harper & Row, Publishers, Inc., 1968.

Cooper, S. Methods of teaching revisited—The nominal group process. *Journal of Continuing Education in Nursing,* 1982, *13*(2), 38–39.

Corsini, R., & Rosenberg, B. Mechanisms of group psychotherapy: Processes and dynamics. *Journal of Abnormal and Social Psychology,* 1955, *51,* 406–411.

Cronenwett, L. Elements and outcomes of a postpartum support group program. *Research in Nursing and Health,* 1980, *3*(1), 33–41.

Dalkey, N. C. *The Delphi method: An experimental study of group opinion.* Santa Monica, Calif.: Rand Corp., 1969.

Dalkey, N. C., & Helmer, O. An experimental application of the Delphi method to the use of experts. *Management Sciences,* 1963, *9*(3), 458–467.

Delbecq, A. L., & Van de Ven, A. H. Nominal group techniques for involving clients and experts in program planning. *Academy of Management Proceedings,* 1970, 208–227.

Deutsch, M. The effects of cooperation and competition upon group process. In D. Cartwright & A. Zander (Eds.), *Group dynamics: Research and theory,* 3rd ed. New York: Harper & Row, Publishers, Inc., 1968.

Dewey, J. *How we think.* Lexington, Mass.: D.C. Health & Co., 1910.

Festinger, L. Informal social communication. In D. Cartwright & A. Zanders, (Eds.), *Group dynamics: Research and theory,* 3rd ed. New York: Harper & Row, Publishers, Inc., 1968.

Fisher, B. A. *Small group decision making: Communication and the group process.* New York: McGraw-Hill Book Company, 1974.

Forsyth, D. M., & Cannady, N. J. Preventing and alleviating staff burnout through a group. *Journal of Psychiatric Nursing and Mental Health Services,* 1981, *19*(9), 35–38.

Goldberg, A. A., & Larson, C. E. *Group communication: Discussion processes and applications.* Englewood Cliffs, N.J.: Prentice-Hall, Inc., 1975.

Jones, S. E., Barnlund, D. C., & Haiman, F. S. *The dynamics of discussion: Communication Groups,* 2nd ed. New York: Harper & Row, Publishers, Inc., 1980.

Klein, R. H. The patient-staff community meeting: A tea party with the mad hatter. *International Journal of Group Psychotherapy,* 1981, *31*(2), 205–222.

Lieberman, M. A., Yalom, I. D., & Miles, M. B. *Encounter groups: First facts.* New York: Basic Books, Inc., Publishers, 1973.

Linstone, H. A. & Turoff, M. *The Delphi method: Techniques and applications.* Reading, Mass.: Addison-Wesley Publishing Co., Inc., 1975.

Loomis, M. E. *Group process for nurses.* St. Louis. The C. V. Mosby Company, 1979.

Loomis, M. E. & Dodenhoff, J. T. Working with informal patient groups. *American Journal of Nursing,* 1970, *70*(9), 1939–1944.

Marram, G. D. *The group approach in nursing practice,* 2nd ed. St. Louis: The C. V. Mosby Company, 1978.

Naisbitt, J. *Megatrends: Ten new directions transforming our lives.* New York: Warner Books, Inc., 1982.

Oberst, M. T. Priorities in cancer nursing research. *Cancer Nursing,* 1978, *1*(4), 281–290.

Osborn, A. F. *Applied imagination: Principles and procedures of creative thinking,* rev. ed. New York: Charles Scribner's Sons, 1957.

Raven, B. H., & Rietsema, J. The effects of varied clarity of group goal and group path upon the individual and his relation to his group. *Human Relations,* 1957, *10,* 29–44.

Schuurmans, M. J. Five functions of the group therapist. *American Journal of Nursing,* 1964, *64*(12), 108–110.

Schutz, W. C. *FIRO: A three dimensional theory of interpersonal behavior.* New York: Holt, Rinehart & Winston, Inc., 1958.

Shaw, M. E. *Group dynamics: The psychology of small group behavior*, 2nd ed. New York: McGraw-Hill Book Company, 1976.

Stech, E., & Ratliffe, S. A. *Working in groups: A communication manual for leaders and participants in task-oriented groups*. Skokie, Ill.: National Textbook Company, 1976.

Steinglass, P., Gonzalez, S., Dosovitz, I., & Reiss, D. Discussion groups for chronic hemodialysis patients and their families. *General Hospital Psychiatry*, 1982, *4*(1), 7–13.

Tubbs, S. L. *A systems approach to small group interaction*. Reading, Mass.: Addison-Wesley Publishing Company, 1978.

Tuckman, B. W. Developmental sequences in small groups. *Psychological Bulletin*, 1965, *63*(6), 384–399.

Van de Ven, A. H., & Delbecq, A. L. The effectiveness of nominal, Delphi and interacting group decision making processes. *Academy of Management Journal*, 1974, *17*(4), 605–621.

Western Interstate Commission for Higher Education. *Delphi survey of clinical nursing research priorities*. C. A. Lindeman, Principal Investigator. Boulder, Colo.: The Commission, 1974.

Yalom, I. D. *The theory and practice of group psychotherapy*, 2nd ed. New York: Basic Books, Inc., Publishers, 1975.

Yalom, I. D. *Inpatient group psychotherapy*. New York: Basic Books, Inc., Publishers, 1983.

Zander, A. F. *Making groups effective*. San Francisco, Calif.: Jossey-Bass, Inc., Publishers, 1982.

7 Communication in Health Care Organizations

The communication system of an organization is an increasingly powerful determinant of the organization's overall effectiveness, and it may have a limiting effect on the ability of the organization to grow, to perform efficiently, or to survive.

—Farace, Monge, and Russell, 1977

Changes in the size and complexity of health care organizations, increased technology in health care, shifts in ethical values, and new types of management strategies have all heightened the need for more effective communication within health care organizations. Leaders who can communicate effectively are needed at all levels in health care organizations, from administrative and management positions to direct patient care areas.

In previous chapters we discussed health communication as it occurs in different types of health care relationships (e.g., professional-client, professional-family) and as it occurs in small groups. Now we will shift our focus and consider communication from a broader perspective—as it occurs in health care *organizations*.

We begin with a discussion of a definition and related model of organizational communication as it applies to health care organizations. Next we provide descriptions of how organizational factors such as philosophy, structure, communication channels, and sources of power affect communication in health care organizations. Then we discuss the important relationship between leaders and followers in health care organizations, giving special attention to communication issues that arise in various leadership situations. The chapter concludes by applying leader-follower concepts to positions in health care organizations.

AN ORGANIZATIONAL COMMUNICATION PERSPECTIVE

Much has been written about organizational behavior (e.g., Argyris, 1960; Katz & Kahn, 1966; Likert, 1961; Mayo, 1933; & Taylor, 1911). For years researchers have analyzed and assessed the nature of organizations in order to understand how organizations function and also to find ways to make them work more effectively. In this chapter certain aspects of organizational research that have direct application to health communication will be discussed. Since organizational communication includes a vast body of research, we will not summarize the entire area but will instead focus on the ideas and research in the area that are particularly useful to understanding communication in health organizations.

Definition of Organizational Communication

In order to define the term *organizational communication,* it is necessary first to answer the question, What is meant by an organization? Rogers and Agarwala-Rogers (1976) state that an organization is a system of individuals who work together, using a hierarchy of ranks and a division of labor to achieve common goals (p. 6). Similarly, King (1981) suggests that "An organization is composed of human beings with prescribed roles and positions who use resources to accomplish personal and organizational goals" (p. 119). Common to both definitions is the idea that organizations involve a system of *people* within a particular structure who are working *interdependently* in their various capacities to attain mutual *goals.* In health care, examples of organizations include hospitals, rehabilitation centers, intermediate health care facilities, nursing homes, hospices, health maintenance organizations, home health care agencies, and public health departments, to name a few. The people within these various health care structures must work interdependently and communicate with each other to achieve various health care goals.

Earlier in the book, communication was defined as the process of sharing information through a set of common rules. We emphasized that human communication is a process that is transactional and multidimensional. Considering this earlier definition of communication and the preceding discussion of organizations, *organizational communication* can be defined as *the process whereby a system of interdependent individuals in various roles and positions share information according to a common set of rules in order to achieve mutual goals.* The following section provides a model of organizational communication based on this definition and relates it to the health communication model presented in Chapter 1.

An Organizational Communication Model

As a specific field of academic study, organizational communication is very new; the first college textbook on this subject appeared in 1973. However, since that time there has been a great deal of writing and research in this field. Goldhaber (1983) has developed a paradigm of organizational communication that visually represents the central components of the organizational communication process (see Fig. 7.1). Although the paradigm is very simplistic, it is helpful in conceptualizing communication in health care organizations in a way that is compatible with the health communication model discussed in Chapter 1. Goldhaber's emphasis on organizations and people-messages parallels a similar emphasis on health care contexts and participants (e.g., professionals, clients) and their health transactions in the health communication model.

The paradigm in Figure 7.1 illustrates three major aspects of organizational communication:

1. Organizational communication occurs within a complex open system which is influenced by and influences its environment;
2. Organizational communication involves messages and their flow, purpose, direction, and media; and
3. Organizational communication involves people and their attitudes, feelings, relationships, and skills. (Goldhaber, 1983, p. 17)

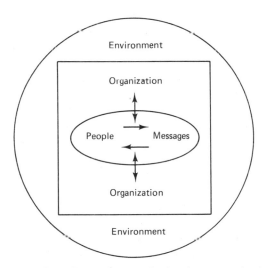

FIGURE 7.1 Paradigm of organizational communication. (From Goldhaber, Gerald M., *Organizational Communication,* 3rd ed. © 1974, 1979, 1983 Wm. C. Brown Publishers, Dubuque, Iowa. All Rights Reserved. Reprinted by permission.)

In health care organizations, *environment,* as represented in Figure 7.1, refers to external factors that can influence health care relationships inside the organization. Government regulations or external economic pressures toward cost containment are examples of environmental factors that have an impact on the personnel and services in health organizations. The *organization* in the diagram refers to the organizational structure such as the hospitals or health care agencies in which health care services are provided. Organizational changes made in response to environmental changes impact on the personnel in health care agencies. *People* and *messages,* which are the focal point of the paradigm, refer to the transactions that occur between individuals in the health care organizations (e.g., professional-professional, professional-client interactions). These interactions may also be affected by changes in agency policies. Health care organizations are not insulated institutions but rather are affected by factors inside and outside of the organization.

In this chapter we will focus on how organizational factors affect the transactions of individuals in health care settings. To make communication in health organizations more effective, it is necessary to be aware of these factors and how they influence communication.

FACTORS THAT INFLUENCE COMMUNICATION IN HEALTH CARE ORGANIZATIONS

There are several factors that can influence the communication within a health care organization. In this section four factors and their impact on communication within an organization will be discussed: (1) organizational philosophies, (2) organizational structures, (3) communication channels, and (4) sources of power.

Organizational Philosophies

The way in which communication functions in health care organizations can be viewed from three different philosophical viewpoints concerning organizational behavior: (1) scientific management, (2) human relations, and (3) systems theory. The *scientific management* perspective, which is based on the early work of Taylor (1911), focuses on structures and ways of maximizing individual output through reward systems. In this approach, the emphasis is on communication that is formal, hierarchical, one-sided, vertical (top-down), and task related (Rogers & Agarwala-Rogers, 1976, p. 34). Although the scientific management perspective is an older approach to organizational behavior, it can still be observed in some health care agencies that have strong authoritarian leadership and that emphasize top-down communication and individual worker productivity.

The *human relations* perspective, which developed after the scientific management school, focuses on satisfying the social needs of employees rather than their economic needs and emphasizes group member satisfaction rather than organizational efficiency (Rogers & Agarwala-Rogers, 1976). According to this approach, attending to the human needs of employees increases productivity. Interpersonal communication is of central importance in organizations that are run from the human relations vantage point. Workers are encouraged to discuss their concerns with each other and with management. Communication flows *between* workers and management rather than *from* management *down to* workers. Health care organizations that minimize hierarchies and authoritarian leadership and maximize democratic leadership, participatory decision making, and employee involvement would be examples of the human relations school.

A third approach to organizational communication is based on general systems theory. The *systems perspective* emphasizes that organizations are composed of many subunits or subsystems (e.g., departments) that are interdependent and that interact with the environment (Katz & Kahn, 1966). From this perspective the organization is considered to be more than just the sum of its parts. Rather than placing the focus on top-down communication or small group communication, systems theory looks at communication in the organization as a whole: Communication is like the connective tissue that holds the organization together. As Rogers and Agarwala-Rogers (1976) point out:

> Communication is the basic process facilitating the interdependence of the parts of the total system; it is the mechanism of coordination. The role of communication is to be a "harmonizer" of the organization, an orchestrator of its parts (p. 57).

A systems perspective gives attention to how communication flows between and within departments of a health care organization and between the organization and the community.

Each organization operates from its own organizational philosophy. Some health care organizations operate from a scientific management perspective, which emphasizes productivity and task completion. Other health care organizations emphasize a human relations perspective and, as a result, place more importance on the satisfaction of their employees. The systems perspective regards organizations almost like complex organisms. These different organizational philosophies set the climate for the types of interpersonal relationships and interactions that will be fostered within the organization.

Organizational Structures

Structure affects process. In organizational settings, the structure of the organization affects the communication that will take place within it. Some organizational structures facilitate communication among people, while other organizational structures hinder it. Two structural facets that can impact on internal communication are (1) the shape of the organizational hierarchy and (2) the span of control given to various individuals in the organization.

Organizational shape

Organizational structures are often categorized as tall or flat. Tall organizations have many different levels in their organizational structure and also many middle-management positions (see Fig. 7.2). The managers in tall organizations frequently serve as "gatekeepers" who regulate the kind and amount of communication that flows up the organizational hierarchy (Sanford, Hunt, & Bracey, 1976). In tall structures, supervisors are able to exert more control over subordinates and they can also maintain a close watch over their activities (Bernhard & Walsch, 1981). Tall structures are advantageous in promoting lines of authority and accountability within the organization but disadvantageous because the many levels hinder people lower in the hierarchy from getting messages through to administrators higher up.

Flat structures, illustrated in Figure 7.3, have fewer intermediate levels in the organization and, as a result, fewer middle-management people.

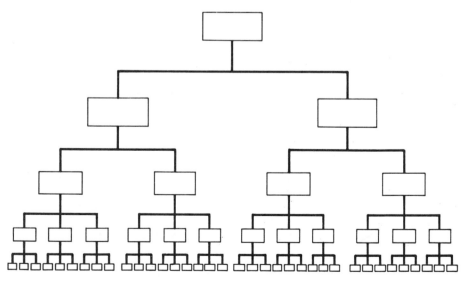

FIGURE 7.2 Tall organizational structure.

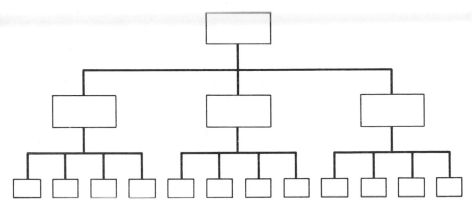

FIGURE 7.3 Flat organizational structure.

Flat organizational structures are often decentralized, giving employees more input into organizing and implementing work activities. The advantages of flat decentralized structures are that employees have more control over their own work, the communication distance between people at different levels in the organization is shortened, and costly middle managers are eliminated (Bernhard & Walsch, 1981; Veninga, 1982). The main disadvantage of flat structures is that the elimination of numerous middle managers leaves the remaining managers to supervise a greater number of employees. Veninga (1982) points out that tall or flat structures are not inherently good or bad, but each structure has advantages in some situations and disadvantages in other situations.

Many hospitals have tall, centralized organizational structures. However, there seems to be a trend for hospitals to decentralize, at least in some areas of their organizational structures. Donovan (1975) reports, for example, that some nursing departments are decentralizing by dividing nursing administration between two assistant directors and eliminating several intermediate supervisors. Similarly, in some patient care areas, there is movement to change from the more hierarchical team management structure to the less hierarchical primary care structure (see Fig. 7.4). This change represents a move toward decentralization that is intended to foster staff members' control and make them more accountable for their services.

Span of control

The number of people a manager is required to supervise is called the span of control. With a narrow span of control a manager may supervise only 2 or 3 people. A manager who has a broader span of control may supervise 30 or more people (see Fig. 7.5). Veninga (1982) reports that at one time 7 employees was considered the ideal number of employees for a manager to supervise, whereas, more recently, the ideal span of control is considered arbitrary and can vary depending on factors such as the work task to be

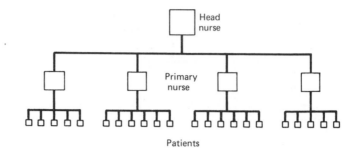

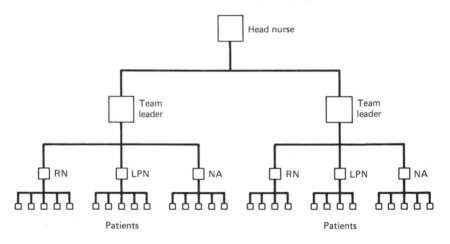

Organization of the primary nursing delivery system

Organization of the team nursing delivery system

FIGURE 7.4 Comparison of two different health care delivery systems. (From L. A. Bernhard and M. Walsh, *Leadership: The Key to the Professionalization of Nursing.* New York: McGraw-Hill Book Company, 1981, pp. 40, 41.)

accomplished. Veninga notes that for simple repetitive tasks a large span of control (one supervisor per 40 employees) may be acceptable. However, when workloads are unpredictable and more interdependence among employees is necessary, then a smaller span of control may be desirable.

Commenting on span of control in nursing departments, Stevens

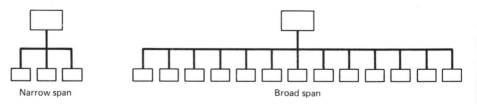

FIGURE 7.5 A comparison of a narrow and broad span of control.

(1983) states that a "nursing executive who has 20 head nurses reporting to her [or him] with no intervening management layer has exceeded the logical span of control unless those persons are exceptionally experienced and need little actual direction" (p. 48). She also notes that a nursing supervisor with only a few head nurses to supervise may not be able to justify his or her position. Obviously a supervisor with a span of 20 employees will have less time to interact with each employee while a supervisor with a smaller span of control would have greater opportunities for interaction. Span of control should be established in such a way that it provides supervisors sufficient time to adequately meet the communication needs of their subordinates.

Communication Channels

Communication channels are a third factor that can exert a strong influence on the nature and quality of the communication within an organization. Communication channels refer to the lines or pathways through which communication flows in an organization. There are two kinds of communication channels that typically exist in an organization: formal and informal.

Formal channels

The flow of communication through formal channels corresponds to the hierarchical structure of the organization or the chain of command. An employee who utilizes the formal channels of an organization would report to the unit supervisor who reports to an area director who reports to a division director and so on up the organizational hierarchy. In a hospital, a staff nurse sends communication messages to the nurse manager of the unit who relays the messages to the nursing supervisor. The flow of communication in each of these instances essentially follows the boxes and connecting lines of an organizational chart.

Communication along formal pathways occurs in three directions: downward, upward, or horizontally (see Fig. 7.6). *Downward communication* occurs as a person at a higher level in the organization sends a message down to a person at a lower level in the organization. The messages sent from a director of a social services department to a staff social worker or from a charge nurse to a staff nurse typify downward communication. Downward communication usually involves giving orders or telling subordinates about new regulations (Downs, Berg, & Linkugel, 1977). It can also include giving job instructions, relaying organizational policies, sending employees information, and transmitting organizational ideology (Katz & Kahn, 1966; Smith, Richetto, & Zima, 1977). Downward communication can take the form of written memos, bulletin board notes, procedure manuals, or face-to-face contact between the supervisor and subordinate.

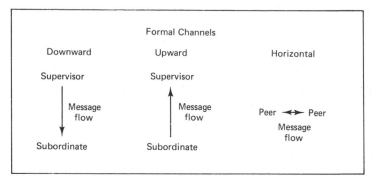

FIGURE 7.6 Direction of communication flow in three formal channels of an organization.

Effective downward communication has been a common concern of managers who want organizational objectives and policies implemented at lower levels. Although some distortion and filtering of messages can occur as messages move down the hierarchy, for the most part downward communication is taken seriously by personnel because it comes through an official channel.

Upward communication is directed from a person on a lower level of the organizational hierarchy to a person at a higher level: from subordinate to supervisor, from unit clerk to unit manager, or from dietary assistant to dietitian, for example. Upward communication often takes the form of seeking clarification, providing requested information, making inquiries, and filing complaints (Smith, Richetto, & Zima, 1977).

For many years, the importance of upward communication to organizational effectiveness was overshadowed by downward communication. For example, organizations based on scientific management principles primarily stressed downward communication. Many managers thought that they could improve organizational planning if they focused on getting their messages across to subordinates. Managers are now realizing that upward communication is equally important and represents an essential form of feedback between people at different levels of the organization. Upward communication also supplies supervisors with information about staff members' attitudes and values, provides information on the degree of task accomplishment, and gives subordinates a sense that their opinions are of value and that their participation in formulating organizational policies is desired (Smith, Richetto, & Zima, 1977).

Although people may agree that effective upward communication is highly desirable, it can be difficult to achieve. Subordinates often hesitate to disclose fully to their supervisors: For instance, subordinates may "filter" the messages in order to please their supervisor. Furthermore, they may hide their anger in front of supervisors so as not to put their jobs in jeopardy. To illustrate, a nurse manager in a meeting with her area director underplayed the problems she was having implementing primary care on her unit. The nurse manager felt that if she told the area director how difficult the transition was for unit personnel, it would reflect poorly on her leadership skills. The nurse manager told the supervisor only that information which reflected well on the manager's leadership skills. In other situations, some subordinates sense the risk of communication with a supervisor and avoid initiating upward communication altogether. For example, a home care nurse, who had previous clashes with the agency supervisor, worked independently on her caseload of clients in the community and had as little contact as possible with the supervisor. When upward communication is filtered or channels are not used, as illustrated in these two examples, supervisors receive overly optimistic reports about how the organization is functioning; subsequent problem solving within the organization will then be based on inadequate or poor-quality information.

Furthermore, the demand on health professionals to provide many important services to clients and families leaves little time for supervisors and subordinates to interact. Also due to the 24-hour services provided in hospitals, members of evening and night shifts seldom have extended contact with head nurses who typically work the day shift. These individuals often communicate upward and downward through notes or messages passed on through other people—practices that hinder feedback and accuracy. In addition, in large organizations the supervisors' offices may be far away from subordinates' work settings, or supervisors may be covering so many different geographical areas in a health center that it is difficult for them to spend time with subordinates in any one area.

To foster more effective communication in health care organizations, supervisors need to be aware that upward communication involves *risk* for some subordinates and therefore supervisors need to try to create a climate in which subordinates feel comfortable communicating both positive and negative information. Planning specific times and opportunities for supervisor-subordinate interaction is also important. Tortoriello, Blatt, and DeWine (1978) believe that sharing coffee breaks or having rap sessions helps to foster effective communication. Too often, they note, supervisors want to spend time with other supervisors and not with subordinates, thereby eliminating this vehicle for communication. Tortoriello, Blatt, and DeWine also outline other practices that can foster organizational communication, especially upward communication. These practices include

Maintaining an "open door" policy that invites ongoing dialogue between supervisor and subordinate

Making grievance procedures available that allow the subordinate to make his or her concern known through a formal procedure

Conducting attitude and opinion surveys in order to tap employees' beliefs or opinions in specific areas of concern

Utilizing exit interviews with employees who are leaving the institution as a means to obtain both positive and negative feedback about the organization (p. 55).

Formal communication within an organization not only occurs in a vertical direction, upward or downward, but it also flows horizontally. *Horizontal communication*, sometimes referred to as lateral communication, takes place among peers at the same level within the organization. Horizontal communication can take place between peers in the same unit or among peers who are at the same level but in different departments of an organization. For example, the interactions between staff nurses on the nephrology unit, or between staff social workers assigned to different units, or between supervisors responsible for different areas in a hospital, all represent horizontal communication. Whereas downward communication often regulates and assigns and upward communication often gives feedback and makes requests, horizontal communication usually focuses on coordinating activities and fostering the social and emotional ties between people (Allen, 1977). Since many employees are more comfortable with their peers or think that their peers will be better able to understand their work concerns, employees often seek emotional support from one another rather than from people above or below them in the organizational hierarchy (Tortoriello, Blatt, & DeWine, 1978).

The horizontal channel of communication was virtually ignored by early organizational researchers, possibly because there was no place for it in their models of organizational hierarchies (Koehler, Anatol, & Applbaum, 1976). Over the years, however, the importance of horizontal communication to the overall effectiveness of communication in the organization has become apparent.

Certain barriers sometimes inhibit effective horizontal communication in organizations. Allen (1977) notes that competition for recognition and promotions among employees at the same level can interfere with cooperative relationships. It can also be difficult for members of highly specialized units to communicate with people in other specialized units (due to different technical jargon) even though they may be in the same level of an organization. Also in some organizational settings effective vertical communication (upward or downward) may be rewarded more than horizontal communication, causing employees to be more sensitive to their communication with superiors or subordinates than with peers (Smith, Richetto, & Zima, 1977).

Nevertheless, health care employees need to communicate with their peers as they attempt to provide quality patient care. Communication is vital for coordinating care when several health professionals (sometimes as many as 30 in a day) are involved in providing care to one client. While there is a clear need for horizontal communication among staff members within the same unit, the importance of communication between people at the same level in different departments (e.g., director of medicine and director of nursing) may be less apparent, but it is very important because departments are often so interdependent; horizontal communication must also take place if organizational goals are to be achieved.

Informal channels

Informal channels, frequently referred to as "the grapevine," often develop among people in an organization who cluster together either because they work close to each other or are friends or have other things in common. Informal channels connect people in an organization who *want* to communicate in contrast to those who *must* communicate (Wofford, Gerloff, Cummins, 1977). Informal channels of communication rarely run parallel to the established authority lines in organizational charts, but they often take on a grapevinelike appearance (see Fig. 7.7). Davis (1981), who has done a considerable amount of work on grapevine networks, suggests that the grapevine can take many patterns but that the most common pattern is the cluster pattern in which one person tends to communicate to a cluster of other persons rather than to just one other person.

The organizational grapevine is often associated with many negative connotations. It is frequently considered a rumor or gossip mill, full of in-

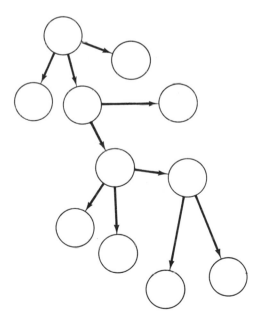

FIGURE 7.7 The flow of communication in the organizational grapevine.

accuracies. Nevertheless, the grapevine can possess high accuracy and low distortion—Davis reports that over 75 percent of the information passed on the grapevine is accurate. He notes, however, that the stories passed are often not complete and are therefore subject to serious distortion even though many of the details are accurate.

Informal communication channels supplement and complement formal channels in an organization and they allow communication to flow in many directions and to cross organizational boundaries that normally would make communication less likely. Informal channels provide another means by which people gain access to information which can help in solving problems and making decisions. Furthermore, grapevines frequently pass information much faster than formal channels (Downs, Berg, & Linkugel, 1977), which can enhance problem solving in times of crises when rapid decisions must be made.

The pitfall of relying on the grapevine for organizational information is that judgments can be made on inadequate or incomplete information. Also grapevines seldom allow for a feedback mechanism that would verify the accuracy of a message between the originator of the message and the numerous receivers of the message.

Health care organizations contain both formal and informal channels of communication. These channels are major factors that influence professional-professional communication within the organization.

Sources of Power

We have discussed the effect that organizational structure and channels of communication can have on organizational communication, but we also need to examine the role that power plays in organizational settings. Power is considered one of the strongest forms of influence and a necessary element in large social systems (King, 1981). Power is also relative and can only be understood when we look at the amount of power held by one person in relation to the power held by another (Kalisch & Kalisch, 1982; Yukl, 1981). To understand communication in organizations, it is necessary to be aware of the various sources of power available to health professionals and how these forms of power can influence professionals' interactions with others.

Power is often used in organizations to influence decision making, to control information, and to persuade others (King, 1981). Administrators use power to lead health care organizations in new directions. Physicians use power at times to control other health care personnel. Patients try to influence staff through power, and staff use power to influence patients (Kritek, 1981). As discussed in Chapters 1 and 2, control or power is built into all human relationships. The way power is used by people in a health care organization is often an indication of how successful the outcomes of health communication will be.

French and Raven (1959) have distinguished five common bases of power: reward power, coercive power, legitimate power, referent power, and expert power. At any given time an individual in a health care setting may be utilizing one, or sometimes more than one, of these bases of power. These five bases of power can also be categorized under two more general sources of power: (1) position power and (2) personal power.

Position power

The power that a person derives from a particular rank or office in an organizational hierarchy is called *position power*. Presidents have greater position power than vice presidents, and supervisors have greater position power than staff personnel.

Reward power and coercive power are often combined and labeled *position power* because they can be used by a person in a higher position to induce others to follow. When a supervisor praises or rewards followers for their behavior, the supervisor is operating from a base of *reward power*. For example, a supervisor who tries to get a staff nurse to work a holiday weekend by offering the nurse overtime pay plus a better work schedule after the holiday is exercising reward power. On the other hand, if a supervisor uses punishment or threats to obtain results, that leader is acting with *coercive power*. If the supervisor just described threatens the staff nurse with negative comments on a job evaluation record unless the nurse works that weekend, the supervisor is exercising coercive power. Coercive power should seldom be used and only in those situations in which other forms of power are ineffective because coercive power often creates resentment and hostility in others (Yukl, 1981).

Both reward power and coercive power are derived from a person's being in a position in an organization that affords him or her the chance to give positive or negative reinforcement to subordinates. Position power is often useful in those situations in which a supervisor is trying to get followers to comply with unpopular plans or procedures (Yukl, 1981).

How does position power influence interactions in health care organizations? In essence, the person with position power has a strong impact on the kind of communication that occurs with subordinates. The person with position power can be more persuasive in interactions with others because he or she has the ability to punish and reward subordinates. Furthermore, the person with position power can use this power to control subordinates by limiting subordinates' access to information. Position power can also be used to inhibit subordinates from openly communicating negative information. As we discussed earlier in the chapter, it can be risky for subordinates to be completely open in their communication with superiors if they perceive their superiors as a threat. As a rule, position power has a less positive effect on interpersonal communication than the types of personal power discussed in the following section.

Personal power

Legitimate power, referent power, and expert power are all forms of what is called *personal power,* a kind of power derived from followers rather than from an organizational position. Effective leaders often utilize personal power, which is based on their expertise and the degree of attraction that followers have toward them, rather than position power (Yukl, 1981).

Subordinates who follow leaders because they "ought to" or "should" follow them are giving the leaders *legitimate power,* power derived from the internalized values of the followers. Parents, priests, police, nurses, and teachers, to name a few, are often given power because followers have learned that they are "supposed" to follow these individuals. These followers believe that it is the appropriate and right thing to do. However, in the discussion of changing roles in Chapter 3 it was suggested that society no longer views health care professionals in the same way it did in earlier times. The increase in malpractice suits and the advocacy for patient rights are evidence that health care personnel are no longer automatically given legitimate power by the public. Also, with increased emphasis on the sharing of responsibility for health care decisions, the health care professional cannot always assume that she or he will have legitimate power in influencing others.

Another kind of personal power is *referent power,* which is based on the identification, affection, and attraction of followers for leaders. Referent power takes time to develop and it depends primarily on the way the leader treats subordinates (Yukl, 1981). A leader who is considerate of followers' needs will engender more personal loyalty from followers than a leader who is insensitive to followers' needs. Rodin and Janis (1979) have hypothesized that referent power is probably the least-used source of power in health care. They suggest, however, that it may be the most effective in situations where it is essential that patients internalize or adopt the recommendations made by a health professional. Professionals can gain referent power by behaving in ways that others perceive as attractive, likable, or benevolent. On the other hand, professionals who have hostile and defensive interpersonal styles will not gain referent power because others (either patients or other professionals) will choose not to emulate them (McFarland & Shiflett, 1979).

The final type of personal power, *expert power,* is held by professionals who are perceived by followers as having knowledge and competence. In highly technological health care organizations, examples of expert power might include technicians who are the only individuals able to direct certain technical procedures, physicians who are specialists in unique areas such as pediatric oncology, and clinical nurse specialists who practice in such areas as intensive care, neonatology, and cardiac surgery.

The expert power of health professionals is undergoing some challenge in health care organizations, in much the same way that legitimate power is being questioned. More and more often clients and families request second opinions regarding medical treatments and procedures. Consumers are also asking for more information from health professionals, so that they can be more active in the decision-making process. It is no longer true that health professionals are granted unlimited power on the basis of their expertise.

Health professionals in most organizations probably draw upon a combination of sources of power. An effective charge nurse may have not only coercive and reward power, but some legitimate and expert power as well. A nurse educator who assumes the new role of head nurse on a unit where she previously worked with students and was highly respected for her professionalism and knowledge will have both legitimate and expert power. In other settings, clinical specialists may have a great deal of expert power, yet they may lack the reward or coercive power (position power) to effect the changes they feel are necessary. It is important for individuals with limited bases of power to be attentive to ways in which they can enhance their power base.

Power is an important concept that is interwoven throughout the fabric of an organization. Power is used to influence others in order to meet both personal and organizational goals. Since power is relational, health professionals need to be aware of the sources of power they have as they interact with others in the organization and they also need to be aware of the power others have to influence their goals and programs. According to Yukl (1981) effective leaders generally use power in a subtle manner and are careful not to overemphasize the status differences between themselves and their followers. In addition, Yukl contends that effective leaders are responsive to the needs of subordinates and keep communication channels open so that two-way interaction and reciprocal influence can occur between leaders and followers. In summary, *the types of power* and *the way that power is exercised* will influence the professional's effectiveness in various organizational situations. Power is an integral part of effective organizational communication.

LEADER-FOLLOWER INTERACTIONS IN HEALTH CARE ORGANIZATIONS

In the previous section, we discussed how certain factors such as structures, channels, and power can influence organizational communication. In this section we are going to turn to another factor, leadership, which has a wide-ranging impact on organizational communication. Effective leadership and the relationship between leaders and followers are crucial components in the overall functioning of health care organizations. According to Goldhaber's organizational communication model presented earlier, leader-follower interaction would be found in the people-messages portion of the paradigm.

Communication is necessary for effective leadership. Leadership does not take place within a vacuum or in isolation from followers; it exists within an organizational system and it is affected by the system. Leadership occurs through the ongoing *transactions* between the individual who is designated as the leader and those who are the followers. *Communication* becomes the means or vehicle that the leader uses to effect change in others. An effective leader will select methods of communicating that are likely to have a positive impact on followers and that will result in progress toward the desired goal (Yura, Ozimek, Walsh, 1981).

In the following discussion of leader-member interaction we will begin by clarifying what is meant by *leadership*. We will also describe three systems approaches to leader-member interactions and discuss how they directly apply to leadership in health care organizations.

Leadership Defined

Leadership can be defined in several different ways. The word conjures up different meanings in different people. The terms *leadership* and *management* are often used interchangeably although they are not synonymous. *Leadership* refers to the process in which one person attempts to influence another person or group in order to attain some goal (Hersey & Blanchard, 1982). Leadership does not depend on an organizational hierarchy; it can be displayed by an individual in any area of a health care setting who attempts to influence or direct others—patients or professionals—in a particular way. Yura, Ozimek, and Walsh (1981) state that "Leadership is free-standing and not limited to the formal organization" (p. 68). *Management,* on the other hand, usually occurs within a structured organization and is concerned with the planning, organizing, and controlling of budgets, time, equipment, and people in an effort to attain organizational objectives (Douglas & Bevis, 1983; Hersey & Blanchard, 1982). While it is highly desirable that a person assigned to a management position be a good leader, managers are not always good leaders. Leadership is not attached to a position but rather to the process whereby individuals influence others.

Probably the oldest and most familiar definition of leadership focuses on the *traits* of the individual who is engaged in leading. In this approach, leadership is defined as a quality or set of qualities that some individuals naturally exhibit that allows them to bring about change in an organization

TABLE 7.1 Traits of Leaders That Appear in Early and More Recent Leadership Research

LEADERSHIP RESEARCH 1904 to 1947	LEADERSHIP RESEARCH 1948 to 1970
Leaders exceed the average person in:	Leaders are characterized by:
Intelligence	Drive for responsibility and task completion
Scholarship	Vigor and persistence in pursuit of goals
Dependability	Originality in problem solving
Activity and social participation	Initiative in social situations
Socioeconomic status	Self-confidence and sense of identity
Sociability	Willingness to accept consequences
Initiative	Readiness to absorb interpersonal stress
Persistence	Willingness to tolerate frustration and delay
Knowing how to get things done	Ability to influence others' behavior
Self-confidence	Capacity to structure social interaction
Cooperativeness	
Popularity	
Adaptability	
Verbal facility	

Adapted from R. M. Stogdill, *Handbook of Leadership: A Survey of Theory and Research.* New York: The Free Press, 1974, pp. 35–91.

or a society. The unique set of inborn traits (or characteristics) that certain individuals are able to show are labeled *leadership.*

Considerable research has been done on the specific traits that leaders exhibit (see Table 7.1). However, identifying the specific traits has presented problems for researchers, who have found that the list of traits is endless and contradictory (Goldberg & Larson, 1975; Jones, Barnlund, & Haiman, 1980). In addition, the traits identified as leadership traits in one situation were not always found to be leadership traits in other situations. Also, persons who had the traits to achieve leadership in one situation were not always individuals who could maintain leadership over an extended period of time (Fisher, 1974, p. 75). For the most part, the trait definition of leadership is considered outdated because it focuses only on the leader's behaviors and overlooks the dynamic interchange between leaders and followers.

Quite different from the trait definition, a more recent approach (McGregor Burns, 1978) regards leadership as a *process* whereby one individual influences the beliefs and behaviors of others in attempting to reach a common goal (see Fig. 7.8). When leadership is defined in this manner, it becomes available to everyone. It is not reserved for a select few with special inborn traits, but rather is a behavior everyone can learn to exhibit.

The process definition implies that the leader affects and is affected by followers. It implies that leadership is not a linear, one-way event but a transactional event occurring between the leader and his or her followers.

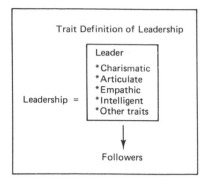 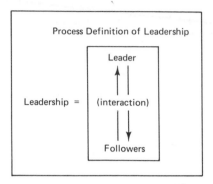

FIGURE 7.8   The different views of leadership based on the trait and process definitions.

A process definition of leadership is more consistent than a trait definition with the basic assumptions of human communication that were discussed in Chapter 1.

In a discussion of leadership it is also necessary to distinguish between two other common definitions of leadership: assigned leadership and emergent leadership. Leadership that is based on a person's occupying a position within an organizational hierarchy is called *assigned leadership*. Team leaders, unit managers, department heads, and administrative heads are all examples of assigned leadership.

However, the person assigned to a leadership position does not always become the real leader in a particular setting. When an individual is perceived by others as the most influential member of a group or organization, regardless of the individual's title, the person is exhibiting *emergent leadership*. The individual acquires emergent leadership through other people in the organization who support and accept that individual's behavior. This type of leadership is not assigned by position, but rather it *emerges* over a period of time through communication.

Fisher (1974) has identified the positive communication behaviors that account for successful leader emergence. Foremost, emergent leaders are verbally active, fluent, and express their thoughts articulately in group interaction. They initiate new ideas in conferences, seek opinions from others, and express their own opinions with firmness but not rigidity. Although this list is not exhaustive, these are the kinds of communicative behaviors that emergent leaders exhibit.

On the negative side, Geier (1967) has identified the behaviors that eliminate individuals from emerging as successful leaders. These negative communicative behaviors included low participation, uninformed contributions, rigid argumentation, overly directive comments, stilted language, and incessant talking. Individuals who engage in these types of communication are less likely to emerge as leaders in health care organizations.

It is not unusual in some health care situations for both assigned leadership and emergent leadership to operate simultaneously. For example, a charge nurse may call together a number of staff nurses to discuss a difficult patient care situation. The charge nurse, who plans for and directs the meeting, would be operating as the *assigned leader*. During the meeting, however, one of the staff nurses may make a number of insightful comments about the patient's condition and may offer many innovative ideas for dealing with the patient's problems. By the end of the meeting, it would become obvious to the group that the staff nurse was the *emergent leader* while the charge nurse remained the *assigned leader*.

In this section we will use a process definition of leadership which views leadership as the *process whereby one individual influences the beliefs and behaviors of others in an attempt to reach a common goal within an organizational setting*. This definition most closely parallels the transactional perspective that has been emphasized throughout the book. Under the process definition, everyone has the *potential* to demonstrate leadership (Cattell, 1951), which makes leadership accessible to many individuals rather than being limited to only a few.

Approaches to Leadership

There are many approaches for understanding effective leadership in an organization. In this section we will discuss three approaches to leadership that take a systems view of leadership: (1) the situational approach, (2) the contingency approach, and (3) the path-goal approach. These approaches are also compatible with the organizational communication perspective presented at the beginning of the chapter. Each of the three theories takes into consideration not only qualities of the leader but qualities of the followers and characteristics of the organizational environment in which the leader-follower interaction occurs.

Situational approach

Many theorists have emphasized the importance of considering the impact of situations on the leadership process (Hemphill, 1949; Bass, 1960; House, 1971). The situational approach to leadership stresses that the leadership process is a function of the leader's style interacting with the demands of the setting. The situational approach looks more closely at the characteristics of the *followers* and the situation than do earlier leadership theories.

Research by Hersey and Blanchard (1969) at the Center for Leadership Studies at Ohio University exemplifies the situational approach. Hersey and Blanchard developed a refined leadership theory called the situational leadership theory (SLT). This theory has many practical implications for understanding the way in which leadership functions in health care organizations.

The situational approach assumes that a leader's effectiveness depends on the leader's ability to adapt his or her style to the *maturity* level of the followers or group members in a particular organizational *situation*. In situational leadership theory, different styles of leadership are prescribed as effective for different levels of subordinate maturity. Maturity is defined as "the capacity to set high but attainable goals (achievement motivation), the willingness and ability to take responsibility, and the education and/or experience of an individual or a group" (Hersey and Blanchard, 1977, p. 161). Levels of maturity, illustrated on the lower portion of the diagram in Figure 7.9, are classified into four categories from very low maturity (M1) to a high level of maturity (M4).

The styles of leadership that have been found to be effective at the different levels of maturity are also classified into four separate categories (see Fig. 7.9). The first style is recommended in situations where followers are very immature. It is a *high* task–*low* relationship style, sometimes referred to as a "telling" approach. In this approach the leader focuses communication on goal achievement and spends little time attending to subordinates' social needs. Style 2 is called a "selling" approach and is a *high*

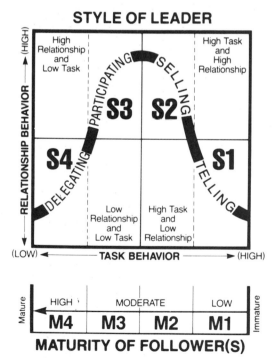

FIGURE 7.9 Situational leadership. (Paul Hersey and Kenneth H. Blanchard, *Management of Organizational Behavior: Utilizing Human Resources,* 4th ed., © 1982, p. 248. Reprinted by permisson of Prentice-Hall, Inc., Englewood Cliffs, N.J.)

task–*high* relationship style recommended for followers of moderately low maturity (M2). In this approach the leader focuses communication on both goal achievement and maintenance of subordinates' social needs. Style 3 leadership is recommended for followers of moderately high maturity (M3). This "participating" approach is a *low* task–*high* relationship style. In this approach the leader does not focus on goals but stresses human relationships among subordinates. Lastly, style 4, which is recommended for very mature (M4) followers, is a *low* task–*low* relationship style, a "delegative" approach (see Fig. 7.9). In this approach the leader takes a lower profile on both task issues and issues related to subordinates' social needs.

In the situational approach, the recommended styles of leadership directly parallel the levels of maturity of followers. At the very lowest level of maturity, leaders should exhibit a directive high task–low relationship style toward followers. As followers become more mature, leaders need to shift their styles and become more relationship oriented while maintaining a task emphasis. Continued growth in maturity by followers should result in leadership that maintains a relationship emphasis and is less task oriented. For followers who are at the highest maturity level, the situational approach suggests that leaders who exhibit reduced task and relationship behavior will have the highest probability of success.

According to the situational approach, there is no single ideal style of leadership. Instead, the key to effective leadership is to diagnose the situation properly (especially the maturity level of group members) and then adopt an appropriate leadership style that adapts to the unique demands of the situation.

To assess a leader's style and diagnostic ability, Hersey and Blanchard have developed a leadership questionnaire that can be self-administered, self-scored, and self-interpreted. It is found in their text, *Management of Organizational Behavior: Utilizing Human Resources* (1977).[1]

The principles of the situational leadership theory can be directly applied to health care settings. For example, a charge nurse on the night shift in the emergency room, with a new group of orderlies, will find a high task–low relationship leadership style to be effective if the orderlies are operating at a low level of maturity. So, too, an inservice coordinator in charge of orientation for new hospital employees may choose to be task oriented because inexperienced employees need more structure. On the other hand, an individual chosen to chair a hospitalwide committee, composed of department heads, could expect the group members to be operating at a relatively high maturity level, indicating that the leader should choose a delegative low task–low relationship approach. In a similar way, the leader in a treatment planning conference composed of the heads of various treat-

---

[1]The questionnaire and scoring manual can also be obtained through University Associates, Inc., 8517 Production Avenue, P.O. Box 26240, San Diego, Calif. 92126.

ment areas would probably be a more effective leader if he or she adopted a delegative approach.

A nurse on a nephrology unit could run into situations where she or he should exhibit a low task–high relationship approach (style 3 in the situational model). There could be times in such a unit when the dialysis patients might be quite mature. The patients might know a lot about their condition and might understand many of the technological procedures involved in dialysis, yet they may have a difficult time coping with the implications of the disease. In cases of this sort, low task–high relationship interaction between the leader and followers would be in order.

Probably the most frequently exhibited leadership style is the high task–high relationship style (style 2 in the situational model). It is used by the nurse who spends considerable time discussing surgery with a group of preoperative patients the night before surgery, or by the hospital social worker who discusses an older patient in a staff discharge planning meeting, or by a unit supervisor as she or he discusses shift problems at a staff conference.

Health care organizations are replete with examples to which the situational leadership theory can be applied. For our purposes, the theory is valuable because it provides a simple model of how effective leadership occurs. Leaders who understand the theory can improve their probability of success by adapting their style to the maturity of their followers.

Contingency approach

Contingency theory, based on the work of Fiedler and his associates, also examines the relationship between leadership styles and situational factors that are present in different settings (Fiedler, 1967, 1974; Fiedler & Chemers, 1978). Effective leadership is viewed as being *contingent* on the *match* between a leader's style and the demands of a situation.

In contingency theory, leadership *styles* are described as task oriented or relationship oriented. Task-oriented leaders are concerned primarily with reaching a goal while relationship-oriented leaders are concerned with developing close interpersonal relations. To measure leader styles, Fiedler developed the least preferred co-worker (LPC) scale (see Fig. 7.10). Leaders who score high on this scale are described as relationship oriented and those who score low on the scale are identified as task oriented.

Three *situational* factors considered in contingency theory are (1) leader-member relations, (2) task structure, and (3) position power. Leader-member relations refers to the degree of confidence, loyalty, and attraction that followers have toward their leader. Task structure describes the degree to which specific tasks are clearly defined, structured, and standardized. Position power refers to the amount of authority that the leader has to reward or punish his or her followers. Together, these three factors determine the "favorableness" of various situations. Situations that

INSTRUCTIONS: Think of the person with whom you can work least well. He/she may be someone you work with now or he/she may be someone you knew in the past. He/she does not have to be the person you like least well, but should be the person with whom you had the most difficulty in getting a job done. Describe this person as he/she appears to you.

Pleasant	: ___ : ___ : ___ : ___ : ___ : ___ : ___ : ___ :	8	7	6	5	4	3	2	1	Unpleasant
Friendly	: ___ : ___ : ___ : ___ : ___ : ___ : ___ : ___ :	8	7	6	5	4	3	2	1	Unfriendly
Rejecting	: ___ : ___ : ___ : ___ : ___ : ___ : ___ : ___ :	1	2	3	4	5	6	7	8	Accepting
Helpful	: ___ : ___ : ___ : ___ : ___ : ___ : ___ : ___ :	8	7	6	5	4	3	2	1	Frustrating
Unenthusiastic	: ___ : ___ : ___ : ___ : ___ : ___ : ___ : ___ :	1	2	3	4	5	6	7	8	Enthusiastic
Tense	: ___ : ___ : ___ : ___ : ___ : ___ : ___ : ___ :	1	2	3	4	5	6	7	8	Relaxed
Distant	: ___ : ___ : ___ : ___ : ___ : ___ : ___ : ___ :	1	2	3	4	5	6	7	8	Close
Cold	: ___ : ___ : ___ : ___ : ___ : ___ : ___ : ___ :	1	2	3	4	5	6	7	8	Warm
Cooperative	: ___ : ___ : ___ : ___ : ___ : ___ : ___ : ___ :	8	7	6	5	4	3	2	1	Uncooperative
Supportive	: ___ : ___ : ___ : ___ : ___ : ___ : ___ : ___ :	8	7	6	5	4	3	2	1	Hostile
Boring	: ___ : ___ : ___ : ___ : ___ : ___ : ___ : ___ :	1	2	3	4	5	6	7	8	Interesting
Quarrelsome	: ___ : ___ : ___ : ___ : ___ : ___ : ___ : ___ :	1	2	3	4	5	6	7	8	Harmonious
Self-assured	: ___ : ___ : ___ : ___ : ___ : ___ : ___ : ___ :	8	7	6	5	4	3	2	1	Hesitant
Efficient	: ___ : ___ : ___ : ___ : ___ : ___ : ___ : ___ :	8	7	6	5	4	3	2	1	Inefficient
Gloomy	: ___ : ___ : ___ : ___ : ___ : ___ : ___ : ___ :	1	2	3	4	5	6	7	8	Cheerful
Open	: ___ : ___ : ___ : ___ : ___ : ___ : ___ : ___ :	8	7	6	5	4	3	2	1	Guarded

SCORING: Sum the numbers under the blanks that you checked for each of the 16 items. Mean score = 60. High LPCs score above 60. Low LPCs score below 60.

FIGURE 7.10 Least preferred co-worker (LPC) scale. (Adapted with permission from F. E. Fiedler, *A Theory of Leadership Effectiveness*. New York: McGraw-Hill Book Company, 1967, p. 41. Copyright ©1967 by McGraw-Hill, Inc.)

are rated "most favorable" are those having good leader-follower relations, defined tasks, and strong leader position power. Situations that are "least favorable" have poor leader-follower relations, unstructured tasks, and weak leader position power.

As was pointed out previously, contingency theory emphasizes the

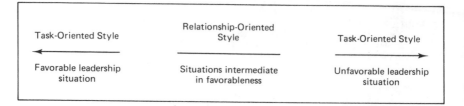

FIGURE 7.11 Leadership styles appropriate for various group situations. (Adapted with permission from F. E. Fiedler, *A Theory of Leadership Effectiveness.* New York: McGraw-Hill Book Company, 1967, p. 14. Copyright ©1967 by McGraw-Hill, Inc.)

match between leader *styles* and the nature of different *situations.* According to Fiedler, leaders who are task oriented work best in extreme situations that are either very favorable or very unfavorable (see Fig. 7.11). Leaders with relationship-oriented styles work best in situations that are intermediately favorable (see Fig. 7.11). These predictions about the success of matching leader styles to situational characteristics are central to contingency theory.

There has been considerable controversy regarding contingency theory (Yukl, 1981) and specifically about the interpretation of the LPC scale's measure of leadership style (Behling & Schriesheim, 1976). The LPC scale has been criticized as an unreliable measure and as an instrument to which it is difficult to attach precise meaning. Regardless of these criticisms of the scale (which were addressed by Fiedler in 1978), the contingency approach provides a very valuable theoretical framework for understanding leadership in health care areas. As Behling and Schriesheim pointed out, "it is still the most completely tested of the situational leadership theories and is viewed by many as one of the better descriptions of the leadership process presently available" (p. 308).

The concept of contingency is valuable because it emphasizes the importance of assessing situational factors (leader-follower relations, task structure, position power) that affect the leadership process. Leadership does not occur in a vacuum; it occurs in real life contexts, and contingency theory provides a framework for understanding how these contexts have an impact on leadership performance.

Second, the contingency approach has a research base from which predictions can be made concerning effective leadership strategies. From this model, we can predict that individuals who are task oriented (who score low on the LPC scale) will be effective in *extreme* situations. Individuals who are relationship oriented (who score high on the LPC scale) will be better suited for leadership in *moderately* favorable contexts.

Finally, contingency theory is valuable in that it provides a rationale for why leaders should not feel that their own styles have to be effective in all situations. Contingency theory is realistic in suggesting that each individual has a style of leadership that can be effective in particular situations but that there is no style which will always be effective.

If we apply contingency theory to health care, we may find useful explanations as to why some leaders are effective in certain situations and others are not effective (Calkin, 1980). For example, when administrators' or supervisors' styles are matched with the unique characteristics (e.g., follower relations, task, and power factors) of the settings in which they work, they will most likely be effective. Individuals who are task oriented would function best in units in which everything is going very well or in units in which there are significant problems. For example, a highly task-oriented nurse would function well in a *very favorable* situation such as a neonatology unit where staff members have good relationships, tasks are clear, and the leader has considerable position power. This same task-oriented nurse would also function well in a *very unfavorable* situation such as a hectic emergency room that has a number of new staff members who are unclear about their roles, who question the leader's authority, and who have not yet developed good working relationships with each other. A relationship-oriented nurse, according to the contingency model, would function better in moderate situations that are *neither* very favorable nor very unfavorable (see Fig. 7.11). This nurse's leadership style might be more suited to a community health agency where tasks are less clearly defined and more emphasis is placed on relationship issues. It should be noted, however, that contingency theory is *seldom* used as a pragmatic tool to assign individuals to various positions: It is used for explanatory purposes after individuals have been assigned.

Contingency theory also has implications for training programs in health care organizations. These organizations have traditionally developed rigorous training programs that are supposed to turn out leaders who can function well in nearly all circumstances. Contingency theory suggests that perhaps training programs should have a different emphasis. Programs could be oriented toward analyzing the styles that leaders exhibit and then matching them to compatible situations in the organization. In addition, training programs could be designed to assist leaders in changing the dynamics of situations in which they function so that the leader-situation match would be enhanced (Calkin, 1980). The point is that contingency theory stresses the need for training programs to teach leaders how to analyze their own styles and to assess the places in the organization into which their styles will fit best—rather than training programs to "build leaders."

Path-goal approach

The final theoretical approach to leader-follower interaction to be discussed in this section is path-goal theory, which was developed by House

(1971) and his associates (House & Dessler, 1974; House & Mitchell, 1974). Path-goal theory is similar to contingency and situational leadership in that it focuses on the interaction between leaders, followers, and situations. As the name of the theory implies, this approach emphasizes how leaders can assist followers as followers *proceed to travel on a path toward a goal.*

The basic principles underlying path-goal theory are derived from motivation theory and focus on the ways leaders can help or *motivate* subordinates to accomplish personal and organizational goals and to feel *satisfied* with task activity. According to Filley, House, and Kerr (1976), "the motivational functions of the leader consist of increasing the personal pay-offs to subordinates for work-goal attainment, and making the paths to these pay-offs easier to travel" (p. 254). Essentially, the leader clarifies paths, reduces road blocks, and increases opportunities for followers to attain personal satisfaction while trying to reach organizational goals. The specific way that leaders help subordinates will depend on followers' needs and the nature of the situation.

An individual who chooses path-goal leadership is concerned with several areas. First, the leader *identifies the personal and organizational goals* and becomes aware of how working toward these goals can be made rewarding for subordinates. By understanding goal requirements of subordinates, leaders can determine how to make subordinates' jobs more fulfilling. Second, the leader attempts to *clarify the route* that the subordinate needs to travel in order to accomplish the goal. This includes using straightforward communication that helps followers understand precisely what they are required to do to reach a certain goal and makes these requirements as free of ambiguity as possible. Furthermore, the path-goal leader tries to *remove the obstacles* that get in the way of subordinates as they work toward the goal. The leader is basically helping subordinates by making their route to the goal smoother, less complex, and unencumbered. Lastly, this approach requires that the leader try to *use a leadership style (task or process) that is best adapted to followers;* depending on the group, this could mean being directive, participative, supportive, or achievement oriented. As the leader adapts his or her style to the special needs of subordinates, the followers will find the task more satisfying and rewarding.

In health care situations, the path-goal theory has specific pragmatic value. For example, Lancaster and Gray (1982) point out that the "Path-Goal Theory has considerable potential for nurses. It is basically a human-relations set of activities that recognizes the need to respect others and to provide guidance, encouragement, and clarity of directions" (p. 90). The health professional who employs this approach must ask these basic questions: What is it I am asking of my staff? How can I help them clarify their goals? How can I make these goals less difficult for them to achieve, and how can I support and assist staff in their efforts? The path-goal approach requires that leaders maintain supportive, trusting, and open communication with subordinates. This approach requires that the vertical lines of communication (both upward and downward) are used freely between leader and followers. The following example illustrates the use of this approach.

> A hospital inservice director used the path-goal leadership approach to assist a group of staff nurses in obtaining further academic degrees. The nurses were uncertain about what type of degree they wanted, what programs were available to them in the area, and how to work through the number of obstacles that stood in the way of their returning to school (e.g., work responsibilities, family responsibilities, financial problems, etc.). Using a supportive style, the director was able to help each nurse identify a type of degree that would fit in with the nurse's future career plans. In addition, the director was able to assist the nurses in thinking about how they could change their work schedules to accommodate class schedules, in finding additional financial support, as well as in making arrangements to meet family responsibilities.

As illustrated in this example, path-goal theory is a very pragmatic approach when used by leaders to assist subordinates in achieving their goals in satisfying ways.

Applying Concepts of Leader-Follower Interaction to Practice

From the preceding discussion on leadership theories, it is clear that there are many ways to view leadership—as a trait of a few select people or as a process occurring between the leader and followers. From our perspective, the leadership theories that seem most useful in describing leadership in health care settings are situational theory, contingency theory, and path-goal theory. Each of these theories is consistent with the transactional communication perspective that has been emphasized throughout this book, and each of these theories directs the health professional to assess three areas: (1) characteristics of the *leader*; (2) characteristics of the *followers*; and (3) characteristics of the *situation*. Effective leadership communication results from an interactive process that blends the style of the leader with the needs of the followers within the context of a specific health care situation. Leadership communication cannot and should not be narrowed down to one or two isolated communication techniques used by the leader.

Health professionals can use the leadership theories discussed in this section in a number of ways. First, these theories can serve as a guide for professionals in assessing leadership needs in specific health care organizations. Health professionals who are knowledgeable about a wide range of theories can select specific theories that are helpful in explaining the leadership issues that they confront on their jobs. In addition, these theories may be helpful for health professionals who are in the process of changing jobs. Leininger (1974) notes that health professionals need to give more thought to matching the skills and interests of the leader with the beliefs and practices of the organization. For example, one or more theories could provide an excellent framework in which to consider a new job possibility. The health professional could ask questions such as, How does my own preferred leadership style fit in with the structure of the organization and the needs of the patients and professionals with whom I would be working? What would I need to be an effective leader in this position?

Second, these theories can be useful in diagnosing leader-follower communication problems. For example, a leader who is having difficulty interacting with team members may find certain theoretical frameworks helpful in explaining his or her interpersonal difficulties. Applying situational theory, the leader may determine that he or she has been too autocratic for the mature, independently functioning members on his or her unit. Third, leadership theories help to break down the myth that only a few select individuals are capable of becoming leaders. The theories emphasize that leadership is a pragmatic process that can be used by many individuals at all levels of the health care organization. Fourth, leadership theories with an interactional focus point to a need for more effective followers as well as effective leaders. The active follower is one who functions in an autonomous role to give responsible, accountable care to clients. By assessing the followers' task and process preferences as well as the leaders' preferences, health professionals may foster better working relationships between both parties. Together the leader and follower will be able to maximize the quality of care provided to clients and families within the health care organization.

Leadership positions in health care organizations

Supervisory leadership.   The role of supervisory personnel is increasingly important in health care organizations. Not long ago, a supervisor was a person who had been promoted to a leadership position on the basis of seniority rather than on his or her management and human relations skills. Now it is becoming apparent that supervisory leaders can no longer be chosen only on the basis of years of service or dedication to the organization. Instead, from an organizational communication perspective, it becomes important to find supervisors whose leadership styles match the needs of followers and the demands of various situations. Supervisors need to assess their interactions with followers and recognize that mature subordinates can handle more responsibility with less direction, while less self-directed individuals will require more supervision. Supervisors also need to foster effective upward and downward communication within health care organizations as well as horizontal communication between and within various departments.

Team leading and primary care roles.   The traditional role of the team leader is being altered as more and more health care organizations move toward primary care models. No matter whether the health professional is leading the team of professionals and paraprofessionals or whether he or she is the primary coordinator of all individuals involved with patient care, both roles require effective communication. While these current roles are evolving, the newer transactional models of leadership appear to be more useful for the professional working with a variety of people than do the earlier and more authoritarian models of leadership. As the problems of the hospitalized client become more complex, a blending of expertise from a variety of professionals will be required. Team leaders and primary care nurses need to foster communication that will allow a variety of health professionals to provide their input.

Administrative positions.   Administrators are required to confront leadership issues daily. Sometimes the criticism is made that health care administrators place staff in new leadership roles without helping them to understand characteristics of the organizational hierarchy which would enhance their effectiveness in the new roles (Calkins, 1980). Administrators can assist new supervisors in carrying out their roles if they orient supervisors to organizational structure and how to use existing channels of formal and informal communication. Health administrators also need to examine the characteristics of various departments and units, then to find personnel whose leadership styles will best fit into those settings. Matching personnel with the unique demands of various situations will enhance the effectiveness of leaders, improve the communication within the organization, and result in better patient care.

Finally, administrators will also need to continue to battle environmental pressures such as cost containment issues. Administrators who give other personnel a chance to have input into these difficult decisions will be more effective than those who issue authoritative directives about budget cuts and the inability to fill positions. Effective leaders of the future must be able to balance the increased demands for services while maintaining the support of their personnel.

Future directions for leadership in health care organizations
Health professions need leaders (Yura, Ozimek, & Walsh, 1981). Whether these leaders assume their roles from assigned or emergent routes, there will be a continued and growing need for effective leader-follower interactions in health care organizations. One question that faces each professional is what his or her role will be in the selection of these new leaders.

What qualities, attributes, philosophies, behaviors, and management styles will we be looking for in our leaders? Although we ourselves may choose not to be an assigned leader in an organization, we will be working with the leaders and we have a responsibility to set standards and expectations for our leadership personnel (Fuller, 1979).

Future health care leaders face the complex challenge of blending innovative and expanded roles of health professionals with authoritarian, organizational hierarchies, and also balancing the humanistic values of service with the pragmatic goals of cost containment. Health care leaders will also have the difficult task of maintaining standards of quality care for patients and families in face of the changing pool of health professionals and the increasing clamor to open new specialized units. Finally, fostering ethical leadership that respects the human dignity of patients as well as personnel in an increasingly technological era is another challenge that health professionals face. Obviously, leadership in the future will not be an easy task. However, as health professionals continue to discuss and clarify their perspectives on effective leadership, it should be possible to identify health care leaders who have the communication ability and the leadership style to adapt to and handle the complex challenges of health care organizations.

SUMMARY

Organizational communication is defined as the process whereby a system of interdependent individuals in various roles and positions share information according to a common set of rules in order to achieve mutual goals. A model of organizational communication was presented which conceptualizes communication in health care organizations from a system perspective emphasizing the interrelationships between the environment, the organization, and the messages between people within the organization.

Among the factors that can influence communication within health care organizations are organizational philosophy, organizational structure, communication channels, and sources of power. Organizational philosophies help to explain the beliefs and communication behaviors that are emphasized within an organization. Organizations that use the scientific management approach emphasize reward systems and formal, one-sided, top-down, task-related communication. Health organizations that operate from the human relations perspective stress communication between workers and participatory decision making in the organization. In the systems perspective, the communication that flows between subsystems of the organization and between the organization and the environment is highlighted.

Organizational structure is another factor that influences organizational communication. In organizations with a tall shape, communication travels through many different levels and through many middle managers. Organizations that have flat structures are typically more decentralized and communication pathways are shorter, giving employees more input and control. Span of control refers to the number of people a manager is required to supervise. Organizations should be designed to give supervisors sufficient time to adequately address the communication needs of all their subordinates.

Communication channels can be formal or informal. Formal communication follows structured pathways that extend downward, upward, or horizontally. Informal channels, which are like a grapevine, transfer messages rapidly and with a relatively high degree of accuracy within the organization.

Five main bases of power are reward, coercive, legitimate, referent, and expert power. Reward and coercive power are considered to be examples of position power, whereas legitimate, referent, and expert power are characterized as personal power.

Leadership has a wide-ranging impact on organizational communication. Leadership is a transactional interpersonal communication process that is strongly influenced by followers and the situation. Although the early approaches to leadership, such as the trait approach, assume that only a few people have the unique qualities to be leaders, the newer approaches to leadership emphasize that any individual has the potential to be an effective leader if he or she utilizes a leadership style that takes into consideration the needs of the followers and the characteristics of the leadership situation. The situational approach views leadership as an adaptive process in which the maturity level of the followers helps to determine the leadership approach that is needed in a particular situation. A similar approach, the contingency approach, utilizes a leader-match theory that pairs task and relationship styles of the leaders with the demands of the organizational setting. The path-goal theory emphasizes how leaders can assist followers as they proceed on their path toward a goal.

Among the many applications of leadership theories in health care settings are assessment of leadership needs, diagnosis of leader-follower communication problems, and recognition of effective follower behavior. Leadership positions in health care organizations include team-leading and primary care roles as well as supervisory and administrative positions.

REFERENCES

Allen, R. K. *Organizational management through communication*. New York: Harper & Row, Publishers, Inc., 1977.

Argyris, C. *Understanding organizational behavior*. Homewood, Ill.: Dorsey, 1960.

Bass, B. M. *Leadership psychology and organizational behavior*. New York: Harper & Row, Publishers, Inc., 1960.

Behling, O., & Schriesheim, C. *Organizational behavior*. Boston: Allyn & Bacon, Inc., 1976.

Bernhard, L. A., & Walsh, M. *Leadership: The key to the professionalization of nursing*. New York: McGraw-Hill Book Company, 1981.

Calkin, J. D. Using management literature to enhance new leadership roles. *Journal of Nursing Administration*, 1980, *10*(4), 24–30.

Cattell, R. B. New concepts for measuring leadership, in terms of group syntality. *Human Relations*, 1951, *4*, 161–184.

Davis, K. *Human behavior at work: Organizational behavior*, 6th ed. New York: McGraw-Hill Book Company, 1981.

Donovan, H. M. *Nursing service administration: Managing the enterprise*. St. Louis: The C. V. Mosby Company, 1975.

Douglass, L. M., & Bevis, E. L. *Nursing management and leadership in action*, 4th ed. St. Louis: The C. V. Mosby Company, 1983.

Downs, C. W., Berg, D. M., & Linkugel, W. A. *The organizational communicator*. New York: Harper & Row, Publishers, Inc., 1977.

Farace, R. V., Monge, P. R., & Russell, H. M. *Communicating and organizing*. Reading, Mass.: Addison-Wesley Publishing Co., Inc., 1977.

Fiedler, F. E. *A theory of leadership effectiveness*. New York: McGraw-Hill Book Company, 1967.

Fiedler, F. E. The contingency model and the dynamics of the leadership process. In L. Berkowitz (eds.), *Advances in experimental social psychology*, Vol. 2. New York: Academic Press, 1978, 60–112.

Fiedler, F. E., & Chemers, M. M. *Leadership and effective management*. Glenview, Ill.: Scott, Foresman & Company, 1974.

Filley, A. C., House, R. J., & Kerr, S. *Managerial process and organizational behavior*, 2nd ed. Glenview, Ill: Scott, Foresman & Company, 1976.

Fisher, B. A. *Small group decision making: Communication and the group process*. New York: McGraw-Hill Book Company, 1974.

French, R. P., & Raven, R. The bases of social power. In D. Cartwright (ed.), *Studies in social power*. Ann Arbor, Mich.: Institute for Social Research, 1959.

Fuller, S. Humanistic leadership in a pragmatic age. *Nursing Outlook*, 1979, *27*(12), 770–773.

Geier, J. G. A trait approach to the study of leadership in small groups. *Journal of Communication*, 1967, *11*, 316–323.

Goldberg, A. A., & Larson, C. E. *Group communication: Discussion processes and applications*. Englewood Cliffs, N.J.: Prentice-Hall, Inc., 1975.

Goldhaber, G. M. *Organizational communication*, 3rd ed. Dubuque, Iowa: William C. Brown Co. Publishers, 1983.

Hemphill, J. K. *Situational factors in leadership*. Columbus, Ohio: Ohio State University, Bureau of Educational Research, 1949.

Hersey, P., & Blanchard, K. H. Life cycle theory of leadership. *Training and Development Journal*, 1969, *23*, 26–33.

Hersey, P., & Blanchard, K. H. *Management of organizational behavior: Utilizing human resources*, 3rd ed. Englewood Cliffs, N.J.: Prentice-Hall, Inc., 1977.

Hersey, P., & Blanchard, K. H. *Management of organizational behavior: Utilizing human resources*, 4th ed. Englewood Cliffs, N.J.: Prentice-Hall, Inc., 1982.

House, R. J. A path-goal theory of leader effectiveness. *Administration Science Quarterly*, 1971, *16*, 321–338.

House, R. J., & Dessler, G. The path-goal theory of leadership: Some post hoc and a priori tests. In J. Hunt and L. Larson (eds.), *Contingency Approaches in Leadership*. Carbondale: Southern Illinois University Press, 1974.

House, R. J., & Mitchell, T. R. Path-goal theory of leadership *Contemporary Business,* 1974, *3,* 81–98.

Jones, S. E., Barnlund, D. C., & Haiman, F. S. *The dynamics of discussion: Communication in small groups,* 2nd ed. New York: Harper & Row, Publishers, Inc., 1980.

Kalisch, B., & Kalisch, P. *Politics of nursing.* Philadelphia: J. B. Lippincott Company, 1982.

Katz, D., & Kahn, R. L. *The social psychology of organizations.* New York: John Wiley & Sons, Inc., 1966.

King, I. M. *A theory for nursing: Systems, concepts, process.* New York: John Wiley & Sons, Inc., 1981.

Koehler, J. W., Anatol, K. W. E., & Applbaum, R. L. *Organizational communication: Behavioral perspectives.* New York: Holt, Rinehart & Winston, 1976.

Kritek, P. B. Patient power and powerlessness. *Supervisor Nurse,* 1981, *12*(6), 26–34.

Lancaster, J., & Gray, C. F. Change agents as leaders in nursing. In J. Lancaster & W. Lancaster. *The nurse as a change agent: Concepts for advanced nursing practice.* St. Louis: The C. V. Mosby Company, 1982.

Leininger, M. The leadership crisis in nursing: A critical problem and challenge. *Journal of Nursing Administration,* 1974, *4*(2), 28–34.

Likert, R. *New patterns of management.* New York: McGraw-Hill Book Company, 1961.

MacGregor Burns, J. *Leadership.* New York: Harper & Row, Publishers, Inc., 1978.

Mayo, E. *The human problems of an industrial civilization.* New York: Macmillan, Inc., 1933.

McFarland, D., & Shiflett, N. The role of power in the nursing profession. *Nursing Dimensions,* 1979, *7*(2), 1–14.

Rodin, J., & Janis, I. L. The social power of health-care practitioners as agents of change. *The Journal of Social Issues,* 1979, *35,* 60–81.

Rogers, E. M., & Agarwala-Rogers, R. *Communication in organizations.* New York: The Free Press, 1976.

Sanford, A. C., Hunt, G. T., & Bracey, H. J. *Communication behavior in organizations.* Columbus, Ohio: Charles E. Merrill Publishing Company, 1976.

Smith, R. L., Richetto, G. M., & Zima, J. P. Organizational behavior: An approach to human communication. In R. Huseman, C. Logue, & D. Fresley (eds.), *Readings in interpersonal & organizational communication* (3rd ed.). Boston: Holbrook Press, Inc., 1977.

Stevens, B. J. *First-line patient care management,* 2nd ed. Rockville, Md.: Aspen Systems Corporation, 1983.

Stogdill, R. M. *Handbook of leadership: A survey of theory and research.* New York: The Free Press, 1974.

Taylor, F. *Scientific management.* New York: Harper & Row, Publishers, Inc., 1911.

Tortoriello, T. R., Blatt, S. J., & DeWine, S. *Communication in the organization: An applied approach.* New York: McGraw-Hill Book Company, 1978.

Veninga, R. L. *The human side of health administration.* Englewood Cliffs, N.J.: Prentice-Hall, Inc., 1982.

Wofford, J. C., Gerloff, E. A., & Cummins, R. C. *Organizational communication: The keystone to managerial effectiveness.* New York: McGraw-Hill Book Company, 1977.

Yukl, G. A. *Leadership in organizations.* Englewood Cliffs, N.J.: Prentice-Hall, Inc., 1981.

Yura, H., Ozimek, D., & Walsh, M. B. *Nursing leadership: Theory and process,* 2nd ed. New York: Appleton-Century-Crofts, 1981.

8 Conflict and Communication in Health Care Settings

What is dispiriting in the modern world is that we neither accept conflict nor know how to resolve it rationally and peacefully. We still want to subdue or silence our opponents, ignorant of the basic human truth that our differences should be our glory, and not our doom.
—Sidney Harris, 1979[1]

Conflict is inevitable in human organizations. In health care organizations the potential for conflict is heightened because within these settings individuals must address life and death issues; they have to function both independently and interdependently within a system containing considerable role ambiguity and complex lines of authority. Health care workers also need to be highly skilled both in technical areas and in human relationships. Other organizations may demand similar qualities from individuals, but seldom to the same extent that they are required of professionals in health care. These demands on health professionals make conflict unavoidable.

Conflict creates the need *for* change and it occurs as the result *of* change. When confronted with conflict, we often feel uncomfortable because of the strain, controversy, and stress that accompany conflict. To manage conflict we have to change our own behavior or we have to change the situation around us. Conversely, change itself can create conflict. Most of us like a degree of consistency in our work and in our relationships; thus when rules or procedures change or when people change, we are thrown

[1]S. Harris, "Every governing idea needs an opposing idea." *Detroit Free Press*, May 19, 1979, p. 7B. Reprinted by permission of Sydney J. Harris and Field Newspaper Syndicate.

off balance and we feel somewhat disoriented. These dissonant feelings that accompany change can in turn lead to conflict.

Although conflict is uncomfortable, it is not unhealthy nor even necessarily bad. Conflict will always be present in health care organizations and it will usually produce change. The important question for us to address is not, How can we *avoid* conflict and *eliminate* change? but rather, How can we *manage* conflict effectively and produce *positive* change? If conflict is managed in effective and productive ways, the result is a reduction of stress, an increase in creative problem solving, and an increase in positive outcomes (Deutsch, 1971; Nichols, 1979).

In this chapter we will approach conflict from a communication perspective. Conflict can be placed at the center of the health communication model presented in Chapter 1. Conflict occurs in the *transactions* between people in professional-professional, professional-client, professional-family, and family-client *relationships* in various health care *contexts*. Throughout the book we have tried to emphasize that health communication is multidimensional and we have stressed the importance of viewing communication in health care relationships as a transactional process. Similarly, conflict is not a static unidirectional event but a process that is transactional.

When conflict exists in human relationships it is recognized and expressed through communication (Brown, Yelsma, & Keller, 1981; Frost & Wilmot, 1978). Communication becomes the means that people use to express their disagreements or differences. Muniz (1981) suggests that conflict is acted out through communication; communication is the observable part of the conflict or the "tip of the iceberg," while the causes of conflict frequently lie somewhere deeper beneath the surface. Communication also provides the avenue by which conflicts can be successfully resolved or by which conflicts can be escalated to produce negative results.

This chapter will emphasize ways to manage conflict. First, we will present selected definitions of conflict. Next, we will discuss two basic kinds of conflict (content and relational), and two theoretical approaches that have been taken in the study of conflict. The chapter will conclude with an examination of different communication strategies and styles of approaching conflict.

CONFLICT DEFINED

When we think of conflict in simple terms, we think of a struggle between people, groups, organizations, cultures, or nations. Conflict involves confrontation—two opposing forces brought face to face. When conflict occurs it is usually painful in some way and causes stress.

Generally, conflict has been investigated from three perspectives:

personal conflict, interpersonal conflict, and social conflict. Personal conflict research has focused on the conflict that occurs *within* individuals, the dynamics of personality that predispose individuals to experience conflict within the self. Psychoanalytic theorists as well as other personality theorists discuss personal conflict at great length. Interpersonal conflict refers to conflict *between* individuals, especially between people who are different. Social conflict refers to clashes between societies and nations, and studies in this field include research on the causes of international conflicts, war, and peace. Our discussion in this chapter will focus on the communication that occurs between individuals who are in conflict—the interpersonal conflict perspective.

A review of the definitions employed in the research literature on conflict provides us with a more explicit meaning for the term *conflict*. Sociologist Coser (1967) provides a frequently cited definition of conflict:

> a struggle over values and claims to scarce status, power, and resources
> in which the aims of the opponents are to neutralize, injure, or elimi-
> nate the rivals (p. 8).

Deutsch (1973, p. 10) suggests that conflict exists whenever there are incompatible activities between people, groups, or nations. An incompatible activity is one that obstructs, interferes with, or prevents another activity. Both Coser and Deutsch stress that conflict need not be destructive but that it can be turned to constructive ends.

Frost and Wilmot (1978), who view conflict from a communication perspective, also emphasize the positive aspects of conflict. They define conflict as

> an expressed struggle between at least two interdependent parties, who
> perceive incompatible goals, scarce rewards, and interference from the
> other party in achieving their goals. They are in a position of opposition
> in conjunction with cooperation (p. 9).

They suggest that conflict should not be viewed as abnormal or undesirable but rather as constructive and growth producing (p. 8).

The approach we will take toward conflict in this chapter incorporates several dimensions of conflict suggested by the authors just mentioned. First, conflict is a *struggle*; it is the result of opposing forces coming together. For example, conflict exists between two community health professionals when they oppose each other on the type of sex education program that could be adopted in a school system. Similarly, conflict occurs when two individuals are arguing opposite positions on an issue such as abortion. Conflict involves a clash between individuals (Nichols, 1979).

Second, there needs to be an element of *interdependence* between individuals for conflict to take place (Booth, 1982; Thurkettle & Jones, 1978).

If health professionals could function entirely independently of each other, there would be no reason for conflict. Everyone could do his or her own work and there would be no area of contention. However, personnel in health care organizations do not work in isolation from one another. In fact, health care personnel often need to function with a high degree of interdependence. Clients depend on nurses, nurses depend on social workers, physicians depend on nurses, administrators depend on staff, and so on. This interdependence among persons sets up an environment in which conflict is very likely.

Third, in conflict there is always an *affective* element. Conflict involves the arousal of feelings (Brown & Keller, 1979; Nichols, 1979). When our beliefs or values on a highly charged issue (e.g., the right to strike or autonomy over professional practice) are challenged or blocked, we become upset and usually feel it is important to defend them or fight for our position. As we mentioned earlier, it is the feelings aroused in these situations that produce the discomfort that surrounds conflict.

Fourth, conflict involves *differences* between individuals that they perceive to be incompatible. Conflict can result from differences in individuals' beliefs, values, and goals (content issues), or from differences in individuals' desires for control, status, and affiliation (relational issues). The opportunities for conflict are almost endless because each of us is unique and each of us has developed a particular set of beliefs, needs, and behaviors (Stern, 1982). These differences are a constant breeding ground for conflict (Booth, 1982; Kalisch & Kalisch, 1977).

Based on these four elements, we will be using the following definition of conflict: *Conflict is a felt struggle between two or more interdependent individuals over perceived incompatible differences in beliefs, values, and goals, or over differences in desires for control, status, and affection.* This definition of conflict will be the base from which we discuss conflict in this chapter.

KINDS OF CONFLICT

There are two major kinds of conflict: conflict over content issues and conflict over relationship issues (see Fig. 8.1). Both kinds are present in health care settings. These two kinds of conflict parallel the communication perspective, which states that all interpersonal messages contain a content and a relational component (see Chapter 1). Conflict over content issues involves struggles between health professionals who differ on issues such as policies or procedures. Conflict over relationship issues involves struggles between health professionals about how they are related to each other. Although both kinds of conflict are distinct, they do have an impact on each other. A closer examination of each kind of conflict will provide us with a clearer picture of each and also give us a basis from which we can discuss theories of conflict and styles of effective conflict management.

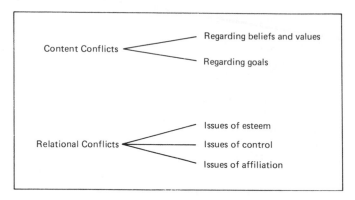

FIGURE 8.1 Different kinds of content and relational conflicts.

Conflict on the Content Level

Debating with someone about the advantages or disadvantages of a particular organizational change is something that is familiar to all of us. In fact, a large portion of the time we spend in discussions with other health professionals is spent talking about the pros and cons of health care issues such as cost containment, allocation of resources, staffing needs, and related topics. Strong disagreements on these topics are not uncommon. These disagreements are considered conflicts on the *content* level when they center on differences in (1) beliefs and values or (2) goals and ways to reach those goals.

Conflict regarding beliefs and values

Each of us has a unique system of beliefs and values that constitutes a basic philosophy of life. We each have had different and unique parents, educational experiences, and work experiences. When we communicate with others, we become aware that others' orientations are often very different from our own. If we perceive what another person communicates as incompatible with our own viewpoint, a conflict in beliefs or values occurs. Meux (1980) contends that value conflicts frequently pervade many aspects of our lives.

In health care, conflict arising from differences in beliefs and values can be illustrated in several ways. For example, patients from certain religious faiths who do not believe it is right to have blood transfusions may be in conflict with health professionals who believe blood transfusions are necessary to maintain the patient's life. Another example of conflict of beliefs occurs when some health professionals believe they should have the right to strike while others feel that health care professionals should not be allowed to withhold services. Still another example would be the conflict that takes place in a discussion when one professional favors national health care while another is vehemently opposed to it. In each of these examples, conflict occurs because one individual feels that his or her *beliefs* are incompatible with the position taken by another individual on the issue. Conflicts over differences in beliefs and values are often manifested in the conversations, debates, or arguments that occur between individuals.

In his play *Whose Life Is It Anyway?* Brian Clark (1978) vividly illustrated a conflict in *values* between a health professional and a client. Clark's play provides a moving account of the experiences of a young sculptor who becomes a quadraplegic as a result of an accident. In the play, the sculptor (Ken) is in conflict with his doctor (Dr. Emerson) over who is to control Ken's destiny. Ken wants to leave the hospital, which means he will die because he cannot care for himself without the help of others. Even though he would die, Ken prefers to leave the hospital because he thinks existing in the hospital would be meaningless. Dr. Emerson wants Ken to remain in the hospital where he can receive continuing care that would sustain his life. The following interaction begins with a nurse (sister) preparing medication for Dr. Emerson to give to Ken.

DR. EMERSON: Have you the Valium ready, Sister?

SISTER: Yes, sir. (*She hands him the kidney dish. Dr. Emerson takes it. Sister makes to follow him.*)

DR. EMERSON: It's all right, Sister. You've plenty of work, I expect.

SISTER: There's always plenty of that. (*Dr. Emerson goes into Ken's room.*)

KEN: Hello, hello, they've brought up the heavy brigade. (*Dr. Emerson pulls back the bed clothes and reaches for Ken's arm.*) Dr. Emerson, I am afraid I must insist that you do not stick that needle in me.

DR. EMERSON: It is important that I do.

KEN: Who for?

DR. EMERSON: You.

KEN: I'm the best judge of that.

DR. EMERSON: I think not. You don't even know what's in this syringe.

KEN: I take it that the injection is one of a series of measures to keep me alive.

DR. EMERSON: You could say that.

KEN: Then it is not important. I've decided not to stay alive.

DR. EMERSON: But you can't decide that.

KEN: Why not?

DR. EMERSON: You're very depressed.

KEN: Does that surprise you?

DR. EMERSON: Of course not; it's perfectly natural. Your body received massive injuries; it takes time to come to any acceptance of the new situation. Now I shan't be a minute. . . .

KEN: Don't stick that ------ thing in me!

DR. EMERSON: There. . . . It's over now.

KEN: Doctor, I didn't give you permission to stick that needle in me. Why did you do it?

> DR. EMERSON: It was necessary. Now try to sleep. . . . You will find
> that as you gain acceptance of the situation you will be able to find a
> new way of living.
> KEN: Please let me make myself clear. I specifically refused permis-
> sion to stick that needle in me and you didn't listen. You took no
> notice.
> DR. EMERSON: You must rely on us, old chap. Of course you're de-
> pressed. I'll send someone along to have a chat with you. Now I re-
> ally must go and get on with my rounds.[2]

Some health professionals place a high value on the patient's right to make choices and exert personal control. Other health professionals, like Dr. Emerson, place a greater value on sustaining and preserving human life by utilizing all the available medical technologies. The value conflict between Dr. Emerson and Ken is acute. At the same time, both individuals are highly interdependent on one another: To carry out his decision to leave the hospital, Ken needs Dr. Emerson's agreement; to give medical care, Dr. Emerson needs cooperation from Ken. Both individuals perceive the other's values as incompatible and this makes conflict inevitable. The communication between Dr. Emerson and Ken illustrates conflict over a particular content area—values.

Conflict regarding goals

A second common type of content-related conflict occurs in situations where individuals have different goals. In a study of the dimensions of interpersonal conflict in small group contexts, Knutson, Lashbrook, and Heemer (1976) identified two types of conflict that occur regarding group goals: (1) procedural conflict and (2) substantive conflict.

Procedural conflict refers to differences between individuals with regard to the approach they wish to take in attempting to reach a goal. In essence it is conflict over the best means to an agreed-upon end. The struggle in procedural conflict is over the *method* that will be used to achieve the goal, not over *what* goal to achieve. In health care, conflicts can be observed in many situations—from the best technique for giving an intramuscular injection to the optimal method for intubating a patient, and from the most effective way to approach a depressed patient to the best approach for teaching a woman how to breast-feed her baby. In each instance, conflict can occur when individuals do not agree with each other on what is the best way to achieve a goal.

Substantive conflict occurs when individuals differ with regard to the substance of the goal or what the goal should be. For example, a hospital administrator whose goal it is to increase the number of available hospital

[2]Reprinted by permission of Dodd, Mead & Company, Inc., from *Whose Life Is It Anyway?* by Brian Clark. Copyright © 1978 by Brian Clark.

beds may have a conflict with a nursing administrator whose goal it is to limit opening hospital beds due to personnel shortages. Two public health professionals may have different viewpoints on whether the goals of a public health agency should be directed to developing more treatment services or to preventing disease. In health care agencies in general, substantive conflicts often occur between administrators whose goals for more accurate record keeping conflict with staff goals to spend more time providing direct services to clients. These illustrations by no means exhaust all the possible examples of substantive conflict; however, they point out that conflict can occur as a result of two or more individuals disagreeing on what the goal or goals are to be in a health care agency.

Conflict on the Relational Level

Have you ever heard someone say, "I don't seem to get along with her (or him); we have a personality clash"? The words *personality clash* are another way of describing a conflict on the relational level. Sometimes we do not get along with another person, not because of *what* we are talking about (conflict over content issues) but because of *how* we are talking about it. *Relational conflict* refers to the differences we feel between ourself and others concerning how we are relating to each other. It is typically caused neither by one person nor the other, but arises in their relationship (Hill, 1977). Relational conflict is usually related to incompatible differences between individuals over issues of (1) self-esteem, (2) control, and (3) affiliation (see Fig. 8.1).

Relational conflict and issues of esteem

The need for esteem and recognition has been identified by Maslow (1970) as one of the major needs in an individual's hierarchy of human needs. Each of us has needs for esteem—we want to feel significant, useful, and worthwhile. We desire to have an effect on our surroundings and to be perceived by others as worthy of their respect. We attempt to satisfy our esteem needs through what we do and how we act, particularly in how we act in our relationships with clients and other health professionals.

When our needs for esteem are not being fulfilled in our relationships, we experience relational conflict because others do not see us in the way we wish to be seen. For example, a nursing technician may have repeated conflicts with a head nurse if the head nurse fails to recognize the unique contributions the technician can make to the overall health care process. Similarly, older staff members may feel hostile and upset when they do not receive the respect they feel they deserve because of their experience. So, too, younger nurses may want recognition for their innovative approaches to problems but older staff may fail to give it.

At the same time that we want our own esteem needs satisfied, other persons want their esteem needs satisfied as well. If the supply of respect we can give each other *seems* limited (or scarce), then our needs for esteem will clash. We will see the other person's needs for esteem as competing with our own or draining the limited resource away from us. To illustrate, consider a situation in which an occupational therapist and a physical therapist are both working with a person who has had a stroke and both staff members feel they have contributed to the progress that the patient has made in her or his rehabilitation. In this instance, if one or both the staff members believe that they are not receiving sufficient credit for their contribution to the patient's recovery, conflict may result. As their conflict escalates, the effectiveness of their working relationship and the quality of their communication may diminish. When the amount of available esteem (praise from others) seems scarce, a clash develops regarding who is to receive credit for the work that has been done.

Health professionals want to receive respect for their competence from other health professionals as well as from clients. When others interact with health professionals in ways that do not give them the recognition they believe they deserve, the result is often conflict.

Relational conflict and issues of control

As we discussed in Chapter 2, effective communication in health care relationships is strongly related to how individuals share control in their relationships. Because many jobs and roles in a health care setting are not always clearly defined, the control or power inherent in any one role is also seldom explicit. Furthermore, the power structures in health care units today are also changing, leading to greater uncertainty about who has how much power over whom (Kalisch & Kalisch, 1977). For example, Booth (1982) points out that

> nurses are assuming leadership roles that only physicians and administrators have occupied in the past. This results in an obvious shift of power and control, and increases the probability of conflict between all the individuals involved. When one group loses territory or resources to another group, the situation becomes ripe for the generation and escalation of conflict (p. 447).

It is no longer true that the lines of authority are simple and straightforward, (e.g., physician-nurse-patient). In recent years power has become more widely distributed among many roles (Booth, 1982; Stern, 1982).

Relational conflict also occurs when individuals in health care roles (e.g., patient, medical social worker, nurse) perceive that the actual control which they have in their relationships is incompatible with the amount of control that they would ideally like to have. Each of us has different needs for control. Some people like to have a great deal, while others are satisfied (and sometimes even more content) with only a little. In addition, our needs for control may also vary from one time to another. For example, there are times when a person's need to control others or events is very high, but at other times this same person may prefer that others take charge. Relational conflict over control issues develops when there is a clash between the needs for control that I have at a given time (high or low) and the needs for control that others have at that same time (high or low). If my need to direct events is compatible with yours, no conflict will take place; however, if I perceive your needs for control to be getting in the way of my control needs, then we will soon find ourselves in conflict. As struggles for control ensue, the communication among the participants will reflect negative, challenging remarks as each person tries to gain control over the other. In addition, considerable undermining can occur as one person tries to usurp the power of the other and obtain control (Chaska, 1979).

A graphic example of a conflict over relational control is provided in the exerpt from *Whose Life Is It Anyway?* which we discussed in the previous section. The patient (Ken) and the health professional (Dr. Emerson) are engaged in a major conflict over who will control Ken's present care and future plans. When Dr. Emerson gives the Valium against Ken's will, he is exerting control over Ken. This behavior of the doctor clashes dramatically with Ken's desire to exert control over the process by refusing treatment. Ken and Dr. Emerson both want control, and this struggle brings out many strong negative feelings and challenging comments toward one another.

Relationships between participants in health care contexts are replete with struggles for control. They are frequent occurrences between health professionals and other health professionals, and between health professionals and clients (see Chapter 3). In the final section of this chapter we will present some conflict management strategies that are particularly helpful in coping with relational conflict that arises from issues of control.

Relational conflict and issues of affiliation

Schutz (1966) has suggested that, in addition to the need for control, individuals also have a need to be included and loved by others. Each of us has a need to be involved in our relationships and to receive affection. If our needs for closeness are not satisfied in our relationships, we feel frustrated and experience feelings of conflict. Of course, some people like to be very involved and very close in their relationships, while others prefer less involvement and more distance. In any case, when others behave in ways that are incompatible with our own desires for warmth and affection, feelings of conflict emerge.

Relational conflict over these affiliation issues is illustrated in the following two examples. In a nursing home setting, conflict can arise between staff members, who have limited time and many responsibilities, and residents, who have a great deal of time and few responsibilities. A resident who is lonely may want staff members to sit and engage in extended conversations. However, if staff members have many residents to care for, they may find extended conversations with any one resident impossible. In this situation, interpersonal conflict may occur between a resident and staff member over their different needs for affiliation. The resident wants the staff member to be close and personal—like a companion. The staff member, who may have affiliation outside the job, may feel flattered but unable to fulfill this need of the resident. Their incompatible desires concerning affiliation create conflict.

Conflict over needs for affiliation is also evident in rehabilitation centers. In this type of setting, patients often develop strong relationships with staff members. For example, a patient who gradually makes big strides in physical therapy may become attached to the physical therapist who is responsible for directing the treatment. As the physical therapist attempts to withdraw from this intense relationship and to shift the primary responsibility for the therapy back to the patient, the patient may feel a loss of warmth and closeness. In this situation the patient's feeling of loss of affection or of rejection can create conflict.

Relational conflicts—whether they are over affiliation, esteem, or control—are seldom overt. Due to the subtle nature of these conflicts, they are often not easy to recognize. In addition, because it is difficult for many individuals to openly communicate that they want more recognition, control, or affection, these relational conflicts are difficult to resolve.

According to communication theorists, relational issues are inextricably bound to content issues, as discussed in Chapter 1. This means that relational conflicts will often surface during the discussion of content issues. For example, what may at first appear to be a conflict between two professionals regarding the *content* of a community-based stop-smoking program may really be a struggle over which of the persons will ultimately have *control* of the program. As we mentioned, relational conflicts are complex and not easily resolved.

Communication remains central to managing different kinds of conflict in health care settings. Health professionals who are able to keep channels of communication open with others will have a greater chance of understanding others' beliefs and values and needs for esteem, control, and affiliation. With increased understanding, many of these common kinds of conflict will seem less difficult to resolve and more open to negotiation. In the next section we will discuss theories that have been advanced to explain content conflicts as well as conflicts on the relational level, and we will discuss how both kinds of conflict can be resolved.

THEORETICAL APPROACHES TO CONFLICT

Many theories have been advanced by researchers to explain human conflict. Game theory and conflict resolution theory are the two major theoretical perspectives that have emerged in the research on conflicts between individuals and between groups. A brief examination of each of these approaches will help to clarify the nature of interpersonal conflict.

At the beginning of this chapter we mentioned that human conflict was inevitable and that it need not be considered bad. As Deutsch (1973) has suggested, "The point is *not* how to eliminate or prevent conflict but rather how to make it productive" (p. 17). Each of the following theoretical approaches emphasizes the ways in which conflict can be used to produce constructive outcomes.

Game Theory

An abundance of research on conflict uses game theory as its basis (Von Neumann & Morganstern, 1944; Rapoport, 1960; Deutsch, 1973; and others). Game theory focuses on the logical aspects of conflict and various strategies that can be employed to win a game. The players use a series of moves during the game that maximize their likelihood of gain and minimize their chance of loss (Steinfatt & Miller, 1974, p. 16). Game theory assumes that individuals will select strategies and make choices that are beneficial to their own self-interest. Because game players' choices are usually interdependent, their self-interests often collide—which produces conflict.

Game theory is a useful approach for studying conflict. It allows researchers to control some of the situational factors surrounding conflict by establishing predetermined payoffs and losses. Frost and Wilmot (1978) point out that engaging in conflict games in a laboratory setting provides new insights for individuals who are learning conflict management skills. In the laboratory, researchers can directly observe how specific conditions foster competition or cooperation, how communication influences the outcomes, and how other variables affect interpersonal conflict. However, as we mentioned in Chapter 2 in our discussion of the Prisoner's Dilemma Game, results based on "laboratory" games cannot always be generalized or applied to real world settings. In real-life situations the complexities of interpersonal conflict are seldom as clear-cut as in the laboratory setting.

Conflict Resolution Theory

A second theoretical approach to conflict, conflict resolution theory, encompasses a large body of research literature. Deutsch's book, *The Resolution of Conflict* (1973), and Jandt's work, *Conflict Resolution Through Com-*

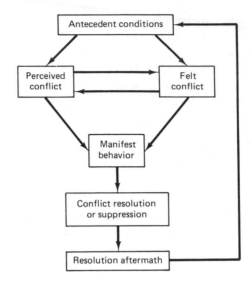

FIGURE 8.2   The conflict process. (From *Interpersonal Conflict Resolution* by Alan C. Filley, p. 8. Copyright © 1975 by Scott, Foresman and Company. Reprinted by permission.)

munication (1973), provide substantive overviews of this theoretical approach. Given the definition of conflict discussed earlier, which process will resolve conflicts? How can conflict be resolved so as to produce positive outcomes?

To answer these and similar questions, Filley (1975) proposed a model of conflict resolution represented in Figure 8.2 which was based on his own research and that of Pondy (1967) and others. Filley argues that the conflict resolution process moves through six steps: (1) antecedent conditions, (2) perceived conflict, (3) felt conflict, (4) manifest behavior, (5) conflict resolution or suppression, and (6) resolution aftermath (see Fig. 8.2 and Table 8.1). Since Filley's model is frequently cited and often used in discussions of conflict, we will describe each of the six steps in more detail in the following sections.

Antecedent conditions

Filley's model suggests that there are several antecedent conditions that set the stage for conflict. The potential for conflict is greater when

Individuals' responsibilities and roles are ambiguous.

There is competition for resources.

There are barriers to communication.

TABLE 8.1   Steps in the Conflict Resolution Process

Antecedent conditions.   Certain conditions exist which *can* lead to conflict, though they do not always do so.

Perceived conflict.   Two or more individuals logically and objectively recognize that their aims are incompatible.

Felt conflict.   Individuals experience feelings of threat, hostility, fear, or mistrust.

Manifest behavior.   Overt action or behavior takes place—aggression, competition, debate, or problem solving.

Conflict resolution or suppression.   The conflict is resolved—or suppressed—either by all parties' agreement or else by the defeat of one party.

Resolution aftermath.   Individuals experience or live with the consequences of the resolution.

From *Interpersonal Conflict Resolution* by Alan Filley, pp. 8–9. Copyright © 1975 by Scott, Foresman and Company. Reprinted by permission.

Individuals are forced to depend on others.

There is a high degree of differentiation in organizational levels and job specialties.

Joint decision making and consensus are a necessity.

There are many rules, procedures, and policies.

There are unresolved prior conflicts (Filley, 1975).

Many of these conditions are present in health care settings. In hospitals, for example, nearly all the antecedent conditions mentioned above are frequently present. First, as we pointed out in Chapter 3, the roles of health professionals in the hospital are not always explicitly defined, and they often overlap with the responsibilities of other health professionals. For example, dietitians' responsibilities overlap nurses', nurses' duties intersect with physicians', physical therapists' responsibilities overlap those of occupational therapists, and social workers' may coincide with nurses', to list a few. Also, in light of hospitals' emphasis on containing costs, the competition for resources between departments and even between professional groups can be intense. Furthermore, barriers to communication in hospitals are created by having rotating shifts for personnel (day, evening, and night shifts) or by placing highly interdependent departments far apart from each other. Moreover, personnel are often required to engage in joint decision making while being governed by a multitude of rules, procedures, and policies. Finally, because hospitals are organizations with many levels of authority and numerous job specialties, the potential for communication difficulties and conflict is increased.

Perceived conflict and felt conflict

Assuming that the conditions necessary for conflict are present, the next steps in the conflict process are *perceived conflict* and *felt conflict* (see Fig. 8.1). Conflict occurs more readily if the perceptions of the opposing parties are very far apart. When person A perceives a problem differently from person B, they are more likely to come into conflict. For example, physicians and nurses may have two very different perspectives on patient care. Physicians often highlight the importance of diagnostic procedures and the *cure* component of health care. Nurses and other health professionals, on the other hand, often highlight the importance of psychosocial interventions and the *care* component of health care. Their perceptual differences about what comprises good patient care can create a *perceived* conflict between professionals. On the other hand, if doctors view their duties as including considerable care and nurses share a concern for correct diagnosis, the perceived conflict is considerably reduced.

Felt conflict refers to the level of emotional involvement in a problem situation. Many times conflict between individuals is not based on rational elements but is the result of the emotional reactions of individuals. In fact, as we mentioned near the beginning of this chapter, it is this *affect* dimension that makes us uncomfortable with conflict, and may even make us try to avoid it at times. One mental health worker commented on the conflict she experienced with the director of her agency.

> I was so angry with her [the director] that I felt like my blood was boiling. I was intensely frustrated at what I felt was a blocking move on her part. I tried to avoid her as much as I could. I was worried that if I saw her I would burst out in anger and put my job in jeopardy.

Clearly, if we can learn to cope with the intense emotions felt in conflict, our ability to resolve the conflict will be enhanced.

Manifest behavior

Manifest behavior refers to the behavior and action of individuals in response to conflict. These are the signs of conflict that are observable to bystanders. Individuals manifest primarily two kinds of behaviors in response to perceived and felt conflict: (1) conflictive behaviors (negative) and (2) problem-solving behaviors (positive). *Conflictive behavior* is characterized by the conscious attempts of one person to compete, dominate, and win over a second person. For example, conflictive behavior would be manifested by a health professional in an interdisciplinary meeting who consciously tries to block the innovative program suggested by another health professional. The dominating professional may try tactics such as discrediting the proposed program or diverting the discussion to a completely different topic in order to prevent program adoption. *Problem-solving* behaviors, on the other hand, are conscious attempts to find mutually acceptable alternatives—to find approaches to problems that have positive outcomes for both parties.

Conflict resolution or suppression

The next step in the conflict model is conflict resolution or suppression. In conflict situations, individuals can either suppress conflict or engage in activity which will lead to its resolution. Behavior directed toward the resolution of conflict can be characterized by three different *communication strategies*: (1) win-lose, (2) lose-lose, or (3) win-win.

Win-lose strategies.   The win-lose strategy of conflict resolution is quite common, and most of us have used it at one time or another. It is not the optimal way to resolving conflict because one of the participants loses. This strategy is characterized by attempts of one individual to control or dominate another so as to obtain his or her own goal(s) even at the expense of another's goal(s). In this type of conflict, the parties (1) frequently see each other as adversaries; (2) define their goals individually rather than mutually; and (3) emphasize the problem rather than the long-term nature of the relationship (Filley, 1975, p. 25). The following case illustrates a win-lose strategy.

> Financial reports indicated that revenues in a large metropolitan hospital were down 10 percent. In light of the reduced income, the vice-presidents of the various departments within the hospital were told to cut their departmental expenditures by 10 percent. (In this particular hospital 68 percent of the overall costs were for personnel.) One of the vice-presidents met with the director of social services and told her to make the necessary cuts within her department.
>
> During their meeting the social service director reminded the vice-president that the administration and medical staff had recently approved a new "open" referral policy to the social service department. Under the new policy, any staff member, patient, or family member could initiate a referral and no longer needed to go through a physician. The director showed the vice-president records that indicated the number of social service referrals had increased by 40 percent during the six months in which the policy had been in effect. The vice-president listened to the director's arguments but said that considering the total hospital situation, the social service department would just have to "make do" with the reduced budget.
>
> The social service director left the meeting frustrated and decided to submit a proposal to the budget committee and get their decision on the matter. The director was well aware that the vice-president, who was on the budget committee, would argue against the proposal.
>
> The conflict between the director and the vice-president evolved into a win-lose situation. If the budget committee approved the pro-

posal, the director would win and the vice-president would lose. If the budget committee rejected the proposal, the opposite would occur. In either situation, there would be long-term implications for both the social service department and the vice-president's reputation, and also for the ongoing working relationship between the director and the vice-president.

Lose-lose strategies.   The lose-lose approach to conflict is obviously one we would all like to avoid when possible. Most people do not intentionally select a lose-lose strategy, but they end up with this outcome when other strategies, such as a win-lose strategy, fail. In lose-lose conflicts both parties try to win over the other but both end up losing to each other. Neither person's goals are achieved and the relationship is weakened. Attempts by individuals to dominate over each other result in mutually destructive communication between the participants and negative outcomes. The following case study illustrates a lose-lose form of conflict resolution.

A school of nursing was seeking a new director. Administrators at the college strongly desired to have an "in-house" person assume the position, since that person would already be familiar with the program and would have faculty support. Two faculty members said that they would like the position and both tried to line up faculty support. In their attempt to gather faculty support, strong disagreements developed between the two candidates and two distinct factions developed within the faculty. Both factions of faculty members threatened to quit if the person of their choice was not selected. In the end, neither in-house candidate was appointed director of the program; instead a person from the outside who was less qualified had to be hired for the position. The tension and conflict that were generated within the two faculty groups produced what could be called a lose-lose, destructive outcome.

Win-win strategies.   Individuals who employ win-win strategies approach conflict in ways that are significantly different from the strategies used by individuals who take win-lose or lose-lose approaches toward conflict. The win-win strategy is an approach that allows both individuals to feel they have accomplished all or part of their goals. This strategy tries to satisfy mutual needs, to solve problems creatively, and to develop relationships. There is no attempt by one party to win over or control another party in this approach.

Win-win strategies are not easy to use because they entail a great deal of time and energy. They also require effective interpersonal communication since an individual must argue strongly for his or her own goal and at the same time listen closely to the thoughts and feelings of the other individual arguing for another goal. When using this approach, individuals have to be attuned to creative alternatives that allow *both* parties to obtain what they want. However, in the midst of interpersonal conflict, when we are absorbed by our own feelings and needs, it is often difficult to perceive or feel the other person's needs. Finding win-win conflict solutions means suppressing but not sacrificing our own needs in order to listen for the needs of others. Whether it be a conflict over a policy or procedure or a conflict for control or esteem, win-win strategies mean both parties communicate in ways that allow each of them to satisfy at least some of their needs.

Win-win solutions strengthen relationships. They make individuals feel better about how they are related to others. Over time, the strengthening of relationships has the advantage of helping individuals in future conflict resolution. The following case study helps to illustrate a win-win strategy for conflict resolution.

> The director of a nursing program at a liberal arts college in a small midwestern community was very concerned about the lack of available nurses with Master's degrees to teach in the program. He also noticed that a number of the Master's-prepared faculty that he did employ were leaving to work in a nearby service setting where the salaries were higher and where faculty could utilize their "rusty" clinical skills.
>
> A director of a large hospital in the same community was concerned about the lack of strong role models for the young staff at her hospital. The director also experienced a constant need for highly educated nurses to offer inservice programs in the hospital.
>
> For a short period of time both directors found themselves competing for the few highly educated nurses who lived in this community. The directors, becoming aware of their similar problems, started to work together to find ways of attracting more specialized professionals into their community and also to make better use of the persons that were already available. After numerous extended dialogues they agreed to design and develop a joint-appointment program in which staff could spend part of their time working for the school of nursing and part of their time working for the hospital. They found that this type of program would benefit both institutions as well as the individual staff members. In the ensuing years the directors not only developed the program, but they were also able to obtain a grant to fund their collaborative program.

Win-win solutions are facilitated if the individuals can engage in *creative problem solving*. This technique, which originated from Dewey's (1910) work on critical thinking, usually involves five steps:

1. Mutually define the problem(s).
2. Identify potential solutions to the problem(s).
3. Assess the advantages and disadvantages of each of the solutions.
4. Select the solution which represents the best alternative to solving the problem.

5. Discuss and evaluate the fit between the selected solution and the problem.

Problem-solving techniques give a structure or set of rules for conflict resolution. The problem-solving process is only a format for arriving at win-win solutions and does not need to be followed exactly. The form of problem solving used should depend on the type of problem being addressed. For some conflicts, identifying the problem will be the most difficult part; in other conflicts, finding the best solution from a series of alternatives will be the primary concern. No matter which segment is highlighted, this process will aid conflict resolution. Each step requires, however, that participants communicate their ideas clearly to one another, listen thoughtfully to the suggestions of others, and evaluate the suggestions and the alternatives that are proposed in an objective, nonjudgmental manner.

Resolution aftermath

The final aspect of conflict in the Filley conflict model is *resolution aftermath* (see Fig 8.1). During this phase, participants experience feelings directly related to the outcome of the resolution process. If the conflict is resolved in a positive fashion, the participants will have good feelings about themselves, about each other and the situation. This was the case in the example involving the director of the school of nursing and the director of the hospital. Participants using a win-win strategy will find that they are strongly committed to the agreed-upon solution and to maintaining a good relationship with other participants. On the other hand if the conflict is resolved in an unproductive style, participants will have negative feelings about themselves, each other, and the relationship. This was evident in the case study about the social service director and the hospital vice-president who were in conflict about budget cuts. In win-lose and lose-lose situations, participants may feel less cooperative, more distrustful, and very prone to further conflicts (Filley, 1975, p. 18). Obviously, the preferred goal of conflict resolution is to arrive at solutions that result in positive feelings, productive interactions, and cooperative relationships among the participants.

STYLES OF APPROACHING CONFLICT

We have discussed the nature of conflict, different kinds of conflict, theoretical perspectives on conflict and strategies for resolving conflict. Now we would like to address the questions, Do individuals have different ways of handling conflict? and, How do the styles employed by individuals affect the outcomes of the conflicts?

Researchers have found that individuals approach interpersonal conflict utilizing basically five styles: (1) avoidance, (2) competition, (3) accom-

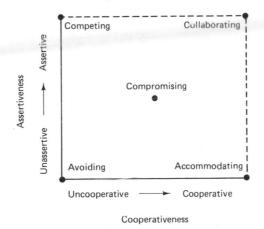

FIGURE 8.3   A diagram depicting the relationship between assertiveness, cooperativeness, and styles of approaching interpersonal conflict. (Adapted with permission of authors and publisher from R. H. Kilmann and K. W. Thomas, *Psychological Reports*, 1975, p. 972.)

modation, (4) compromise, and (5) collaboration. This five-category scheme for classifying conflict was developed by Kilmann and Thomas (1975, 1977) and is based on the work of Blake and Mouton (1964). Each of the styles in the category system is unique and can be applied to conflicts that are typical in health care settings. To measure conflict styles, Thomas and Kilmann (1974) have developed a conflict mode instrument that assesses individual behavior in conflict situations.[3]

A model developed by Kilmann and Thomas (1975) illustrates the interrelationships between the conflict styles (see Fig. 8.3). As you can observe, the model describes conflict styles along two dimensions: assertiveness and cooperativeness. Each conflict style is characterized by how much assertiveness and how much cooperativeness an individual shows when confronting conflict. *Assertiveness* refers to attempts to satisfy one's own concerns while *cooperativeness* represents attempts to satisfy the concerns of others. In conflict situations, both sets of concerns are present. Effective conflict management is a mix of assertiveness and cooperativeness—it involves attending to concerns for self and others simultaneously.

In the model, five commonly observed styles of conflict are identified along the assertiveness and cooperativeness dimensions. In conflict situations, a person's individual style is usually a combination of these different styles. "Each of us is capable of using all five conflict-handling modes; none of us can be characterized as having a single, rigid style of dealing with con-

[3]The Thomas-Kilmann Conflict Mode Instrument can be obtained through XICOM, INC., Sterling Forest, Tuxedo, N. Y. 10987.

flict" (Thomas & Kilmann, 1974, p. 13). Nevertheless, because of past experiences of situational factors, some persons may have a tendency to rely more heavily on one conflict style than on others. *Successful conflict resolution occurs when individuals select the conflict style that most appropriately meets the demands of the situation.*

In the next section, each of the five conflict styles will be discussed in more detail. As you read the descriptions of these styles, perhaps you can identify which style of conflict management you most commonly use in your communication with others. Is that style productive or counterproductive? Of all the styles described, is there one or more that you could develop to enhance your conflict-handling skills?

Avoidance

Avoidance is both an unassertive and uncooperative conflict style. As the word suggests, avoidance is a style characteristic of individuals who are passive and who do not want to recognize conflict. These persons generally prefer to ignore conflict situations rather than confront them directly. In conflict-producing circumstances, these individuals are not assertive about pursuing their own interests nor are they cooperative in assisting others to pursue their concerns.

Avoidance as a style for managing conflict is usually counterproductive and often leads to stress and further conflict. However, there are some situations in which avoidance may be useful—for example, when an issue is of trivial importance or when the potential damages from conflict would be too great. King (1982) points out that overemphasis of minor conflicts can be counterproductive, costly, and time consuming. Avoidance can also provide a cooling-off period (Thomas & Kilmann, 1974). Generally speaking, though, it is better if individuals confront conflict and attempt to resolve it, if at all possible.

In health care settings, avoidance is not an uncommon conflict style. In fact, there are times when avoidance may almost be necessary. For example, one department in a hospital may frequently be in conflict with another department that is always slow in responding to requests. If the request is directly related to the survival of a patient, the interdepartmental conflict becomes less important than just getting the service immediately— and avoiding conflict may be the best way. Health care practitioners are frequently dealing with life and death decisions for patients; consequently they often need to suppress their own concerns or conflicts with other staff members in order to perform the necessary services. In these critical situations, avoidance of conflict may facilitate the health care delivery process.

In general, however, avoidance is not a constructive style of confronting conflict. Health professionals who are continually required to avoid conflict experience a great deal of stress. They bottle up their feelings of irritation, frustration, anger, or rage inside themselves, creating more anxiety, instead of expressing them or resolving the situation. Furthermore, avoidance is essentially a static approach to conflict: It does nothing to solve problems or to make changes that could prevent conflicts. In health care organizations, the problems that exist will seldom be alleviated or resolved if avoidance is employed in conflict situations.

Competition

Competition is a conflict style characteristic of individuals who are highly assertive about pursuing their own goals but uncooperative in assisting others to reach their goals. These individuals attempt to resolve a struggle by controlling or persuading others in order to achieve their own ends. A competitive style is based on a win-lose conflict strategy.

Competition is widespread in our culture and it can produce solutions to conflicts that are more effective and more creative than if competition were not present. For example, in a community in which hospitals are competing to provide specific services, the quality of the services will be higher, and the cost to the public will usually be lower than if there were no competition. In the area of cost containment, a competitive approach to conflict can generate innovative cost-saving solutions to complex problems. Similarly, on the interpersonal level, when two professionals compete to provide quality care, the outcomes can be very positive for clients. In effect, competitive approaches to conflict can challenge participants to make their best efforts, and this can have positive results.

Generally, though, competitive approaches to conflict are not the most advantageous approach to conflict because they are more often counterproductive than productive. In failing to take others' concerns into account, we do others a disservice. When we attempt to solve conflict with dominance and control, communication can easily become hostile and destructive. Too much competition among health professionals can direct energy away from patient care objectives toward unnecessary interprofessional struggles. Too much competition between health care facilities can lead to a duplication of services within communities (e.g., two CAT scans, two dialysis units, etc.) and duplication increases health care costs. Competitive approaches to conflict create unstable situations as one party is constantly striving to attain or maintain dominance over the other party. Finally, competition is disconfirming; in competition individuals fail to recognize the concerns and needs of others.

Accommodation

Accommodation is a conflict style that is unassertive but cooperative. It is an approach to conflict that is "other-directed." An accommodating individual attends very closely to the needs of others and ignores her or his own needs. Using this style, individuals confront problems by deferring to others.

In the beginning of this chapter we defined conflict as a felt struggle between individuals over incompatible differences. Accommodation is one way for individuals to move away from the uncomfortable feelings of struggle that conflict inevitably produces. By yielding to others, individuals can lessen the frustrations that conflict creates. In accommodating, an individual essentially communicates to another, "You are right, I agree; let's forget about it." The felt struggle is reduced through acquiescence.

The problem with accommodation is that it is in effect a lose-win strategy. Individuals who accommodate may lose because they fail to take the opportunity to express their own opinions and feelings. Their contributions are not fully considered because they are not actively expressed or forcefully advocated. This style is primarily a submissive style which allows others to take charge. To illustrate accommodation, consider the following conflict between a nurse and a physician regarding the use of pain medication with a terminally ill cancer patient. The physician believes that pain medication should be given no sooner than every four hours. In contrast, the nurse believes that the patient should be allowed to request pain medication as necessary and should not have to adhere to a rigid four-hour schedule. After only a brief discussion of their differences, the nurse decides to give in—to accept the physician's approach to the situation. The nurse in this situation suppresses his or her values regarding pain management in order to maintain an amicable nurse-physician relationship and in order to prevent further conflict. Although the accommodating approach to conflict probably resolves conflict faster than some of the other approaches, the drawback of this approach is that the accommodator sacrifices his or her own values and possibly the quality of care in order to maintain smooth relationships with others.

From a positive perspective, accommodation can be useful in situations in which preserving harmony is necessary. For example, if two professionals differ on an issue but one professional is deeply interested in the particular issue while his or her colleague is less involved in the issue, then it can be useful for the professional who finds the issue less important to go along with the concerned professional in order to maintain good personal relations. Accommodation can also be effective in conflict-arousing situations such as staff scheduling. If individuals accommodate others in schedule conflicts it helps to reduce tension among staff members and it enhances the overall quality of their professional-professional relationships. In general, accommodation can at times be an effective means of eliminating conflict. As a rule, however, accommodation is not a preferred conflict style.

Compromise

As Figure 8.2 indicates, compromise occurs halfway between competition and accommodation, which means it includes both a degree of assertiveness and a degree of cooperativeness. In using compromise to approach conflict, an individual attends to the concerns of others as well as to her or his own concerns. On the diagonal axis of Figure 8.2, compromise occurs midway between avoidance and collaboration. This means that persons using this approach do not completely ignore confrontations but neither do they struggle with problems to the fullest degree. Thomas and Kilmann (1974) point out that this conflict style is often chosen because it is expedient and provides a quick means to find a middle ground. It partially satisfies the concerns of both parties.

While growing up, children are often taught that it is important to be able to compromise when a fight or conflict occurs with others. Although it was never easy to compromise, we were taught that we should strive for it. To a certain extent this is correct; compromise is a positive conflict style because it requires that individuals attend to others' goals as well as their own. Compromise reminds us of the golden rule: "Do unto others as you would have them do unto you." The problem with compromise is one of degree. It does not go far enough in resolving conflict. As two persons give in to one anothers' demands, both individuals also pull back from fully expressing their own demands. Both individuals suppress personal thoughts and feelings in order to reach solutions that are not completely satisfactory for either side.

In health care, the compromise strategy may sometimes be seen in the communication among health professionals in interdisciplinary team meetings. One person may quickly agree with another person in order to resolve a problem so that each of them can get back to other responsibilities. Although this may be efficient and conserve time, innovative solutions are sacrificed in favor of quick solutions. In compromising, individuals also make themselves submissive to others and they squelch their uniqueness. The need for harmony supersedes the need for optimal solutions to conflict.

Collaboration

Collaboration, the most preferred of the conflict styles, requires both assertiveness and cooperation. It involves attending fully to others' concerns while not sacrificing or suppressing one's own concerns (see Fig. 8.2). Collaboration is the ideal conflict style because it recognizes the inevitability of human conflict. It confronts conflict, and then uses conflict to produce constructive outcomes.

Although collaboration is the most preferred style, it is the hardest to achieve. Collaboration requires energy and work among participants. To resolve incompatible differences through collaboration, individuals need to take enough time to work together to find mutually satisfying solutions. This often involves extended conversation in which the participants search for entirely new alternatives to existing problems. For example, individuals who collaborate may think or say things such as; "Is there any way we can resolve this problem that we haven't thought of up to now? Have we thought of every angle to this conflict?" The work of collaboration requires sharing control in an effort to obtain innovative solutions that are mutually acceptable. The results of collaboration are positive because both individuals win, communication is satisfying, relationships are strengthened, and future conflicts can be resolved more easily.

The five styles of approaching conflict—avoidance, competition, accommodation, compromise, and collaboration—can be observed in various conflict situations. Although there are advantages and disadvantages to each style, the conflict-handling style that meets the needs of the participants while also fitting the demands of the situation will be most effective in resolving conflict. Interpersonal conflict is transactional and will depend on people consciously choosing a style for handling conflict that is likely to result in optimal outcomes for both people in the conflict. An effective style such as collaboration and productive strategy such as the win-win approach both require that participants attend closely to one another's opinions and proposals and interact in ways that result in solutions acceptable to all parties. Effective communication is the pivotal element that prevents differences among individuals from escalating and facilitates constructive resolution to conflict situations.

SUMMARY

In human relationships, interpersonal conflict is inevitable. Conflict is defined as a felt struggle between two or more individuals over perceived incompatible differences in beliefs, values, and goals, or over differences in desires for control, status, and affection. If it is managed in appropriate ways, conflict need not be destructive but can be constructive and used to positive ends. Communication plays a central role in the conflict.

Conflict occurs between individuals on two levels: content and relationship. Conflict on the content level involves differences among people in beliefs, values, or goal orientation. Conflicts regarding goal orientation can be further divided into procedural and substantive conflicts. Procedural conflicts involve differences regarding the best way of approaching a goal and substantive conflicts occur over struggles about the nature of the goal itself. Conflict on the relational level refers to differences between individuals with regard to their desires for esteem, control, and affiliation in their relationships. Relational conflicts are seldom overt, which makes them difficult for people to recognize and resolve.

The major theoretical approaches advanced by researchers to explain human conflict are game theory and conflict resolution theory. Game theory focuses on the payoffs and losses that people encounter in trying to resolve conflict in a game situation. Game theory is most useful in understanding conflict in laboratory settings. Conflict resolution theory, based on Filley's model, is helpful in describing conflict in real-life situations. This model identifies six steps that occur in conflict resolution: antecedent conditions, perceived conflict, felt conflict, manifest behavior, conflict resolution or suppression, and resolution aftermath.

To resolve interpersonal conflict, there are basically three strategies: win-lose, lose-lose, or win-win. Individuals attempt to dominate or control one another in the less effective win-lose and lose-lose conflict strategies. Win-win strategies are constructive because they emphasize mutual satisfaction of needs and relationship development, with no attempt by one party to control another. Win-win strategies are facilitated by the process of creative problem solving which includes (1) mutually defining a problem, (2) identifying solutions, (3) assessing the merits of each solution, (4) selecting the best solution, and (5) evaluating the fit between the solution and the problem.

Five styles of approaching conflict are avoidance, competition, accommodation, compromise, and collaboration. Each of these styles characterizes individuals in terms of the degree of assertiveness and cooperativeness they show when confronting conflict. The most constructive approach to conflict is collaboration, which requires that individuals recognize, confront, and resolve conflict by attending fully to others' concerns without sacrificing their own. Managing conflicts effectively leads to stronger relationships among participants and more creative solutions to problems.

REFERENCES

Blake R. R., & Mouton, L. S. *The managerial grid.* Houston: Gulf Publishing, 1964.

Booth, R. Z. Conflict resolution. *Nursing Outlook,* 1982, *30*(8), 447–453.

Brown, C. T., & Keller, P. W. *Monologue to dialogue: An exploration of interpersonal communication.* Englewood Cliffs, N.J.: Prentice-Hall, Inc., 1979.

Brown, C. T., Yelsma, P., & Keller, P. W. Communication-conflict predisposition: Development of a theory and an instrument. *Human Relations,* 1981, *34*(12), 1103–1117.

Chaska, N. The "cooling out" process in a complex organization. *Journal of Nursing Administration,* 1979, *9*(1), 22–28.

Clark, B. *Whose life is it anyway?* New York: Avon Books, 1978.

Coser, L. A. *Continuities in the study of social conflict.* New York: The Free Press, 1967.

Deutsch, M. Toward an understanding of conflict. *International Journal of Group Tensions,* 1971, *1,* 42–54.

Deutsch, M. *The resolution of conflict.* New Haven and London: Yale University Press, 1973.

Dewey, J. *How we think.* Boston: D. C. Heath & Co., 1910.

Filley, A. C. *Interpersonal conflict resolution.* Glenview, Ill.: Scott, Foresman & Company, 1975.

Frost, J. H., & Wilmot, W. W. *Interpersonal conflict.* Dubuque, Iowa: William C. Brown Co. Publishers, 1978.

Harris, S. Every governing idea needs an opposing idea. Detroit Free Press, 1979, May 19, p. 7B.

Hill, R. E. Managing interpersonal conflict in project teams. *Sloan Management Review,* 1977, *18*(2), 45–61.

Jandt, F. E. *Conflict resolution through communication.* New York: Harper & Row, Publishers, Inc., 1973.

Kalisch, B. J., & Kalisch, P. A. An analysis of the sources of physician-nurse conflict. *Journal of Nursing Administration,* 1977, 7(1), 50–57.

Kilmann, R. H., & Thomas, K. W. Interpersonal conflict-handling behavior as reflections of Jungian personality dimensions. *Psychological Reports,* 1975, *37,* 971–980.

Kilmann, R. H., & Thomas, K. W. Developing a forced-choice measure of conflict handling behavior: The "mode" instrument. *Educational and Psychology Measurement,* 1977, *37,* 309–325.

King, B. W. Teamwork/personnel conflicts. *Journal of Emergency Nursing,* 1982, *8*(1), 51–54.

Knutson, T., Lashbrook, V., & Heemer, A. The dimensions of small group conflict: A factor analytic study. Paper presented to the annual meeting of the International Communication Association, Portland, Oregon, 1976.

Maslow, A. *Motivation and personality,* 2nd ed. New York: Harper & Row, Publishers, Inc., 1970.

Meux, M. Resolving interpersonal value conflicts. *Advances in Nursing Science,* 1980, 2(4), 41–70.

Muniz, P. Conflict and strategies for conflict management. *Management of Conflict.* New York: National League for Nursing, 1981.

Nichols, B. Dealing with conflict. *Journal of Continuing Education in Nursing,* 1979, *10,* 24–27.

Pondy, L. R. Organizational conflict: Concepts and models. *Administration Science Quarterly,* 1967, *12,* 296–320.

Rapoport, A. *Fights, games, and debates.* Ann Arbor: University of Michigan Press, 1960.

Schutz, W. C. *The interpersonal underworld.* Palo Alto, Calif.: Science and Behavior Books, Inc., 1966.

Steinfatt, T. M., & Miller, G. R. Communication in game theoretic models of conflict. In G. R. Miller and H. W. Simons (Eds.), *Perspectives on communication in social conflict.* Englewood Cliffs, N. J.: Prentice-Hall, Inc., 1974.

Stern, E. Collective bargaining: A means of conflict resolution. *Nursing Administration Quarterly,* 1982, *30*(8), 447–453.

Thomas, K. W., & Kilmann, R. H. *Thomas-Kilmann conflict mode instrument.* New York: XICOM Inc., 1974.

Thurkettle, M. A., & Jones, S. L. Conflict as a systems process: Theory and management. *Journal of Nursing Administration,* 1978, *8*(1), 39–43.

Von Nuemann, J., & Morganstern, O. *The theory of games and economic behavior.* Princeton, N. J.: Princeton University Press, 1944.

Author Index

Subject Index

Member behavior, 210, 212, 220–221, 223, 243
Member-group relationships, 227
Member roles, 213, 221–223, 232
Members. See Family members
Membership:
  unstable, 218
Messages, 13, 32–33, 133–135, 158, 161, 168
  by touch, 158–159, 168
  See also Relational messages
MHLC. See Multidimensional Health Locus of Control
Midrange groups, 208
Missed meanings, 94
Models, 11, 12, 16, 26, 40
  health-related, 16–22
  of responsibilities, 123
  See also Authoritarian models; Baker model of silence; Compensatory model; Conflict model; Developmental model Enlightenment model; Health belief model; Health communication model; "Hypodermic needle" model; Interaction model; Interdisciplinary health team model; King interaction model; Leary model; Models of helping and coping; Moral model; Organizational communication model; Reflexive model; Rogerian model; Shannon-Weaver model; SMCR model; Speech communication model; Therapeutic model
Model of silence. See Baker model of silence
Models of helping and coping, 86–88
Modifying factors, 18–19
Monitoring, 143
Moral model, 87, 88
Motivation theory, 274
Multidimensional communication, 8, 11, 26
Multidimensional Health Locus of Control (MHLC), 38
Myths. See Isolation myth; Key to success myth; Single meaning myth; Transparency myth

"Near or far," 236
Networks. See All-channel communication network; Communication networks; Social networks
Noise, 12, 164–166
Nominal group technique, 239–241, 244
"Noncontact" cultures, 157
Nondirective interviewing, 177–179, 202
Nonfunctional roles, 222
Nonverbal accuracy, 145–146
Nonverbal assessment, 131
Nonverbal behavior, 129–130, 136–140, 145, 150, 168
  decode, 145
  See also Adaptors; Affect displays; Emblems; Illustrators; Regulators; Unintentional nonverbal behavior
Nonverbal communication, 24, 89, 120, 129–137, 141, 143, 151, 168, 243

definitions, 132, 168
dimensions of, 137–168
environmental factors, 137, 162
and family members, 130
feelings and emotions, 133, 168
functions of, 134, 139
importance of, 130
interaction, 133, 134, 168
modes, 131
nature of, 132
and patients, 130–131
physical factors, 137
and professionals, 130–131
purposes of, 133
relationships, 135
self-image, 134, 168
verbal messages, 134, 168
See also Environment; Intentional nonverbal communication; Kinesics; Myths; Nonverbal behavior; Nonvocal nonverbal communication; Paralinguistics; Proxemics; Touch, Unintentional nonverbal communication; Vocal nonverbal communication
Nonverbal cues, 133, 135, 137, 141, 146
Nonverbal dimensions, 134, 137
Nonverbal facial cues. See Facial cues
Nonverbal movements, 139
  See also Regulators
Nonvocal nonverbal communication, 132, 168
Norming phase, 236
Norms, 213, 215–217, 232, 243, 274
  covert, 215, 243
  enabling, 215–216
  overt, 215, 243
  restrictive, 216
Nursing departments, 253–255
Nursing station. See Communication station

Open communication, 122
Open questions, 190, 191, 192, 193, 203
Opinion giver, 221
Opinion seeker, 221
Organizational communication, 5, 247–250, 260, 263–264
  definitions, 248, 278
  factors influencing, 250
  paradigm of, 249
  See also Channels, Power
Organizational communication model, 249, 264, 278
Organizational philosophy, 247, 250–251, 278
Organizational rationality, 97–98
Organizational shape, 252–253
Organizational structures, 247, 252–253, 263, 278
Organizations:
  definition, 248
  See also Health care organizations
Orientation phase, 232–234, 238, 243
Orientor, 221
"Other-directed" approach, 303
Overfunctioning roles. See Roles, overfunctioning
Overlap. See Role overlap